Da

Indust

Devices and Desires

A HISTORY OF CONTRACEPTIVES

IN AMERICA

Andrea Tone

HILL AND WANG

A DIVISION OF FARRAR, STRAUS AND GIROUX

NEW YORK

Hill and Wang
A division of Farrar, Straus and Giroux
19 Union Square West, New York 10003

Library of Congress Cataloging-in-Publication Data

Tone, Andrea, 1964–
    Devices and desires : a history of contraceptives in America / Andrea Tone.
        p. cm.
    Includes index.
    ISBN 0-8090-3817-X (hardcover : alk. paper)
        1. Birth control—United States—History.   2. Contraceptives—United
States—History.   I. Title.

HQ766.5.U5 T66 2001
363.9'6'0973—dc21
                                                              00-050547

Designed by Jonathan D. Lippincott

Parts of chapter 2, "The Limits of the Law," were first published in the *Journal of American History* 87, no. 2 (September 2000). Parts of chapter 7, "Feminine Hygiene," were first published in the *Journal of Social History* 29 (March 1996). Parts of chapter 11, "Searching for Something Better," were first published in Michael Bellesiles, ed., *Lethal Imagination: Violence and Brutality in American History* (New York University Press, 1999).

Contents

List of Illustrations

Acknowledgments

I decided to write this book in 1992, when I was fortunate enough to be working at the Feminist Women's Health Center, a nonprofit reproductive health clinic in Atlanta. I wish to thank the committed individuals there who first fueled my interest in the history of contraceptives and to express my abiding admiration for the important work they do.

Much of this book focuses on the history of bootleg birth control, a topic that imposed research challenges that might have been insurmountable were it not for the expertise, support, and timely intervention of numerous archivists and scholars. My research began at the National Archives in Washington, D.C. Aloha South guided me through postal records there, and Tab Lewis of the College Park branch located Federal Trade Commission transcripts—and registered an appropriate combination of enthusiasm and alarm when decaying diaphragms and condoms appeared glued to the transcript pages! Trevor Plante and Richard Peuser made my foray into the archives' military records both productive and entertaining. Thanks are also due to Jeffrey Flannery at the Manuscripts Division of the Library of Congress and to the staffs of the National Archives Regional Centers in Atlanta and Manhattan, especially Richard Gelbke.

My research also took me to the American Medical Association Health Fraud Archives in Chicago, where Jane Kenamore helped track down the records of several early birth control firms, and to the Rockefeller Archive Center in Tarrytown, New York, where Thomas Rosenbaum and Catherine Keim provided expert help. I am also grateful for the assistance I received from Susan McElrath at the National Archives for Black Women's History; George Griffenhagen at the American Pharmaceutical Association Library; Dauce Taube at the Regional History Collection of the University of Southern California; Katherine Donahue at the History and Special Collections Division of UCLA's Louise M. Darling Biomedical Library; Brent Sverdloff at the Historical Collections of the Harvard Business School's Baker Library; Allan Jutzi at the Huntington Library; Patricia Gossel at the Division of Science, Medicine, and Society of the Smithsonian; and Suzanne White-Junod at the History Office of the Food and Drug Administration. At Georgia Tech, Bruce Henson and Mary-Frances Panettiere found information on inventions and inventors. I am also indebted to the staffs of the Schlesinger Library, the Countway Library of Medicine, the Massachusetts College of Pharmacy and Allied Health Sciences, the Sophia Smith Collection at Smith College, the New York Public Library, the Moorland-Spingarn Research Center of Howard University, and the National Museum of American History. Special thanks go to Haven Hawley, Rose Holz, Helen Lefkowitz Horowitz, Richard John, Judith Leavitt, Lara Marks, Leslie Reagan, Tom Sitton, Carroll Smith-Rosenberg, Sandra Thornton, and James Harvey Young for fruitful research suggestions.

I began writing this book in January 1998 as a fellow at the Huntington Library, a scholar's dream. Surrounded by acres of lush flowers and fragrant orange groves, I benefited from the counsel of research director Roy Ritchie, from rigorous walks and lively debates with Timothy Breen, and from the excellent company of Hal Baron, Susan Breen, Mary Coomes, Clark Davis, Barbara Donagan, Philip Goff, Sally Gordon, Colleen Jaurretche, Cheryl Koos, Karen Lystra, Lois Nettle, Charles Royster, Gordon Wood, Walt Woodward, and the late Carrie Saliers, whose incandescent spirit I miss. I consider myself particularly lucky to have met in California Bill Deverell and Jenny Watts, whose friendship I treasure.

Research for this project was funded by the Georgia Tech Foundation, Simon Fraser University, the Rockefeller Archive Center, and the Huntington Library and by a summer stipend and Fellowship for University Teachers from the National Endowment for the Humanities; I extend my heartfelt thanks to each of these organizations for its generosity. I am also indebted to Bob McMath, Greg Nobles, and Michael Bellesiles, whose faith in me and this study helped make these fellowships possible.

Portions of this book were first presented to the Southern History Association; the American Association for the History of Medicine; the American Society for Legal History; the Hagley Center for the History of Business, Technology, and Society; the California Institute of Technology seminar on Public Policy, Science, and Ethics; the Caltech-Huntington Committee for the Humanities; and the George Dock Society in the History of Medicine. I have profited from the comments I received on each of these occasions.

Numerous physicians answered questions, granted interviews, and practiced good medicine; thanks especially to James Caillouette, David Hewitt, Maggie Mermin, Earl Nation, Angela O'Neal, Miriam Ziemen, and Bob Hatcher, whose crusade to make quality contraceptive information and supplies available to all I so admire.

Mike Allen, Clark Davis, Bill Deverell, Lawrence Friedman, Lou Galambos, Gus Giebelhaus, Paul Gilmore, Philip Goff, Sally Gordon, Karen Lystra, Margaret Marsh, Greg Nobles, David Nord, Charles Royster, David Thelen, Steve Usselman, Steven Vallas, and Liz Watkins read drafts of chapters and gave excellent advice. My friend and former colleague Phil Scranton read the entire manuscript in record time and with typical insight and precision, ironing out inconsistencies and asking all the right questions. My mother, Elke Kluge, drew on years of lawyering and experience as a literature professor to fine-tune my legal arguments and polish my prose. My grandmother Waltraud Freyer helped translate Victorian love letters cross-written in archaic German and, along with my grandfather, aunt, and uncle, lodged and fed me during frequent trips to Boston.

Friends indulged endless contraceptive anecdotes and raised nary an eyebrow when I announced that I had begun to collect antique condom tins. For their companionship I thank Michael Fellman, Doug Flamming, Deb Johnson, Daniel Kleinman, Joy Parr, Jonathan Prude, Helen Rozwadowski, Sharon Strocchia, and especially Joan Sokolovsky. I am most grateful for the wise words, common sense, and irrepressible energy of my neighbor and friend the historian Michael Bellesiles. Thanks, too, to his partner, Kate Dornhuber, and their daughter, Lilith Claire, who rightly reined in my exuberant dinnertime storytelling with withering looks and pithy remarks.

I am lucky to work in a department, the School of History, Technology, and Society at Georgia Tech, where many of my colleagues are also my closest friends. For years of good conversation I thank Mike Allen, Gus Giebelhaus, Greg Nobles, Jonathan Schneer, Steve Usselman, and Steven Vallas.

It was Greg who suggested I contact Lauren Osborne at Hill and Wang, and I am glad he did. Lauren has been a dream editor. Her sound advice shaped this project at every stage. I especially came to appreciate her insistence that one can craft a good story that forsakes jargon without sacrificing analysis, and her taking the time to show me how. Thanks, too, to Catherine Newman, to my agent Ronald Goldfarb, and to Dan Kevles for putting me in touch with Ron.

My daughter, Sophia, is only three weeks old as I write this, but already she has taught me that in addition to being a choice, parenthood is a precious gift.

Finally, my husband, John, a historian of Spain, came into my life right around the time this project did. He has heard more academic analyses of sex and contraceptives than some would say a spouse should, and yet not once has his support wavered. He read the manuscript multiple times, improving it on every occasion. For his encouragement, insight, humor, and shared passion to get the story right I dedicate this book to him with thanks and love.

Introduction

I grew up at a time and in a family fortunate enough to take quality medical birth control for granted. Like a bad flashback, the memory of my mother dragging me to the office of our family practitioner for a precollege checkup is still vivid. It was the summer of 1982. The Pill was old news. I left the doctor's office with a year's supply stashed in a brown paper bag. I didn't think I would need them, but I tucked them in my luggage and took them to college. Just in case.

Today an astounding 80 percent of all American women born since 1945 have used oral contraceptives—suggesting both a pharmaceutical basis for the "bonds of womanhood" and the extent to which contraceptive technology has become the doctor's domain.[1] It was not always this way. Until very recently, most American men and women got contraceptives not from physicians but "direct" from the marketplace through mail-order buying and purchases made at pharmacies, five-and-dime stores, gas stations, and vending machines and even from door-to-door peddlers. How this market operated, how it changed, and how it affected the lives of millions of Americans are the subjects of this book.

In *Devices and Desires*, I examine the evolution of the modern birth control industry from 1873, when passage of the federal Comstock Act classified contraceptives as obscene, to the 1970s, when problems with the Dalkon Shield, the nation's best-selling intrauterine device, made front-page news. This book introduces a cast of characters whose stories have been hidden from history: men such as Julius Schmidt, a struggling sausage-casing worker by day who turned surplus animal intestines into a million-dollar condom empire, and women such as Antoinette Hon, a Polish immigrant whose brisk trade in "womb suppositories" and "douching powders" was sustained by working-class dollars. I have attempted to write a book that balances big-picture events like the invention of the Pill with the stories of ordinary people who experienced these events firsthand. Nineteenth-century inventors who fashioned cervical caps out of watch springs; Victorian lovers who celebrated the wonders of rubbers; a mother of six who kissed the photograph of Gregory Pincus, the inventor of the oral contraceptive, at a Planned Parenthood meeting: these are the people who make this story of innovation, regulation, and economic change compelling.

Scholars who have studied birth control in the United States have typically framed its history as a tale of physicians, lawmakers, and political activists. As a result, we know a lot about activists such as Margaret Sanger and the legal obstacles to reproductive rights for women but surprisingly little about the technological and industrial developments that have been equally important in transforming Americans' lives. *Devices and Desires* is the story of what it was like to make, buy, and use contraceptives during a century when the contraceptive industry was transformed from an illicit trade operating out of basement workshops and pornography outlets to one of the most successful legitimate businesses in American history. Why was the ineffective Lysol douche the best-selling contraceptive during the Depression? How can we explain the hostile reaction of many African-American leaders to the invention of the Pill? How did the federal government, once charged with eradicating contraceptives, come to police and promote their scientific efficacy? In tackling these questions and others, I hope to broaden our understanding of birth control while contributing to the histories of sexuality, technology, commerce, medical practice, and criminality.

For much of the twentieth century, the contraceptive industry was illegal. My focus here is less on the law than on the lawbreakers—that is, on the people who came to define prohibitions against birth control on their own terms. To exhume the history of a business that operated illegally, we must examine laws as they were enforced and broken in a variety of settings: from the merchant's supply room, to a Navy vessel's canteen, to the matrimonial bedroom during a night of passion. What we find when we do this is a thriving bootleg trade that accommodated a range of budgets and inclinations. From small-scale businesspeople to large corporations, contraceptive makers have endeavored throughout American history to meet women's and men's birth control needs. This is not to romanticize the dependability of the wares they supplied. Without regulations to protect consumers, many contraceptives—from condoms with holes to one-size-fits-all diaphragms—permitted pregnancy and/or caused pain and untold hardship. But the greatest continuity in the history of modern birth control is the extent to which sexually active individuals have turned to the marketplace to meet their contraceptive needs, irrespective of the legal and medical status of birth control.

Americans' long-standing use of contraceptives has important policy implications for our society today. In recent years, innovations in contraceptive technology have proceeded at an exciting pace, promising a veritable smorgasbord of options in the years ahead. Yet with millions of Americans without health care or prescription drug coverage, too many people have been forced to cut corners with their fertility control, often with devastating results. One health care worker recently shared with me the story of a woman who, unable to afford to see a doctor but determined not to have children, fashioned a makeshift intrauterine device out of a chunk of raw potato. It sprouted *in utero*, causing acute pain and pelvic inflammatory disease. Experiences such as these are preventable. In the years ahead, we must strive to ensure that Americans of all backgrounds have access to the devices that best fulfill their desire for safe and effective birth control.

PART ONE

Comstockery

ONE

1873

The citizens of Washington, D.C., prepared feverishly for Ulysses S. Grant's second inauguration on March 4, 1873. Shopkeepers hung brightly colored fabrics on store windows. Construction crews scrambled to build viewing platforms and string streamers and flags along the procession route, which extended from just outside Georgetown to the Capitol. A week before the official festivities were scheduled to begin, the crowds started to arrive. Trains brought in well-wishers and invited guests: noisy West Point cadets sporting new gray uniforms; a car of musicians and soldiers from New York; a fire company from Philadelphia. By March 3, hotels and boardinghouses in the nation's capital had filled to capacity.[1]

In the midst of this excitement, a distracted Congress hurried to complete unfinished business before it adjourned on March 4. A series of scandals involving financial schemes profiting prominent Republicans and their business cronies had cast a pallor over Washington politics and fueled the reformer Horace Greeley's unsuccessful bid for the presidency in 1872. Laboring under a cloud of suspicion, the Forty-second Congress now worked overtime to end the session with a spate of creditable legislation, as presumably befitted hardworking politicians worthy of the public trust. In the final hours of the term, Congress passed some 260 acts, the precise provisions of which remained unknown to many members.[2] So impressed with their industriousness were these gentlemen that one of the last things they did before adjourning was to vote themselves a pay raise of twenty-five hundred dollars, retroactive for two years.[3]

One measure passed in this last-minute frenzy was an anti-obscenity bill approved in the early-morning hours of Sunday, March 2. Commonly called the Comstock Act after its chief proponent, the morals crusader Anthony Comstock, the statute, embedded in a broader postal act, passed after little political debate and was signed into law along with 117 other bills on March 3. The Comstock Act defined contraceptives as obscene and inaugurated a century of indignities associated with birth control's illicit status. Invoking its authority to regulate interstate commerce and the U.S. postal system, Congress outlawed the dissemination through the mail or across state lines of any "article of an immoral nature, or any drug or medicine, or any article whatever for the prevention of conception."[4] At the time, the act largely eluded public comment. Over the next century, however, its impact on birth control would be profound.

It was not the first time Congress had made obscenity a crime or had sought to regulate what was sent through the mails. In 1835, President Andrew Jackson, courting slaveholder support, recommended that Congress prohibit "the circulation in the Southern States through the mail of incendiary publications intended to incite slaves to insurrections."[5] Seven years later, Congress enacted its first anti-obscenity law, passing without explanation a tariff act authorizing customs officials to seize "obscene or immoral" imported prints and pictures (but not printed matter).[6] Implicitly identifying pornography as a foreign, primarily European, phenomenon, the 1842 statute strove to protect republican virtue from the sexual wickedness presumed to be festering overseas.

By the 1860s, a lively domestic trade in tawdry novels, pamphlets, and photographs had revealed not only that the Tariff Act had failed but also that native, not foreign, hands were to blame. Those who doubted Americans' complicity in the pornography boom that swept the country in the 1850s and 1860s had only to survey return addresses on mailed matter to know better; most hailed from New York, not London or Paris. Improvements in printing technology and reductions in postal rates had made possible the widespread diffusion of titillating publications, and the migration of single men to cities had created an expanding urban market for their consumption.[7] Leisure patterns during the Civil War exacerbated the trend. Divided in their politics, soldiers shared common ground in making mail-order pornography a vibrant part of camp life.[8]

By 1865, Congress had become fed up. Senator Jacob Collamer of Vermont, postmaster general during the Taylor administration, demanded that the power of the federal government be harnessed to stop this spreading social menace. "Our mails," he seethed, "have been made the vehicle for the conveyance of great numbers and quantities of obscene books and pictures . . . and that is getting to be a very great evil."[9] Collamer's bill, enacted on March 3, 1865, made the mailing of any "obscene book, pamphlet, picture, print, or other publication . . . [of] vulgar and indecent character" a misdemeanor punishable by a fine not to exceed five hundred dollars or by imprisonment for no longer than a year. It was left to individual postmasters, who could scrutinize return addresses and look inside printed publications (typically sent open at one end, enabling one to discern the contents without breaking the seal), to exclude materials they considered offensive.[10] In 1872, Congress strengthened the 1865 law, adding envelopes and postcards to its list of "suspicious" articles.[11]

The Comstock Law thus continued a policy of federal obscenity regulation that in 1873 was more than thirty years old. It expanded the scope of the 1872 law by eliminating loopholes and codifying an extraordinarily long list of "obscenities." Ominously, contraceptives made the list for the first time. The decision to include them was Anthony Comstock's.

Comstock was born in 1844 in the countryside of New Canaan, Connecticut, about eight miles east of the New York state line. His father was a prosperous farmer, his mother a devout Congregationalist who died when Comstock was ten. After his mother's death, Comstock remained a zealous devotee of the church, attending services and Sunday school regularly. Throughout his life, he clung to the austere, fire-and-brimstone faith of his childhood. The devil was real, omnipresent, and ready to suck souls into the fiery pits of hell. Abstaining from all things evil was one's only hope for salvation. Impure thoughts and behavior—anything that might derail one from a straight-and-narrow path—were as ruinous in Comstock's eyes as lack of faith. Even church-inspired worldliness was suspect. Once, after attending a Catholic midnight Mass out of curiosity, he confided in his diary that he was "disgusted. Do not think it right to spend Sunday morn. in such manner. Seemed much like Theater."[12]

After his older brother died at Gettysburg, Comstock enlisted in the Seventeenth Regiment of the Connecticut Infantry. He passed most of his one and a half years in the Union Army in a peaceful section of Florida, far removed from the skirmishes of battle. Perhaps he felt, as many men who came of age after the Civil War would later, a hollowness for having missed the "good fight." Perhaps it was this void that turned him into a lifelong crusader. He certainly loved to battle, and nothing could restrain him if he believed Satan, masked as a Confederate, a pornographer, or a bottle of gin, was his foe.[13]

Freed from combat with Confederates, Comstock launched a private war against tobacco, alcohol, gambling, and atheism. He joined the Christian Commission, an organization that distributed temperance and religious tracts to soldiers, and established prayer meetings for his regiment, which he attended four to nine times a week. Although some recruits appreciated formal opportunities for worship, most felt differently about Comstock's refusal to drink whiskey and, even worse, his uncharitable habit of pouring his ration onto the ground. When Comstock left the Army in 1865, he did so, by his own admission, an unpopular man.[14]

After holding short-term posts in Connecticut and Tennessee, Comstock moved to New York City seeking fortune. There, the Connecticut farm boy entered a world radically different from anything he had previously encountered. New York in the 1860s and early 1870s was the center of commercialized sex in the United States, home to a wide array of erotica well integrated into the city's economy and public culture. Once sequestered in brothels, assignation houses, and isolated residential districts, commercial sex in postbellum New York had gone public. Sex was easily viewed and consumed on streets and in hotels, shops, and saloons throughout the city. Prostitutes roamed neighborhoods freely, and posted pictures, window modeling, and even newspaper ads promoted their specialties and rates.[15] Local printers sold pornographic books, pamphlets, drawings, and photographs. Stage shows in concert saloons combined alcohol, food, dance, loud music, and heterosexual and homosexual pleasures. Alone or in groups, entertainers would dance, strip, gyrate suggestively, or insert accoutrements like rubber dildos or cigars into various orifices to tease and tempt the crowds. Masked balls, which enjoyed their peak in popularity after the Civil War, permitted men and women of varying social status to transgress traditional boundaries of public sexual behavior.[16] As they danced about the hall, participants would take advantage of their anonymity to engage in flirting, touching, kissing, and even group sex.

Alone and jobless, the newly arrived Comstock rented a room in a cheap lodging house on Pearl Street near City Hall. He soon found work: first as a porter, then as a salesman for Cochran, McLean and Company, a dry-goods notion house. Nights passed in unkempt boardinghouses and days spent walking the streets gave Comstock firsthand exposure to the traffic in sex. His travels took him around Broadway and Pearl, Warren, Nassau, and Grand Streets, areas where the sale of contraceptives, abortion services, and erotica thrived.[17] What he saw disgusted him, as did the behavior of his young business associates, who gawked at pornographic books and pictures.

Comstock's reactions to this sexualized economy influenced his anti-vice campaign. To ignore that the sex trade was first and foremost a *trade* is to miss an important part of the Comstock story. Vice, as he understood it, would forever be entangled in the commercialized state in which it was consumed. Weeding it out meant destroying an industry.

In 1868, Comstock went on the offensive, making the first of what would be hundreds of arrests during his lifetime. Largely through the efforts of the Young Men's Christian Association (YMCA), the New York legislature had recently passed its own anti-obscenity statute. With this for ammunition, Comstock went vice hunting. When a friend blamed a lewd book for luring him to a brothel, where he contracted a venereal disease, Comstock became furious. He pursued the supplier, a book dealer named Charles Conroy, whose business was headquartered in a basement a block away from where Comstock worked. Comstock bought one of Conroy's sexually explicit books and showed it to the captain of the local police precinct; together they arrested Conroy and seized his stock. As he would with other "vice entrepreneurs" he apprehended, Comstock monitored Conroy's subsequent business dealings and in 1874 arrested the book dealer for the third time. An irate Conroy fought back, slashing the face of the man whose relentless pursuit of vice criminals had already become legendary.[18]

In January 1871, Comstock married Maggie Hamilton, a woman ten years his senior. In December, she bore a daughter, Lillie, who died the following summer. She never became pregnant again.[19] After Lillie's death, the Comstocks adopted a young girl. Comstock's desire for a family and the couple's personal tragedy likely amplified his anger toward women who, in his estimation, casually terminated pregnancies.

In 1872, Comstock's activities were brought to the attention of Morris Ketchum Jesup, a founding member of the New York YMCA and a wealthy merchant and financier.[20] Comstock had contacted the YMCA requesting funds to purchase the equipment and stock of a recently deceased surgeon, book dealer, and pornography printer, William Haynes. Comstock viewed Haynes's death as a golden opportunity to seize the printing technologies used to create pornography before they fell into another's hands. Haynes's stock, valued at thirty thousand dollars, was vast and included steel and copperplate engravings, electroplates, woodcuts, and bookplates. The YMCA gave Comstock the requested sum as well as a temporary storage site for the plates. On April 6, 1872, the engravings were taken to a laboratory at the Polytechnic Institute in Brooklyn, where, under Comstock's supervision, they were methodically destroyed by hand-poured acid.[21]

Jesup was impressed by Comstock's thoroughness and introduced him to other luminaries in the YMCA. Like Jesup, they were wealthy men from devout Protestant families—financiers, lawyers, and clergymen occupying a social stratum different from that of the merchants they aspired to destroy. Like Comstock, many had been raised in small towns and farming communities. Benefiting financially from the transformations that had given rise to an industrial economy, they bemoaned the loss of cohesion and social surveillance that seemed to accompany such change. Supporting Comstock's cause, these gentlemen patrons of reform gave the struggling clerk financial backing and instant credibility. They also provided an organization within which Comstock could respectably wage his war, the New York Society for the Suppression of Vice (NYSSV).[22]

Incorporated on May 16, 1873, the New York Society for the Suppression of Vice was part of a larger social purity movement that joined thousands of upper- and middle-class men and women in a nationwide campaign to enact laws to eliminate social problems such as prostitution, alcoholism, gambling, and narcotics abuse. Before the Civil War, reformers had placed their faith in moral or religious suasion as a strategy for

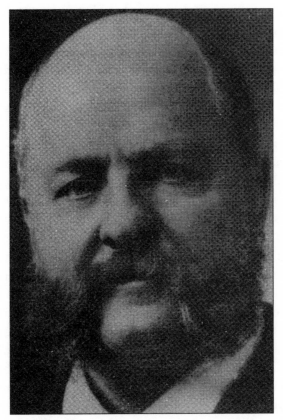

1. Anthony Comstock (Courtesy of the Sophia Smith Collection, Smith College)

coaxing people into exercising self-restraint. As growing numbers of immigrants and working-class people began to settle in urban areas, however, reformers increasingly questioned their ability to regulate the
behavior of "the masses" through personal appeals and sought, instead,
the more authoritative power of government-backed control. Social
purists lobbied hard at the municipal, state, and federal levels, often
working through reform organizations such as the YMCA. The NYSSV,
the YMCA's offshoot, would be one of many urban anti-vice societies
founded after the Civil War. The first of its kind in the country, the
NYSSV was soon joined by parallel organizations in Boston, Chicago,
Cincinnati, Cleveland, Detroit, Louisville, Philadelphia, St. Louis, and
San Francisco.[23]

The public character of the sex trade is what worried reformers most. The Victorian era is often regarded as the height of American prudery, a time of widespread sexual repression. But policy makers at this time reflected far more interest in suppressing public indecency than clandestine acts. This distinction between public and private would have been anathema to Puritans, who strived to unmask and stamp out concealed sin. But it underlay state and municipal measures adopted in the nineteenth century to rein in egregiously public passion. By mid-century, several states had redefined adultery as a crime only when it was "open and notorious." By 1900, most cities had carved out red-light districts for prostitutes, accepting sex for hire in designated areas. As Lawrence Friedman has noted, many social purity reformers accepted vice as an unfortunate but permanent part of society. They sought not to eradicate it but to "build dams and containments: structures of justice and social order that encouraged self-control." Vice was grudgingly tolerated so long as it "remained in the shadows."[24] Certainly, an undercurrent of social control was behind this containment strategy. Public displays of sexuality, reformers warned, would corrupt the innocence of youth, destroy female purity, and inflame the passions of working-class men, whose self-control was already considered weak. Hence Comstock abhorred public nudity, even in the form of high art, because of the dangers it imposed on the uncultivated mind. The crime inhered not in the body itself—"there is nothing else in the world so beautiful as the form of a beautiful maiden," he averred—but in its unveiling: "Let the nude be kept in its proper place and out of the reach of the rabble."[25] Of course, the belief that sexuality was too dangerous to be exposed to the lascivious masses did not prevent even the most zealous vice crusaders from cultivating private pleasures. Comstock's Boston counterpart was Godfrey Lowell Cabot, a leading figure in the New England chapter of the Society for the Suppression of Vice, founded in 1882. In public, Cabot fought the good fight. In private, he penned explicit sexual fantasy letters to his wife.[26]

NYSSV incorporators were some of the wealthiest and most powerful men in the city, including financier J. Pierpont Morgan, copper magnate William E. Dodge, lawyer William C. Beecher (son of Henry Ward Beecher), and head of the Colgate soap empire, Samuel Colgate, who served as NYSSV president for twenty years.[27] But it was the irrepressible Comstock, employed full-time as the NYSSV's agent at a monthly salary of one hundred dollars, who put the organization on the national map. Until his death in 1915, he devoted most of his waking hours to battling the foes of virtue. His latitude for waging this war was great, especially when we consider his background. Here was a man whose station in life (in a society that made much of social distinctions) differed little from that of thousands of other farmers' sons trying to eke out a living in the big city. Only in Comstock's case a few years of struggle and an undistinguished employment record had resulted in direct access to the inner corridors of influence and wealth. Comstock's enforcement powers, authorized by the New York legislature and Congress, were vast. The Society's articles of incorporation, adopted after the Comstock Act had gone into effect, deputized NYSSV agents to assist police in the "suppression of the trade in and circulations of obscene literature and illustrations, advertisements, and articles of indecent and immoral use, as it is or may be forbidden by the laws of the State of New York or of the United States."[28] In 1875, the newly revised New York Criminal Code confirmed the legality of these civilian powers.[29] Comstock received added enforcement privileges directly from Congress, which appointed him special agent of the U.S. Post Office three days after enacting his bill.[30] Because the statute's main enforcement mechanism was the policing of the mails, the position, which Comstock accepted without pay, catapulted him into the ranks of a small band of national law enforcers. All in all, these were extraordinary powers for a struggling-clerk-turned-reformer to wield.

Yet the federal law's nickname was no accident; from the beginning, the campaign for a new anti-obscenity statute had been Comstock's show. His crusade began in earnest in the fall of 1872. In *Frauds Exposed*, the first of his two books, he recalled the circumstances that pushed him into federal politics. "When I undertook the great and all-important work of suppressing by legal process this hydra-headed monster," he wrote, "what did I find? I found a business systemized and systematically carried on. I found newspapers teeming with the advertisements of these bold and shameless criminals. I found laws inadequate, and public sentiment worse than dead, because of an appetite that had been formed for salacious reading."[31] Comstock knew that vice was a national industry sustained by a network of entrepreneurs and agents who used the federal postal service to contact men and women in the farthest reaches of the country. Stopping such a large-scale and intricate business necessitated far-reaching prohibitions. As he explained in a letter to one of his political backers, there were scores of vice entrepreneurs whom "I cannot touch for want of law. There are men in Philadelphia, in Chicago, in Boston, and other places, who are doing this business, that I could easily detect and convict if the law was only sufficient."[32]

After being assured of Jesup's continued financial support, Comstock traveled to Washington in December 1872 to lobby for a statute more inclusive than the 1872 federal anti-obscenity law. Comstock knew firsthand the shortcomings of the 1872 measure. His attempts to prosecute the uninhibited Victoria Woodhull and Tennessee Claflin, sisters and woman's rights activists, for a story on the sexual ruin of two young maidens published in *Woodhull and Claflin's Weekly* came to nought when the presiding judge declared newspapers exempt from the 1872 law.[33] Not one to buckle in the face of adversity, Comstock went to Washington

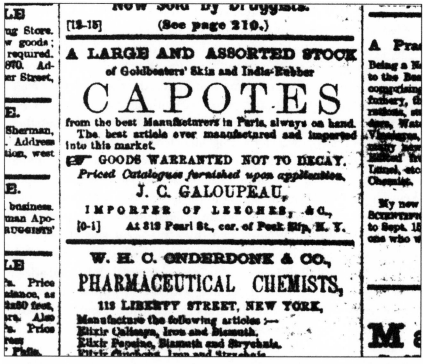

2. Advertisements for birth control, such as this one for skin and rubber condoms published in the January 1871 edition of the *Druggists' Circular and Chemical Gazette*, heightened the public visibility of the contraceptive trade

with a draft of his own bill in tow. Even at this early stage, it included a ban on contraceptives.

Too often, historians have characterized Comstock's bill as a measure whose sole objective was to control women by banning contraceptives and abortion; Comstock's successful criminalization of the fertility control business, moreover, has fanned the belief that he was little more than a nineteenth-century stumbling block on women's path to progress. We need not declare Comstock a champion of woman's rights to recognize that the man's motives and the legislation he authored were more complex than some detractors have suggested. The 1873 act was not a law dealing exclusively with fertility control but an anti-obscenity statute that included birth control and abortion among a long list of commercial "obscenities." To disaggregate the measure, to consider contraception and abortion as isolated components, is to remove them from the political context in which their criminalization was sought and secured. Comstock rallied against contraceptive devices bought and sold in commercial spaces, not against natural forms of birth control such as abstinence and the rhythm method used privately at home. In making this distinction, he articulated the views of many Victorians who publicly supported family limitation only when it was achieved by dignified, "ethical" means.

Comstock's demonization of contraceptives was a direct response to their newfound commercial visibility, not to their invention or use. Women and men have been using birth control since ancient times. The oldest guide to contraception, the *Petrie Papyrus*, an Egyptian medical papyrus dating to 1850 B.C., recommended vaginal suppositories made of crocodile dung, gum, or a mixture of honey and sodium carbonate.[34] Aristotle, writing in the fourth century B.C., noted the tendency of women of his day to coat their cervixes with olive oil before intercourse. Women in preindustrial West Africa made intra-vaginal plugs of crushed root, Japanese women made tampons of bamboo tissue, and women of Easter Island made algae and seaweed pessaries.[35] (A pessary is a substance or device inserted into the vagina that blocks, repels, or otherwise neutralizes sperm.) Although many early techniques undoubtedly made sexual relations awkward and uncomfortable, not all were devoid of contraceptive properties. Honey-based suppositories likely impeded sperm motility. And although crocodile dung probably did not, elephant dung, recommended in thirteenth-century Islamic guides, was more acidic and thus offered women more protection. The olive oil applications of Aristotle's day likely helped prevent pregnancy, too; a 1931 study of birth control by the expert Marie Stopes found a zero percent pregnancy rate in two thousand cases where olive oil had been the only contraceptive.[36]

In early America, women and men built upon and perpetuated this culture of fertility restriction. Prolonged lactation, male withdrawal, abstinence, suppositories, and douching solutions made out of common household ingredients were the mainstays of birth control practice in preindustrial America. Condoms made from linen and the intestines of animals and fish were imported from Europe, where waste from slaughterhouses provided a ready supply of raw materials. More popular than condoms were abortifacients, orally ingested compounds that induced miscarriage. Popular abortifacient ingredients such as savin and pennyroyal grew wild, but as early as the mid-eighteenth century, standard and "female" preparations, advertised in local newspapers, could be purchased in urban centers along the Eastern Seaboard.[37]

The sale of condoms and abortifacients in early America marked the existence of a fledgling contraceptive industry. Developments beginning in the 1830s enhanced its visibility. Vulcanization technology invented by Charles Goodyear in 1839 gave rise to the domestic manufacture of condoms, intrauterine devices, douching syringes, womb veils (the nineteenth-century term for diaphragms and cervical caps), and male caps, shields that covered only the tip of the penis, offering less protection from pregnancy than condoms but greater stimulation to the wearer. Goodyear himself mentioned self-acting syringes, pessaries, and "gonorrhea bags" as examples of the many uses of his discovery in his 1853 book, *Gum-Elastic and Its Varieties*. The vulcanization of rubber expanded birth control options even as it increased individuals' dependence on the market to acquire them. In the early 1870s, condoms, douching syringes and solutions, vaginal sponges, diaphragms, and cervical caps could be purchased from mail-order houses, wholesale drug-supply houses, pharmacies, and dry-goods and rubber vendors. Not just in New York but in cities across the country, vendors of condoms and diaphragms also sold other rubber articles like dildos. The same printers who peddled guides on how to use a douching syringe for contraception sold photographs of naked men, women, and children. Inexpensive, sensationalist, and sporting publications of "questionable character" promoted impotence cures, pornography, and contraceptives simultaneously.[38]

Established firms and respected physicians and druggists also distributed birth control devices. But what Comstock and his cronies found so threatening was the prominence of contraceptives in the vice trade—a robust and increasingly visible commerce in illicit products and pleasures that seemed to encourage sexual license by freeing sex from marriage and childbearing. Entrepreneurs advertised contraceptives in newspapers, broadsides, home medical manuals, and private cards placed strategically on street corners, in railway and steamship depots, and in hotel lobbies. Advertisements on the front page of the *Cleveland Plain Dealer* on July 1, 1863, for "Dr. Wadsworth's Uterine Elevators for Sale, Wholesale and Retail" and "The Great French Preventive Pill" typified how advertising brought the commerce of reproductive control directly into people's homes.[39] According to one observer, in 1872 there was "hardly a newspaper that does not contain . . . open and printed advertisements, or a drug store whose shelves are not crowded with nostrums publicly and unblushingly displayed."[40]

Moralists denounced the increasingly public face of the birth control trade. In his 1867 tract, the aptly titled *Serpents in the Doves' Nest*, the Congregationalist minister John Todd, alarmed at the growth of single-child families, observed, "There is scarcely a young lady in New England—and probably it is so throughout the land—whose marriage can be announced in the paper without her being insulted within a week by receiving through the mail a printed circular, offering information and instrumentalities, and all needed facilities, by which the laws of heaven in regard to the increase of the human family may be thwarted."[41] Others registered similar complaints. In 1872, the Syracuse physician Ely Van de Warker condemned newspaper and magazine publishers for printing "pernicious advertisement[s]" of gynecological nostrums, spurring the growth of a "trade which, without stretching a single existing law, may be called illegal and illicit, carried on in open daylight, in the full knowledge of [the] newspaper-reading public."[42]

In the complex matrix of Victorian sexuality, condemnations of contraceptives did not automatically denote opposition to all forms of family limitation. Rather than universally supporting or denouncing both birth control and abortion, most discussants of reproductive control occupied a contested middle ground in which the two strategies were separately assessed.[43] Although women often relied on both methods to limit family size, physicians, legislators, and social purity reformers made much of the difference. This bifurcation was reflected in the realm of criminal law. Between 1821 and 1841, ten states passed laws criminalizing abortion, making it a statutory offense for the first time in the nation's history. Not until the Comstock Act, however, did legislation deal explicitly with contraception.[44]

Comstock's views on abortion were clear. Abortion was permissible only when a woman's life was in danger. But Comstock's views on birth control were more conflicted. He professed to support contraception when it was "natural" and to oppose it when it was not. When asked by a journalist if contraception was desirable when pregnancy might endanger a woman's life, he agreed that it was. But, he queried, "can they not use self-control? Or must they sink to the level of the beasts? . . . God has set certain natural barriers."[45] Comstock clung to a typology of birth control common in the late nineteenth century that distinguished between natural and artificial (man-made) methods. Although he never defined natural birth control in writing—to have done so likely would have constituted an obscenity in his eyes—he undoubtedly meant, as did others at the time, abstinence or the rhythm method, in which intercourse was avoided during times of suspected ovulation. For Comstock, such acts of self-restraint were permissible when they occurred between wedded men and women in the sanctity of the marriage bed. Indeed, given his affection for sexual self-control, he may have believed them to be character building.

Far from being marginal, Comstock's views on fertility control reflected the sentiments of the majority of his contemporaries who openly discussed birth control and abortion. Although many were complicit in the practice of abortion, its only true proponents were *abortionists* themselves.[46] Sexual radicals such as Ezra Heywood, who condemned marriage as an institution giving men free rein to force themselves sexually on women, and Victoria Woodhull, who advocated free love and female suffrage, despised Comstock, but, like him, they sanctioned only natural birth control. Heywood recommended periodic abstinence. Barrier methods (condoms, douches, and pessaries), male withdrawal, and anything that might tamper with intercourse's journey from erection to ejaculation he deemed "unnatural, injurious, or offensive." "These artificial means of preventing conception," Heywood insisted, "are not generally patronized by Free Lovers." Tennessee Claflin, Woodhull's sister, declared the "washes, teas, tonics, and various sorts of appliances" used for contraception to be nothing short of a "standing reproach upon, and a permanent indictment against, American women."[47]

Other activists also distinguished between strategies of family limitation. Women purity reformers tended to support natural family planning methods but not contraceptives, which they associated with promiscuity, particularly with men's license to have sex outside the bonds of marriage. Their opposition to contraceptives was part of a larger defense of female sexual purity that protected women's roles as guardians of the nation's morals at a time when women's economic and political opportunities were limited. Prostitution, the saloon, and other examples of male licentiousness were condemned as assaults on the sanctity of the home. By uncoupling sex and procreation, contraceptives challenged a critical tenet of the reformers' maternalist campaign: the belief that women's moral authority derived from their distinctive attributes as current and prospective mothers. By promoting the desirability of non-procreative sex, the contraceptive market tacitly endorsed the subversive notion that intercourse could be "just for fun." Suffragists likewise tended to view contraceptives as an inducement to promiscuity or, like the irreverent Woodhull, as physically unnatural, but they supported voluntary motherhood, because it gave women the right to say no and to choose the circumstances under which they became pregnant.

This typology of good and bad contraception, anchored in the belief that couples who elected to have intercourse should not tamper with its result, was also embraced by most physicians of the day. One was Nicholas Cooke, whose 412-page tome, *Satan in Society*, written in 1870, is often considered emblematic of the anti-birth-control extremism of his time. Cooke described the diaphragm as "the invention of hell," but even he believed there were times when pregnancy prevention was medically necessary and considered it his duty to educate readers about what to do under such circumstances. "There are but two legitimate methods of avoiding increase of family," Cooke instructed. The first was total abstinence. The second was partial continence, "absolute avoidance of the conjugal act for the term of fourteen days after the cessation of the last monthly period." All other methods "are disgusting, beastly, positively wrongful, as well as unnatural and physically *injurious*."[48]

The preoccupation with the natural that marked discussions of birth control meant different things to different groups. In the hands of free lovers, the celebration of the natural acknowledged female sexuality to be vital to a woman's spiritual and physiological well-being. For physicians like Cooke, it promoted a reproductive essentialism that upheld traditional roles for women by trumpeting the scientific basis for separate spheres. Like contraceptives, the medical profession had undergone its own market revolution in nineteenth-century America. Through professional organization, state accreditation, and formal training, physicians had buttressed their claim to a monopoly of legitimate medical knowledge and discredited lay practitioners as charlatans and quacks. Claiming science as their ally, licensed physicians (known as regulars) had made axiomatic in medical thinking the view that women were controlled by their reproductive organs. Horatio Storer, the American Medical Association's most vocal anti-abortionist, succinctly summarized this school of thought when he asserted in 1871 that woman was "what she is in health, in character, in her charms, alike of body, mind and soul because of her womb alone."[49]

The flip side to the medical glorification of the womb was the insistence that women who denied its primary task, to bear children, courted disaster. What doctors deemed unprocreative, and hence unnatural, behavior included the desire to stay unmarried, pursue a college degree, or remain childless. In 1873, the Massachusetts physician Edward H. Clarke, arguing against women's participation in higher education, warned that disrespect for "the peculiarities of a woman's organization" hastened the onset of "those grievous maladies which torture a woman's earthly existence, called leucorrhoea, amenorrhoea, dysmenorrhoea, chronic and acute ovaritis, prolapsus uteri, hysteria, neuralgia, *and the like*."[50] Doctors warned women that contraceptive use could induce cancer, sterility, insanity, or "deranged" bladders and rectums. Men, too, were urged to defer to Mother Nature or pay the penalties of disobedience. To deposit one's semen in its natural place was one thing; to disperse it randomly rendered a man weak and susceptible to disease. Masturbation and male withdrawal, cautioned Cooke, "being *against Nature*, she revenges herself for her violated laws in diseases of the brain and spinal marrow, functional disorders, organic diseases of the heart, lungs, and kidneys, wasting of the muscles, blindness, and frequently by impotence."[51]

Remonstrations against contraceptives in public should not be confused with their frequent use in private, which contributed to the steadily falling birthrate in America after 1820 and turned the contraceptive industry into the "hydra-headed monster" Comstock deplored. Karen Lystra's study of romance and courtship in nineteenth-century America has revealed a rich private culture of fertility control and sexual expression at odds with public advocations of passionless sex and repression.[52] Rather, public debate illustrates the need to understand Comstock's opposition to birth control devices within a larger intellectual climate in which activists and professionals whose politics were otherwise opposed found common ground in their denunciation of contraceptives as socially disruptive, morally offensive, and physically dangerous.

In addition, Comstock believed that sexual vice operated according to a domino effect: one evil inevitably led to another. The availability of contraceptives, he believed, encouraged lewdness and lust. By the same token, lust being "the boon companion of all other crimes," it was a short leap from pornography to intercourse in which sexual partners used manmade gadgetry to override God's and nature's plans.[53] In the NYSSV's 1876 annual report, Comstock expounded on the seamlessness of the vice economy:

> We can only hint at the *nature* of this literature. It consists
> of books, pamphlets, tracts, leaflets, of pictures engraved on
> steel and wood, of photographs, cards, and charms, all de-
> signed and cunningly calculated to inflame the passions
> and lead the victims from one step of vice to another, end-
> ing in utmost lust. And when the victims have been pol-
> luted in thought and imagination and thus prepared for the
> commission of lustful crime, the authors of their debase-
> ment present a variety of implements by the aid of which

they promise them the practice of licentiousness without its direful consequences to them and their guilty partners.[54]

The danger in partaking of such pernicious commercial pleasures was that there could be no turning back. Invoking the imagery of infection, Comstock described vice as an aggressive and incurable disease. Once a person was contaminated, vice grew, festered, and finally became all-consuming. "This cursed business of obscene literature works beneath the surface," he explained, "and like a canker worm, secretly eats out . . . moral life and purity." In 1868, he had seen firsthand the inevitable trajectory of vice and arrested Conroy for the ruin of the friend whose pornography purchase had led to the use of prostitutes, disease, and damnation. For Comstock, buying a diaphragm was dangerous, not only because its use was an offense against God but also because it put men and women on the streets and inside shops where vice knew no bounds.

Comstock's understanding of the integrated state of the sexual economy and his views on the contagion of evil led him to condemn commercial birth control. But no evidence suggests that his bill, an antibusiness measure, was designed primarily to compel women to bear children. Nor is there evidence of congressional support for this position. Indeed, the historical record indicates little discussion of birth control and plenty of apathy and confusion.

Arriving in Washington in December 1872, Comstock convinced two Republicans, Representative Clinton L. Merriam, a banker from Locust Grove, New York, and Senator William A. Buckingham of Connecticut, the state's former war governor, to introduce his bill in their respective houses.[55] In January, he visited the House with Merriam and lobbied for his bill by displaying, to the chagrin of a number of representatives, an "exhibit" of pornographic books, pictures, postcards, and contraceptive and abortifacient devices. By the time his traveling stash of horrors made it to the Senate on February 6, the bill had already been brought before both chambers.[56]

But Comstock's was not the only proposal aimed at tightening legal sanctions on the transmission of obscenity. Several other bills were also under consideration. One, instigated by the secretary of the local Wash-

ington YMCA, sought to end the obscenity traffic in the District of Columbia and U.S. territories. Another endeavored to increase the penalty
of the 1872 law without broadening its scope. General Benjamin F. Butler of the House Judiciary Committee had introduced a bill to amend the
interstate commerce law to prohibit common carriers from sending obscene materials across state lines. In the interests of expediency, it was
decided to combine these bills with Comstock's.

The new bill, which included Comstock's ban on birth control, encountered unanticipated obstacles. On February 7, Butler, who had already exhibited a special interest in the topic, took the refurbished bill
home with him and made so many revisions that it had to be reprinted
and reconsidered by committee. A frustrated Comstock sought the
support of Senator William Windham of Minnesota, whom he knew
through their mutual acquaintance the Supreme Court justice William
Strong. Windham introduced the revised bill and had it entrusted to the
Committee on Post-Offices and Post Roads, which recommended it
unanimously. Unfortunately for Comstock, when the bill came out of
committee on February 14, Senator George Edmunds of Vermont took
objection and had it amended to include a clause to permit birth control
or abortion with "the prescription of a physician in good standing." A
suspicious Comstock, ever mindful of the profitability of the sex trade,
wondered in his diary: "Has he friends in this business that he desires to
shield?"[57] Fortunately for Comstock, Senator Buckingham intervened
and quietly quashed Edmunds's amendment through a stream of vaguely
worded substitutions. So deft in his subterfuge was Buckingham that
when the time arrived to discuss the amendments to Edmunds's version,
a confused Republican senator Roscoe Conkling of Utica, New York, admitted that "no Senator is able to get any intelligent idea of the substance of this amendment as contrasted with that which it is to take the
place of."[58] Hoping to quiet Conkling, Buckingham lied. Without mentioning his deletion of the clause exempting physicians from prosecution,
he assured Conkling that no substantive alteration had been made. Although Conkling's continuing concern resulted in yet another reprinting
of the revisions, the bill passed the Senate on February 21 without further discussion, and it did so (as it would later in the House) without a
clause permitting doctors to prescribe birth control. In the long run, this
had special consequences for the legal status of contraceptives. Because

most state abortion regulations contained therapeutic clauses permitting licensed physicians to perform abortions when a mother's life was in danger, the federal law ironically made pregnancy *prevention* the more serious crime.

The brevity of the debate in the Senate was outdone by that in the House, where discussion was virtually nonexistent. On February 22, the House received word that the Comstock bill had cleared the Senate. Around one a.m. on Sunday, March 2, Merriam, hoping for a speedy House concurrence, moved "to suspend the rules to take from the Speaker's table and put upon its passage the bill for the suppression of trade in and circulation of obscene literature and articles of immoral use."[59] Representative Michael Kerr of Indiana, alarmed at the bill's regulatory scope, urged instead that it be referred to the Judiciary Committee. The bill's "provisions are extremely important," he implored, and "they ought not to be passed in such hot haste."[60] But "hot haste" is exactly what Kerr's colleagues fancied in those early-morning hours. Merriam's motion to suspend the rules was approved, and the House, shortly before recessing, passed the Comstock bill by a vote of one hundred to thirty-seven.

The wording of the final act casts birth control as a small but vital part of a diabolical, national trade motored by mail-order commerce. It specifies that

> no obscene, lewd, or lascivious book, pamphlet, picture, paper, print, or other publication of an indecent character, or any article or thing designed or intended for the prevention of conception or producing of abortion, nor any article or thing intended or adapted for any indecent or immoral use or nature, nor any written or printed card, circular, book, pamphlet, advertisement or notice of any kind giving information, directly or indirectly, where, or how, or of whom, or by what means either of the things mentioned may be obtained or made . . . shall be carried in the mail; and any person who shall knowingly deposit, or cause to be deposited, for mailing or delivery, any of the hereinbefore-mentioned articles or things, and any person who . . . shall take, or cause to be taken, from the mail any such letter or

package, shall be deemed guilty of a misdemeanor, and, on
conviction thereof, shall, for every offense, be fined not less
than one hundred dollars nor more than five thousand dollars, or imprisoned at hard labor not less than one year nor
more than ten years, or both, in the discretion of the
judge.[61]

An additional clause authorized the seizure and destruction of obscene
items. Another forbade the importation of contraceptives and abortifacients. Another banned the manufacture, advertisement, and sale of
obscene articles in the District of Columbia or U.S. territories, places
within the exclusive jurisdiction of the United States. With these words
two days before its adjournment, the Forty-second Congress made the
birth control business illegal.

Although how aware many congressmen were of what they were endorsing in those early-morning hours is questionable, Comstock himself
harbored no doubts. His diary captured his mood: "O how can I express
the joy of my Soul or speak of the mercy of God."[62]

The Comstock Act and the reign of sexual censorship it inaugurated
did not go unnoticed in other countries. In Ireland, the playwright
George Bernard Shaw coined the term "Comstockery" to describe the
new puritanism, calling it the "world's standing joke at the expense of
the United States. . . . It confirms the deep-seated conviction of the
world that America is a provincial place."[63] Shaw was right on at least
one count: U.S. laws on birth control stood unique among those of the
Western world. Not until 1892 did Canada make the advertisement or
sale of contraceptives an indictable offense "liable to two years' imprisonment," and even then lawmakers exempted physicians serving the interests of the "public good" from prosecution.[64] European countries were
even slower to act, and the legislation they adopted was less restrictive.
By 1915, Holland and Switzerland had passed statutes to curb contraceptive advertising, and England had adopted a measure reserving contraceptives for individuals who were married or about to be. Italy, France,
and Russia had no restrictions at all.[65]

The federal government's abandonment of a laissez-faire approach to
birth control facilitated comparable state initiatives. Twenty-four states
enacted so-called mini Comstock acts proscribing the sale and advertise-

ment of contraceptives and contraceptive information within state lines. In 1879, Connecticut earned the distinction of criminalizing the very *use* of contraceptives, a prohibition not overturned until the Supreme Court's monumental *Griswold* v. *Connecticut* ruling almost a century later.[66]

But in March 1873, such legislative affirmations of his work still lay ahead for Anthony Comstock. The crusader from New York had come a long way. Only seven years earlier, he had been alone in the great metropolis, scouring the streets in search of work. Now, with the support of some of the country's wealthiest and most powerful men, he had changed national law. Equipped with a new statute and post and an expanded mission, the country's newly ordained vigilante of vice left Washington confident of his ability to destroy the contraceptive trade. In this, he would be wrong. Like Representative Kerr, many Americans questioned the advisability and constitutionality of such far-reaching congressional interference. Others simply refused to consider contraception in any form a crime. After 1873, the "sins" Comstock had conflated would be disaggregated and judged, one by one, where it mattered most—in the marketplace and in the court of Americans' conscience.

TWO

The Limits of the Law

Comstock was excited. Postal agents had caught contraceptive entrepreneur George Brinckerhoff red-handed. On March 12, 1873, Brinckerhoff, sole owner of the Eugenic Manufacturing Company, specializing in the production of "several different styles of Ladies Rubber Goods," sent contraceptives from his Brooklyn office to an undercover postal agent in Washington, D.C. In New York, Comstock arranged for Brinckerhoff's arrest. With correspondence and mail-order merchandise as evidence of wrongdoing, it seemed an open-and-shut case. It was not. In the U.S. circuit court, Brinckerhoff pleaded not guilty, insisting that "he did not know the dangers of the article complained of in his case." To Comstock's chagrin, the prosecutor dismissed all charges, returning Brinckerhoff to the streets, where the entrepreneur resumed his trade. Five years later, he was still in business and, according to credit reporters, doing well.[1]

The ability of people like George Brinckerhoff to violate the law with impunity underscores the need to think of the criminalization of birth control not only as a statutory event decreed by legislators but as a fluid, dynamic process shaped by manufacturers, retailers, consumers, and the justice system. Scholars have often characterized the period between criminalization in the 1870s and Margaret Sanger's movement in the second decade of the twentieth century as birth control's bleakest chapter, a time when only a privileged few could afford the services of sympathetic doctors or of a dwindling number of merchants who would ignore the law for the right price. Sanger herself was among the first to voice this interpretation, stating that an almost yearlong search for information on contraceptives in 1913 yielded "no information more reliable than that exchanged by any back-fence gossips in any small town."[2]

Yet an abundance of evidence—from arrest and Post Office Department records to credit reports, trade catalogues, trial transcripts, advertisements, patents, medical literature, and private letters between lovers and friends—points to a very different scenario in which legal leniency, entrepreneurial savvy, and cross-class consumer support enabled the black market in birth control to thrive. Such findings hardly point to a hitherto unrecognized golden age of safe or effective birth control. They do, however, call into question assumptions of draconian enforcement of birth control restrictions and shed new light on sexual practices as they were defined by ordinary Victorians, not just politicians and moralists. Not openly endorsed, contraceptives were nonetheless accepted as Americans of all backgrounds created a zone of tolerance in which birth control was routinely made, sold, bought, and used.

From the beginning, enforcers of the new law faced many obstacles, including the scope of the regulations and inadequate funding. The Comstock Act banned the distribution of contraceptives and dozens of other obscenities, from lewd photographs to pornographic trinkets. Under the law, the policing of each was accorded equal status. Because the anti-obscenity provisions were embedded in a postal statute, the herculean task of enforcing them became the responsibility of Post Office inspectors, also called special agents. In 1873, their duty roster, which included the enforcement of other postal laws as well as interstate commerce regulations governing the transport of goods by common carrier, was full. With the Comstock Act, it swelled further. Had Congress insisted on the hiring of dozens of additional agents, the law might have been successfully enforced. But Congress did not. Between 1872 and 1873, the postmaster general hired four new inspectors nationwide, increasing the total number from fifty-nine to a still-paltry sixty-three. Few in number and strapped for time, inspectors could only do so much. Of the 410 arrests made by all Post Office agents in the United States between May 1,

1875, and April 30, 1876, only 27 were for violations of the Comstock Law.[3]

The difficulty of eliminating the birth control trade was exacerbated by the balance of federal and state regulatory power. Despite the passage of "mini" Comstock acts in twenty-four states, the regulation of the contraceptive trade was principally a federal matter. Because the birth control business depended on interstate commerce and the U.S. Post Office, its regulation by federal authorities was recognized and accepted. Tellingly, the majority of persons arrested for birth control crimes in post-1873 America were indicted, tried, or sentenced in federal courts for breaking federal law.[4] Designating the contraceptive industry a federal issue, state legislatures made its regulation a federal burden.

The most successful apprehender of birth control "criminals" was Comstock himself. His zeal, ridiculed in the press, coupled with his Post Office colleagues' chronic overwork, ensured that he and fellow NYSSV agents, deputized by the New York state legislature to enforce state and federal obscenity laws, performed the lion's share of obscenity policing. Because agents painstakingly catalogued details of each arrest, including charges filed, the outcome of each legal proceeding, and the arrestee's business address, aliases, inventory, and occupation, we have a remarkable repository of information about contraceptive entrepreneurship and criminality in late-nineteenth-century America.

Although a little over half (54 percent) of those arrested resided in the state of New York, it would be a mistake to assume that this is only a New York story. NYSSV agents typically detected entrepreneurs who advertised in New York's myriad sensationalist and working-class tabloids, media that privileged local merchants. Moreover, contraceptive entrepreneurs, especially those who advertised in newspapers, depended on mail-order commerce and used the postal system to transcend regional and rural obstacles to birth control buying. Indeed, NYSSV arrestees included dozens of contraceptive purveyors who advertised in New York papers but whose mail-order outfits were based in states as far away as Iowa and Tennessee.[5] Surviving records, including newspaper advertisements, private letters, court cases, and patents, support Comstock's fear that New York's contraceptive "troubles" paralleled those of the nation.

What is astonishing about NYSSV records is the infrequency of contraception-related arrests. Notwithstanding the Society's broad discretionary powers, its chief's devotion to the task, and the existence of a vibrant bootleg market, NYSSV agents arrested only 105 men and women between March 1873 and March 1898 for the crime of birth control, fewer than 5 per year.[6] One explanation for this thin harvest was the variety and volume of offenses claiming agents' time. But equally significant was the inspectors' tunnel vision. Ignoring the intricacies of the contraceptive industry, agents pursued a select group of birth control sellers—those whose activities most closely resembled their stereotypes of smut peddling—but left other, equally important participants in the trade alone. In theory, anti-obscenity legislation applied to all purveyors of contraceptives. In practice, smaller players were more likely to be investigated. Investigators viewed contraceptive entrepreneurs not only as businesspeople breaking the law but as a criminal class.

Such elitist understandings of sexual criminality, spawned by a virulent amalgamation of nativism, sexism, and elitism, were not new. It was the social purity movement's success in linking contraceptives to sexual licentiousness, brothels, and bars that had prompted Comstock to classify contraceptives as an obscenity in the first place. Once the law went into effect, contraceptives continued to be tied to a street-and-saloon culture profiting men and women presumed to be devoid of scruples and class: "bad" men, "sly" Jews, "moral-cancer-planters," and "old she villains." Purity crusaders' compartmentalization of the world into separate spheres of vice and virtue encouraged inspectors to view the elimination of the rubber vendors and "infidel quacks" who advertised their wares in tabloids and circulars as key to the suppression of the industry. Such entrepreneurs were disparaged as soulless vermin, "ghouls and vampires" of the lowest sort. By contrast, patrons of the NYSSV who sought their arrest were, in Comstock's words, "honest, brave men."[7]

Ironically, Comstock need have looked no further than his "honest" men to detect a crime in progress. The perpetrator was none other than Samuel Colgate, president of the NYSSV and millionaire heir of Colgate and Company, a New Jersey–based soap firm. Colgate held exclusive U.S. distribution rights to Vaseline and in the mid-1870s launched an aggressive campaign advertising the substance's therapeutic value. The cornerstone of his initiative was a twelve-page promotional pamphlet that included a doctor's endorsement of Vaseline's contraceptive benefits. Reminding readers that "prevention is better than cure," the practitioner observed that "Vaseline, charged with four to five grains of salicylic acid, will destroy spermatozoa, without injury to the uterus or vagina."[8]

Colgate's hypocrisy—serving as president of an organization that opposed contraceptives while attempting to profit from their sale—exemplified the class bias undergirding enforcement efforts, and it did not go unnoticed. The anarchist and free-love advocate Ezra Heywood, who was arrested four times between 1878 and 1890 for violating obscenity laws, correctly identified enforcement, NYSSV-style, as a class issue. There was no justice, he argued, in a world where ordinary people had to "lie and cheat like the devil in order to get an honest living" but privileged men such as Colgate got "rich making and selling Vaseline for preventing conception." Nor was Colgate the only entrepreneur whose crimes were conveniently ignored. Heywood charged that the contraceptive trade was teeming with " 'pure' Shylocks [who] make and vend tons of syringes to prevent conception, yet are unmolested [because they are] well-beloved fellow members of Brooklyn Churches with Comstock [and] Colgate!" Freethinkers dubbed the NYSSV the "Society for the Manufacture and Suppression of Vice" and boycotted Colgate's products for years.[9]

The NYSSV spared Colgate but arrested Morris Glattstine. The twenty-six-year-old Polish Jew, described by Comstock as "shrewd and lazy," bought condoms and diaphragms from the Milwaukee-based Stuart Rubber Company. Most of his stock was reserved for resale to outlying retailers, but Glattstine also sold birth control devices directly to consumers at his druggist's sundries and rubber goods store on 77 East Broadway in New York City. In March 1878, Comstock paid a visit and arrested Glattstine, seizing his inventory—a damning "6 womb veils and 15 caps and capotes"—for evidence. Comstock reported to his superior in the Post Office that he had "discovered where [Glattstine and his clerk] get their stock, of a manufacturer in the West." But he left the Stuart Rubber Company alone.[10]

The legal handling of Colgate, Glattstine, and the Stuart Rubber Company illustrates the selective enforcement of laws against contraceptives. In theory, anti-obscenity legislation applied to all purveyors of contraceptives, including established rubber and pharmaceutical houses that manufactured and distributed items commonly used for birth control. In practice, smaller players were more likely to be arrested. Investigators viewed contraceptive entrepreneurs not only as businesspeople breaking the law but also as members of a criminal class.

Because we cannot enumerate the large and small firms that participated in the contraceptive trade, we cannot be certain of the statistical *extent* of enforcement bias. No census or even informal inventory of bootleg birth control outfits exists. What we *can* say is that established companies that made, distributed, and advertised contraceptives were not prosecuted. Catalogues circulated by B. F. Goodrich, Goodyear, Sears, Roebuck & Company, and wholesale drug-supply houses such as McKesson & Robbins advertised a full line of contraceptives, from intrauterine devices to vaginal pessaries, douching syringes, toilet sponges, and male caps. Like Samuel Colgate, however, these companies had reputations as ethical medical and pharmaceutical vendors that shielded them from prosecution. Intriguingly, the only contraceptive mentioned by brand in the Mosher report, a survey of the marital relations of forty-five women at the turn of the century, was a "Good-year rubber ring," worn by a woman for two years following the birth of her first child. Though that woman had no difficulty associating birth control devices with dignified commerce, law enforcers did. It was more comforting to declare the vice trade something other than business as usual.[11]

In the 1930s, regulations enforced by the Food and Drug Administration and the Federal Trade Commission and the expense of new manufacturing technologies would shut smaller players out, concentrating contraceptive production and profits in the hands of a few. But in the age of Comstock, small entrepreneurs held their ground. They knew they were being hunted. Adopting strategies of concealment, they resisted the criminalization of their trade.

Purveyors disguised their products through creative relabeling. Classified ads published in the medical, rubber, and toilet goods sections of dailies and weeklies indicate a flourishing contraceptive trade in post-1873 America. The hitch was that contraceptives were rarely advertised openly as preventives. Condoms were sold as sheaths, male shields, capotes, and, as one 1889 ad in the weekly crime tabloid the *National Police Gazette* read, "rubber goods . . . [for] gents. 25 cents each." Women's pessaries were advertised as uterine elevators, ladies' shields, protectors, womb supporters, "married women's friends," and "copper molds. You know. $1."[12] Because many of these labels had figured in advertisements published before the Comstock Law was enacted, their reappearance after 1873 signaled to consumers what was being sold. The more discernible shift after criminalization was in advertised uses. Birth control previously marketed openly for the prevention of conception was repackaged under legal euphemisms—"protection," "security," "safety," and "reliability for married women"—that highlighted contraceptive properties while shielding retailers from criminal prosecution.

Inventors resorted to similar acts of subterfuge to disguise their activities. Late-nineteenth- and early-twentieth-century patent records are replete with birth control devices that, in contrast with descriptions from earlier years, omit explicit mention of the inventions' contraceptive uses. Take the case of the Texas inventor Uberto Ezell. In 1904, Ezell applied for a patent for his recently designed condom, which he referred to only as a "male pouch." The item illustrated on his application certainly looked like a condom, and it functioned like a condom as well. According to Ezell, whose patent was approved in 1906, there was only one place his rubber pouch was meant to go: on "the male organ to catch and retain all discharges coming therefrom."[13] An intrauterine device (IUD) patented in 1895 is equally suggestive of inventors' abilities to respond to consumer desire for birth control in the face of legal and medical opposition. It included a streamlined retaining feature and a self-insertion device that required "the exercise of a minimum degree of skill," freeing users from dependence on medical experts.[14]

Camouflaging their products, contraceptive entrepreneurs concealed themselves too. Most adopted commercial aliases, forcing Post Office inspectors to work harder to discover their true identity. Of the 105 men and women arrested for birth-control-related offenses by the NYSSV between 1873 and 1898, 91 (87 percent) had used aliases. Although those aliases did not prevent arrest, their widespread adoption indicates the importance entrepreneurs assigned to them and suggests that subterfuge may help account for low overall arrest rates. Harriet Losey of Louisville, Kentucky, sold contraceptives as Madame Zelaski; Orson Robb, a health officer in West Troy, New York, sold them under the name Madame L. Colton. Many birth control entrepreneurs used multiple aliases. Henry Hunter of New Hampshire, who was arrested on September 22, 1873, admitted to twenty-six.[15]

Retailers also relied on geographic concealment to disguise their stock and trade. Hiding inventory was astute: stock on hand at the time of arrest supplied evidence of criminal activity during statutory prosecutions. Edward Bliss Foote sold birth control in Manhattan but sequestered his inventory elsewhere, filling orders only twice a month. Francis Andrews operated a fancy goods and auction store in downtown Albany but kept five thousand condoms—most of his stock—stashed in a room off his bedroom. When credit reporters tracked down George Brinckerhoff, they found his office "arranged for privacy" and its cautious inhabitant unwilling "to make any disclosure of his financial condition."[16]

Such subterfuge forced inspectors to struggle to catch birth control purveyors in the act. Adopting aliases of their own, agents posed as consumers in search of black-market birth control. They perused "suspect" publications—commercial circulars, lowbrow dailies, and sensationalist sex-and-crime weeklies like the New York–based *National Police Gazette*—and investigated formal complaints. Having identified probable offenders, they contacted them, purchased advertised items, and made arrests once the contraband was in hand. In court, the original ad, follow-up correspondence, and the articles themselves were used as evidence that the accused had broken the law.[17] The detection, hunt, and capture could take weeks, even months.

The endeavor was not only time-consuming; it was often unrewarding. Among entrepreneurs' allies were the prosecutors, judges, and jurors who decided their fate. Of all NYSSV-initiated arrests in the late nineteenth century, those made for reproductive control crimes were the least likely to result in conviction.[18] Had Comstock had his druthers, every arrestee would have received a five-thousand-dollar fine and ten years' imprisonment, the maximum sentence allowed under federal law. But the wheels of justice turned differently.

The leniency accorded Sarah Chase, first arrested in 1878, exemplifies the obstacles law enforcers faced. Since 1874, Chase had been selling contraceptives in Manhattan and Brooklyn without incident. A graduate of the Cleveland Homeopathic College, Chase had moved to Manhattan with her eight-year-old daughter, Grace, in 1874, earning a living giving talks on physiology and sexology at church and meeting halls. She quickly developed a reputation as a gifted and knowledgeable lecturer; with Peter Cooper's permission, she even offered a twelve-session course on "manhood" at the esteemed Cooper Union academy for the advancement of science and art. At the conclusion of her lectures, Chase sold birth control, which she also advertised in circulars sent through the mail.[19]

In 1878, her activities caught Comstock's attention after he was contacted by "a prominent physician, who had been called to treat a young woman terribly ulcerated from repeated use of [Chase's] vile article." The woman had attended one of Chase's lectures, purchased a "sponge swab and syringe," and, following Chase's instructions, used them "immediately after copulation . . . with a solution of sulphuric acid to wash out the parts and destroy the sperm."[20]

Recognizing a crime when he saw it, Comstock sprang into action. Only two months earlier, he had ended the career of Madame Restell, the best-known abortionist in nineteenth-century America. Posing as an

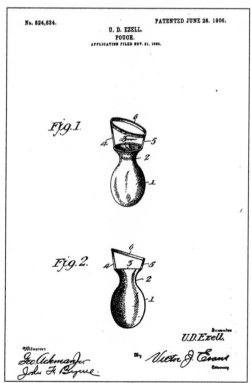

3. Uberto Ezell's pouch was intended to be "applied to the male organ to catch and retain all discharges coming therefrom"

indigent father who could not afford to have more children, Comstock asked Restell for birth control. When she obliged, he had her arrested. Inspectors raided her office and seized "10 dozen condoms, 15 bottles for abortion, 3 syringes, 2 quarts pills for abortion . . . 500 powders for preventing conception"—more than enough to substantiate contraceptive *and* abortion charges. Rather than risk the indignity of a trial and possible imprisonment, the sixty-seven-year-old millionaire, clad in a diamond-studded nightgown, cut her throat in the bathroom of her Fifth Avenue mansion while out on bail. Newspapers scolded Comstock for his unsavory tactics, but he was unmoved. "A bloody ending to a bloody life" was the epitaph he scribbled onto the NYSSV arrest blotter.[21]

With Sarah Chase, Comstock again sought to put his decoy tactics to good use. Adopting the pseudonym Mr. Farnsworth, he wrote Chase and arranged a meeting at her home to purchase a douching syringe for his wife. The day after the sale, Comstock returned to Chase's dwelling with the detective James G. Howe of the Twenty-sixth Precinct, who pretended to need a syringe for his wife, too. When Chase sold him one, Howe disclosed his true identity, served her with an arrest warrant, and seized six other syringes found on the premises. Comstock and Howe escorted Chase to the Tombs, the city jail, where she was released on fifteen hundred dollars bail. In a letter to his boss, the chief special agent of the U.S. Post Office, Comstock derided Chase's gullibility. The contraceptive vendor had misjudged her ability to "keep out of the clutches of the law."[22]

But it was Comstock who had miscalculated. At Chase's hearing, an all-male grand jury decided there was insufficient evidence to warrant a trial. One juror, hearing Comstock compare Chase's crimes with Restell's, lashed out at the vice hunter, asking Comstock if it was his intention to "drive Dr. Chase to suicide" too. Comstock was outraged and demanded a second hearing. The prosecuting attorney refused. Not to be thwarted, Comstock sneaked into the grand jury room and persuaded the foreman to sign two bills of indictment Comstock had prepared. The prosecutor reprimanded him and then entered a *nolle prosequi* for both indictments at Chase's arraignment, formally dismissing all charges. Chase picked up where the prosecutor left off. She filed a ten-thousand-dollar civil suit against Comstock for false arrest.[23]

Although Chase lost the countersuit, it was she, not Comstock, who emerged the victor in their frequent skirmishes. Between 1878 and 1900, Chase was arrested five times. Only once, when a patient died following an abortion, did arrest lead to a jail term; that conviction was not for birth control but for abortion. Significantly, Chase's imprisonment did not affect her views or business practices. On June 4, 1900, she was again arrested by Comstock on the charge of circulating articles to prevent conception. Once again, a grand jury refused to indict her. As in the past, Chase's brush with the law left her free to continue her trade in black-market birth control.[24]

As they did with Sarah Chase, grand jurors let many arrested suspects go free. More frequent than outright acquittals were indictments that did not go to trial. Fully 38 percent (40 of 105) of the individuals arrested by NYSSV agents between 1873 and 1898 for birth control crimes were not convicted. Even those convicted rarely faced stiff sentences. Judges gave 4 of the 65 convicted entrepreneurs suspended sentences and fined and released another 45. Only 16 of the 65 persons convicted on birth control charges went to prison. Prison terms varied in length from ten days to three years, but most were for one year or less. At the time of Comstock's death in 1915, not a single person convicted for the crime of birth control in the United States had received the maximum sentence allowed under federal law.[25]

During his lifetime, Comstock came to regard the justice system as almost as formidable a foe in his war against vice as the criminals he tried to put behind bars. At the 1878 annual meeting of the NYSSV, he declared that the "most serious drawback" the organization faced was the "failure of the New York State courts to perform their duty."[26]

Although the decisions of jurors, prosecutors, and judges were unique to each case, court rulings suggest some of the common themes that supported tolerance of birth control. One was the right to privacy. After 1873, judges upheld the Comstock Act, confirming Congress's jurisdiction over the mails and interstate commerce. But, raising the specter of unchecked centralized power, they set limits on how far federal regulation could go. In 1877, in *Ex parte Jackson*, the Supreme Court ruled that Congress's right to regulate the mails could not abridge the First and Fourth Amendments, which protect free speech and defend citizens from unreasonable searches and seizures. The privacy of the mails was sacrosanct. "No law of Congress can place in the hands of officials connected with the postal service," the Court stated, "any authority to invade the secrecy of letters and sealed packages in the mail." Insisting that sealed materials deposited in the mails remain "as fully guarded from examination . . . as if they were retained by the parties forwarding them in their own domiciles," the Supreme Court insulated mail-order commerce from the very inspection that could have curtailed the traffic of contraceptive contraband.[27]

Applying similar logic, judges challenged the legitimacy of decoy methods used by postal inspectors to apprehend those selling contraceptives. Courts distinguished between the detection of criminal wrongdoing and its inducement through entrapment. Decoy letters sent by agents posing as consumers threatened both the privacy of the mails and the rules of fair commerce. In 1894, an Oregon district court condemned the methods used by a postal inspector to demonstrate the guilt of Mrs. C. J. Adams, a contraceptive entrepreneur in Portland. To encourage Adams to break the law, the agent had written and begged her for contraceptives, falsely assured her, "You can correspond with me with absolute secrecy," and enclosed for her "convenience" postage stamps for her return correspondence. After several increasingly desperate letters, Adams sold the agent a "preventive remedy." The court decided that although Adams had broken the law, it was the agent's actions that had triggered the crime. Citing previous federal rulings denouncing "the practice of decoying or conniving with persons suspected of criminal designs," the Oregon district court declared the agent's conduct "reprehensible" and found Adams not guilty.[28]

Courts also invoked the principle of federalism. In the 1873 case *United States v. Bott*, the first test of the Comstock Act, a federal court in New York upheld the conviction of John Bott for "depositing in the mail a certain powder designed and intended for the prevention of conception." But it warned that although Congress could prohibit the use of the mails "for the transmission of any article," only the states could make "the intent to prevent conception an offence."[29] An 1878 ruling from a federal court in Missouri, *United States v. Whittier*, went a step further. The case involved the indictment of a St. Louis contraceptive proprietor, Clarke Whittier, who, responding to a decoy letter from the NYSSV agent Robert McFee, sent instructions on buying birth control to a Miss Nettie G. Harlan of Butler, Georgia, a fictitious identity established by

McFee. Granting the motion to quash Whittier's indictment, the circuit court ruled that Congress has "no power to make criminal the using of means to prevent conception."[30]

Both rulings distinguished between commerce and use, delineating a careful division of power that allowed the federal government to regulate the importation and dissemination of contraceptives but reserved to the states the right to criminalize their use. Yet only Connecticut enacted such a ban. Revealing, here, was the political path not taken. Connecticut's singularity was not the consequence of political inertia. After 1873, most state legislatures enacted new or revised obscenity statutes mindful of, even inspired by, congressional action. In choosing not to outlaw contraceptive use, even after federal courts had sanctioned such legislative activity, lawmakers paid silent tribute to the legitimacy of birth control as a private matter and individual choice.

Navigating the boundaries between personal and entrepreneurial privacy, on the one hand, and the power of Congress, on the other, courts also struggled to define contraceptives. What was the legal status of an article that prevented pregnancy but had "legitimate" uses as well? This was the central question in the obscenity trial of Ezra Heywood, arrested in October 1882 after he advertised a vaginal syringe in his newspaper, *The Word*. Heywood had long denounced contraceptives as physically dangerous and aesthetically revolting. But he loathed Comstock, whom he referred to during his trial as a "religio-monomaniac," and he was appalled by Comstock's classification of douche vendors as criminals, given the widespread use of syringes by women for hygienic purposes. To assert a principle and to bait his foe, he advertised "the Comstock syringe for Preventing Conception" in three editions of *The Word*. The label "Comstock," though deliberate, was not Heywood's invention; New York vendors had previously advertised Comstock syringes to signal the device's contraceptive attributes. An editorial note explained the ad's appearance: "The publishers of the Word inserted an advertisement of 'The Comstock Syringe' . . . [because] its intelligent, humane and worthy mission should no longer be libeled by forced association with the pious scamp who thinks Congress gave him legal right of way to and control over every American Woman's Womb." As predicted, Comstock arrested Heywood. Thus the test case began.[31]

The crux of Heywood's defense was the multiple uses of a vaginal sy-

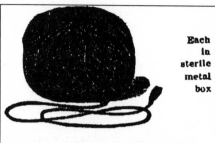

Each
in
sterile
metal
box

Sanitary Sponges for Ladies

The above picture is the exact size of one of our soft silk netted sponges when perfectly dry. They are enclosed in a silk netting. When moistened it expands about one-half more than shown. These are extensively used by ladies—when immersed in a good antiseptic and inserted well up into the vagina the passage is kept germ free. Full grown Turkey sponges as fine in texture as velvet.

— Prices —
½ dozen — $1.25
1 dozen — $2.00

— Post Paid —

4. In the language of antisepsis, sperm became a germ and sponges a tool to keep a woman's body "germ free" (Courtesy of the American Medical Association Archives, Chicago)

ringe. There was nothing about the technology of a syringe that made it inherently a preventive, he argued. "Thousands of physicians and druggists in the States . . . declare [it] invaluable, indispensable in the treatment of female diseases and for applying local remedies to preserve personal health and purity," he asserted. Supporting the contemporary belief in the therapeutic value of douching (which had gained credibility with the popularization of the germ theory of disease), Heywood asked: "Of the seven clefts, apertures, opening in a woman's body the vagina is one; who says it may not need cleansing as well as the ear, or the nostril?" As a health tool, the syringe had become nothing less than a "necessary accompaniment of every lady's toilet." Seen in this light, the syringe was no different from and at least as beneficial as other popular hygiene items, "like a tooth brush or towel."[32]

The logic of Heywood's argument was compelling, especially to a sympathetic judge. From the beginning of the trial, Judge T. L. Nelson had supported Heywood, permitting him to conduct his own defense and to use the courtroom as a soapbox by calling more than three dozen witnesses to the stand to relate the obscenity charge to broader issues such as woman's rights, free speech, and government conspiracy. In his charge to the jury, Nelson specified, "Whatever the words of the advertisement may mean, unless the [Comstock syringe] is designed or intended for [the prevention of conception] the charge has not been proved."[33] The jurors, unable to view the syringe as exclusively a preventive, found Heywood not guilty. Heywood's acquittal muddied the legal waters, making it significantly harder to indict and convict makers and distributors of contraceptives. Almost every contraceptive—syringes, sponges, condoms, intrauterine devices, vaginal pessaries—could be said to possess medicinal or therapeutic value. As the birth control advocate Edward Bond Foote proclaimed in 1889, "Articles themselves . . . will not be possible to suppress . . . while there remains a legitimate use for such things as syringes, sponges, cotton, pessaries and Vaseline."[34] It became the prosecutor's job to prove a seller's guilty intentions and, to be certain of conviction, the advertised article's proprietary use.

Even U.S. presidents rejected Comstock's rigidity. Ulysses S. Grant, who had signed the Comstock Law, pardoned five of the twelve individuals sentenced to jail on birth control charges during his term. Two of the five were Seth Hunsdon and James Patterson, former operators of the Albany Medical Institute who had originally been sentenced to one year of hard labor each. Arrested by Comstock on April 24 and 26, 1873, respectively, they were pardoned by Grant in late November of the same year. Comstock viewed the decision as an error. "O, that I had known of this in time to have got the facts before Grant," he wrote in his diary. "It would not have been granted." Yet the facts were precisely the issue. After Hunsdon's and Patterson's convictions, a petition signed by a local clergyman and their congressman, Lyman Tremain of Albany, insisted that the two had been convicted on a misrepresentation of facts. Grant, reviewing the file, agreed. Five years later, President Rutherford B. Hayes pardoned Heywood, who before his "syringe" trial had been sentenced to two years of hard labor for circulating *Cupid's Yokes*, a pamphlet defending free love and fertility limitation. In Hayes's eyes, the pamphlet advocated "wrong ideas," but it was hardly "obscene, lascivious, lewd or corrupting in the criminal sense." Evaluating Heywood's guilt through his own moral lens, Hayes let Heywood go.[35]

After 1873, others, too, let their own views on morality and privacy guide their assessments of contraceptive criminality. Although Comstock took solace in blaming repeated acts of clemency on the ineptitude of officials or the treachery of his enemies, it was the reasoned deliberation of those who made up the court system, not its corruption, that returned birth control proprietors to the streets. To be sure, the leniency accorded birth control offenders may have been related to widespread loathing of Comstock, the man. Comstock's belligerence and courtroom histrionics offended judges, alienated prosecutors, and provoked a steady stream of derogatory editorials, cartoons, and poems in turn-of-the-century newspapers and journals. But although the frequent ridiculing of Comstock may help to explain support for violators of the Comstock Law in general, it cannot account for the special leniency granted birth control offenders in particular.[36] Rather, those entrusted with enforcing contraceptive laws made choices that bespoke a tolerance of birth control and compassion toward those who sold it, a willingness to see as gray what Comstock could see only as black-and-white. The judicial decisions of an age when popular attitudes toward criminal behavior and reproductive control are often difficult to discern suggest broadly based support of bootleg birth control. Favoring acquittal almost as much as conviction and light sentencing as a rule, judges and jurors created an environment in which black-market birth control could thrive.

And so it did. Although the industry's illegal operation in post-1873 America makes an accurate measure of its economic status impossible, we can gauge its commercial vigor from a variety of sources. Credit reports, for example, indicate that most birth control proprietors did well after 1873; for many, the trade provided decisive, long-term upward mobility. Because the trade required little start-up capital, individuals of limited means could enter it with ease. Such was the case with George Brinckerhoff. In 1863, Brinckerhoff, aged thirty-five, was a member of the firm Groom, Brothers, and Company, a grocery and tea business. The firm borrowed so heavily that in June 1867 it failed, eighty-five thousand dollars in debt. The collapse initially ruined Brinckerhoff's professional reputation. When he tried to resume the business alone, "he found he had no credit" because of the "unfavorable impression entertained by the community relating to his failure in the Tea business." In 1871, he retired from the grocery business and founded the Eugenic Manufacturing Company. After criminal charges initiated by Comstock were dropped in 1873, Brinckerhoff's profits and confidence grew. In August 1878, credit reporters described Brinckerhoff as a man whose business in rubber articles "yields him fair profits" and who "pays promptly and is considered good for small lines [of credit]."[37]

Equally telling is the frequency with which men and women who crossed paths with Comstock returned to their criminal ways. Multiple arrests of birth control purveyors such as Sarah Chase suggest something more than bad luck. They reflect a determination among contraceptive entrepreneurs to stay with a business whose financial benefits outweighed its legal risks. Chase, a single mother, sold birth control and ran a boardinghouse to provide for her family's needs. In an economic culture that restricted opportunities for female entrepreneurship and branded businesswomen deviant, the contraceptive business (like prostitution and abortion, two kindred illicit trades) was more welcoming of women than other businesses.[38] Like other contraceptive purveyors who ran afoul of the law, Chase refused to give up her enterprise. Instead, she took extra precautions to keep herself and it out of harm's way: she moved to the small town of Elmira, New York.

Unscathed by his legal encounter, Morris Glattstine followed a similar trajectory. After Comstock arrested him for selling diaphragms and condoms, Glattstine returned to the criminal trade. Financially, he did well. Between 1881 and 1884, reporters for Dun and Bradstreet consistently awarded him a favorable credit rating. Nonetheless, during the same period, Glattstine became a merchant on the move, selling rubber goods at four separate New York locations. He was not arrested again.[39]

Consumers sustained contraceptive entrepreneurs with their hopes and their dollars. Inventory listings hint at the traffic of articles involved. Horace Brown was arrested with five thousand condoms on hand, Martin Phillips with 150 womb veils. Although these figures cannot tell us how many contraceptives were sold daily, they communicate retailers' expectations that such stock was needed to keep pace with consumer demand.

Arrest records occasionally reveal more precise statistics that corroborate this assessment. When Glattstine was arrested on March 1, 1878, he admitted to selling 432 diaphragms in the previous five weeks. Henry Hunter's annual profits were estimated to be as high as seventeen hundred dollars per year in 1873. Each day, he received an average of three hundred to four hundred letters of inquiry from prospective customers across the country. After the diaphragm vendor Henry Hymes was arrested, he confessed that as many as "500 Brooklyn ladies were using his article."[40]

Medical commentary likewise attests to the existence of a flourishing contraceptive business. Many physicians, guided by their own beliefs rather than the American Medical Association's policy against birth control, supported contraceptive use, but those who did not found plenty to condemn in post-1873 America. "American people," observed one physician in 1880, "suppress the family increase by every device that the arch fiend can suggest."[41] The Boston physician H. S. Pomeroy, author of the 1888 manual *The Ethics of Marriage*, found Americans' preoccupation with childlessness so widespread that he termed it simply "the American sin." Certain that those who casually broke the law must be ignorant of its existence, he concluded his book with a thirteen-page appendix cataloguing contraceptive and abortion restrictions.[42]

Letters confirm the casualness with which sexually active individuals discussed the intended and actual procurement of contraceptives after birth control became a crime. The correspondence of Violet Blair Janin and her husband, Albert, is illustrative. The couple were married on May 14, 1874, fourteen months after the Comstock Act was passed. From Albert's boasts of "hymen breaking" we can surmise that Violet's first experience of intercourse occurred that night. From then on, the bride awaited the onset of her menstrual period with new anxiety, as a fear of dying during childbearing because of long-standing gynecological problems had forged in her mind a resolve to stay childless. Begrudgingly, Albert supported Violet's goal. Since May, the couple had been using the rhythm method, with Albert carefully recording what he believed were Violet's safe and unsafe days. But Violet, who lived in Washington, D.C., did not trust the technique, and her letters to Albert, who worked in New Orleans as a lawyer much of the year, were plagued with worry. At a time when the safe period was generally believed to be the midpoint in a woman's menstrual cycle (the very time when, we now know, conception is most likely to occur), too many women and men had seen this and other natural methods of birth control fail. In Violet's case, only the arrival of her menstrual period could put her mind at ease, and yet its appearance invariably set the stage for a new monthly drama to begin.[43]

By November, she had had enough. When a female homeopath confirmed Violet's suspicions that pregnancy could be fatal, she wrote Albert, "It is best that we should have no children. . . . So I renounce all ideas of it." Renouncing children was one thing, renouncing sex another. Opting for a middle ground, the couple discarded the maligned rhythm technique for condoms, a commercial method they both considered more reliable. On November 26, Violet discreetly asked Albert: "Would it be possible for you to find something you told me about?" By the time her letter arrived, Albert, willing to forgo intercourse until Violet's health improved but preferring not to, had already stocked a supply. "I have managed to procure some things I have once or twice spoken to you about. Can you guess what they are?" he wrote playfully. "I have often wished since the 14th of May [their wedding night] that I had some of them."[44] Buying condoms in New Orleans apparently presented no obstacles worth mentioning.

What emerges from the Janins' prose is not pangs of guilt for breaking the law but a shared resolve to keep Violet from getting pregnant, whatever the cost. And achieving this goal was a joint endeavor. Albert's letters, which frequently refer to birth control, should make us wary of generalizations about family planning in nineteenth-century America as chiefly women's work. The diaries of middle- and upper-class women that encourage such a view of gender relations have been invaluable sources for women's history. At the same time, their self-referential character has obscured men's involvement in intimate affairs pertaining to reproduction. Violet kept a diary too, but it is only through the exchanges penned by the Janins as a couple that we learn about Albert's role in pregnancy prevention. Ironically, the Janins' voluminous correspondence, the result of an atypical living arrangement, suggests just how typical frank discussions of reproductive control may have been among men and women in late-nineteenth-century America.

Whether Violet and Albert knew about the new prohibitions is unclear. Both were ardent followers of national politics, but the Comstock

Act was not headline news, and it would have been easy for them to miss. On the other hand, whenever her writings became especially intimate, multilingual Violet wrote in German. This might have been a strategy to shield their "obscene" missives from censorship, but most likely it was not, for Albert, also multilingual, penned most of his intimacies in English. Violet prided herself on her linguistic prowess, and she had only recently learned German. Using it may have reflected a proud demonstration of newfound mastery or a sexual playfulness enhanced by her ability as a genteel woman to couch naughty words in a foreign tongue.

Whatever their knowledge of the law, Violet and Albert turned to the contraceptive market because they believed purchased birth control meant better birth control. In post-1873 America, they represented two of many women and men who felt that way and acted accordingly. Contraceptives were discussed in private correspondence not as bootleg goods but as a useful bedroom commodity whose availability and efficacy were worth noting to lovers and friends. In 1885, Rose Williams wrote to her newly wed friend Allettie Mosher, "You want to know of a sure preventative. . . . They are called Pessairre or female preventative. . . . They cost one dollar. . . . The Directions are with it."[45] In the same spirit, Mary Hallock Foote of Idaho advised Helena Gilder of New York in 1876 about "a sure way of limiting one's family. . . . [They] are called cundums and are made either of rubber or skin. They are to be had at first-class druggists." About a year later, Mary provided her friend with an update. She and her husband found condoms unpleasant, Mary admitted, but they continued to use them anyway, for good reason: condoms worked, whereas the rhythm method did not. Mary knew whereof she spoke. She had become pregnant counting her "safe days." "The 'French shields' have saved me," she told Helena. "Everything is dreadful except nature and Nature is like the letter of the law which faileth."[46]

Such letters offer more than a touching tribute to the determination of women and men in late-nineteenth-century America to restrict their fertility. They remind us that, as moral reformers found in other attempts to restructure behavior in the nineteenth century, a law did not necessarily work the fundamental change its proponents desired. The volume of smut traffic, the limited number of agents assigned to police it, and contraceptive purveyors' own cunning thwarted efforts to apprehend birth control offenders. People who were arrested, moreover, frequently discovered that those who broke and those who enforced the law were often on the same side. From jurors to prosecutors to judges to presidents of the United States, the men who would interpret the legal meaning of contraceptive criminalization let birth control offenders go free.

The social, sexual, and economic landscape of post-1873 America was populated by individuals who defined contraceptive criminalization on their own terms. There was the Honorable T. L. Nelson, whose charge to the Boston jury specified that Ezra Heywood was guilty only if the government could prove the impossible: that the "Comstock syringe" was exclusively a contraceptive. There was Sarah Chase, who defied convention, Comstock, and the law by lecturing on and selling contraceptives. In Texas, there was Uberto Ezell, who, with thoughts of commercial grandeur, invented the "male pouch." And then there was Albert Janin, who could scarcely wait to try out his New Orleans condoms with his Washington, D.C., wife. These individuals did not cast their votes on the Comstock bill. Yet through their actions—some quiet, others overt—they made their views known. Collectively, they helped sustain a trade Congress had declared a crime.

THREE

Contraceptive Entrepreneurs

Joseph Backrach struggled to earn a decent living, and he knew a good opportunity when he saw one. The German-born immigrant and father of seven sold rubber devices for sexual pleasure and contraception. In his Brooklyn home, he made condoms, ticklers, and male caps; his 1885 inventory included more than twelve thousand such devices. Although most of his products were designed for men, Backrach was not indifferent to women's needs. He also made womb veils, more than three hundred of which he kept stashed in his daughters' bedroom for safekeeping.[1]

Backrach's competition was not the large rubber manufacturers that came of age in the late nineteenth century, powerhouses such as Goodyear and B. F. Goodrich. Until contraceptives became legal, companies with national reputations to protect shunned the manufacture of such obviously sexualized wares. Instead, Backrach's competition came from smaller players, many of whom cobbled together birth control devices in their homes and became central players in the illicit world of contraceptive manufacture. Many entrepreneurs were immigrants, women, or Jews. Few whose records remain possessed a formal education. Denied the credit and social or educational credentials needed to claim professional respectability or ascend the financial ladder, they were drawn to a trade whose illegitimate character and low-capital requirements made it welcoming to ordinary people. At the turn of the twentieth century, an era of trusts and tycoons, contraceptives were as much the business of common folk as of the rubber giants rapidly becoming household names.

Industrial development in the 1870–1920 era is often described as inevitably progressing from small workshop to looming factory, but the evolution of the contraceptive industry followed a different trajectory. The Comstock Act outlawed contraceptive manufacture and thus dissuaded large firms, already in the public eye, from the exclusive production of merchandise of questionable repute. Such hesitancy thwarted the development of a contraceptive "trust" and nurtured a rich entrepreneurial culture in which small-scale production thrived. Throughout the black-market era, the birth control business operated not as a distinct sector of the economy but as a patchwork quilt of outfits, large and small, that straddled several industries, notably rubber, patent medicine, and drugs and chemicals. Located in a variety of settings, from established firms and one-room workshops to the bedrooms and kitchens of entrepreneurs, this collage of commercialism united women and men at the bottom of the economic ladder with reputable manufacturers at the top.

After 1873, established pharmaceutical and rubber firms made devices and chemicals known to have contraceptive benefits but did not market them as birth control. IUDs were sold to correct prolapsed uteri. Carbolic acid, an antiseptic commonly used for contraceptive douching, was marketed for burns, scalds, whooping cough, diphtheria, and morning sickness. Companies' reputations as vendors who sold "therapeutic" devices principally to licensed doctors, druggists, and reputable mail-order houses gave firms legal cover, and the diversity of their product line helped camouflage articles' illicit uses. U.S. Rubber made diaphragms along with tires and footwear; H. K. Mulford Company, manufacturing chemists, produced antiseptic tampons saturated with spermicidal chemicals but only, purportedly, to facilitate vaginal cleaning.[2]

Matters might have been different if manufacturing priorities had shifted, if birth control had become the sole focus of a company's energies. But no reputable company was reckless enough to make contraceptives its primary articles of commerce. Nor was there a need. IUDs sold well, but so did other rubber products, such as seamless gloves and hot-water bottles. Until the 1920s, when court decisions modified legal prohibitions against contraceptive production and distribution, no reputable firm made birth control its main concern. Before that time, some of the country's most august manufacturing companies relegated birth control to a small part of an otherwise ordinary product line. Joining the fray were lesser-known proprietors who hoped that the cloak of legitimacy shielding established manufacturers' activities would protect them too.

More audacious small entrepreneurs—folk such as Backrach—tackled the taboo, producing skins, rubbers, and womb veils clearly intended for contraception. One reason they did so is simply that they *could*. Making commercial birth control involved a range of technologies as diverse as contraceptives themselves. But until the use of mass production and latex in the late 1920s and the 1930s, birth control devices were never so costly or elaborate that individuals could not make them in small shops or in the home. The simplicity of contraceptive production lured entrepreneurs into the commercial vacuum created by the aversion of large firms. With a few ingredients, a little know-how, and a dash of daring, a birth control business could be born.

Probably no sector of this black market was as welcoming to the ambitious as the condom trade. After condoms became legal and government-regulated in the late 1930s, Julius Schmid and Youngs Rubber—the makers of Ramses, Sheiks, and Trojans—came to control the market. Prior to that time, the American condom trade was fiercely competitive, crowded, and replete with bootleggers.[3]

The condom business was doubly tarnished by illegality and sexual connotation, for long before they were outlawed, condoms had been culturally stigmatized as inducements to sexual promiscuity and prurience. Condoms protected users from venereal disease, but the fact that these diseases were acquired *sexually* precluded the acceptance of condoms as medically legitimate devices. Only after the U.S. Army spent more than a million dollars battling the human and financial costs of sexually transmitted diseases in World War I did court rulings and public opinion begin to cast condoms in a more flattering light.[4] Until the convergence of government support and heightened public health concern shattered the veneer of Victorian prudery, working in the condom trade meant battling both the condom's criminal status and its controversial past.

This made condoms off-limits to the industrial giants that emerged from the consolidation of the rubber industry in the late nineteenth century—Goodyear, B. F. Goodrich, U.S. Rubber, and Firestone—but seductive to smaller players like Julius Schmidt. Like other contraceptive entrepreneurs, Schmidt came from a socially marginal background and probably felt he had little to lose entering a trade of questionable repute. Born into poverty in the town of Schorndorf in southern Germany in 1865, Schmidt was a paralytic who walked only with the aid of two wooden crutches. He took these, a few extra clothes, and little else to America in 1882, when his grandfather generously paid his passage to New York. America's quintessential Gilded Age city, New York was less glamorous or welcoming to the Jewish newcomer than he or his grandfather had imagined. Finding employment in a city teeming with fit and qualified aspirants was tough for anyone, but it was especially difficult for an immigrant youth marked by a disability. Alone and jobless, Julius passed miserable nights in Manhattan's Battery district on benches and in cellars. Only the sale of his extra clothes—his shirt went for a dime— gave him the money he needed for food.[5]

Schmidt eventually found work cleaning animal intestines at a sausage-casing firm for seven dollars a month. Although sausages had been around for centuries, artificial casings made out of cellulose or plastic had not yet been invented. That made Schmidt's job time-honored but messy. To create casings, he first had to remove the fat, manure, muscle layers, and mucosa attached to the large and small intestines of slaughtered livestock. After being thoroughly stripped, washed, and cleaned, the intestines were transformed into yards of resilient, membranous tubes, ready to be cut to size and stuffed to eat. Seven dollars a month were decent wages for a working man, but it was probably easy for Schmidt to imagine his cases being transformed into something more lucrative. As perhaps Schmidt knew, slaughterhouse workers had been making condoms out of animal waste products since the Renaissance. In 1883, with surplus intestines, he launched a side business in "skins" at his residence on Forty-sixth Street at the northern edge of Manhattan's notorious Tenderloin district. Once the homes of wealthy New Yorkers, many of the district's signature brownstones had recently been converted to brothels and multifamily dwellings for working-class and immigrant tenants like Schmidt, whose condom business would have meshed easily with other sexual services for sale in the Tenderloin. On September 18, 1890, Comstock raided Schmidt's home and found 696 skins and "one form for manufacturing same." Released on five hundred dollars bail, Schmidt was found guilty of "selling articles to prevent conception" on October 28 and fined fifty dollars. Though a large sum for the average wage earner, it was not a financial obstacle for Schmidt, now a successful bootlegger. He paid the fine and resumed his life of condom crime.[6]

Schmidt's enterprise made him part of a long line of condom producers whose wares had been worn by men around the world for centuries, although not always for contraception. Egyptians in the Twelfth Dynasty (1350–1200 B.C.) donned linen penis sheaths as a sign of social status, as protection against insect bites and tropical diseases, and even as amulets to *promote* fertility.[7] In the 1560s, however, none of these uses was mentioned in the first written description of a condom, penned by the Italian anatomist Gabriel Fallopius. Instead, Fallopius, credited with the discovery of the Fallopian tubes, described a linen sheath presoaked in an herbal decoction used to prevent the transmission of syphilis.[8] It was not long before people recognized that what prevented sexually transmitted disease probably prevented pregnancy too. In the early eighteenth century, condoms made from oiled silk, fish bladders, and the intestines of goats, lambs, sheep, and calves were bought and used as contraceptives, making condoms the first modern birth control to acquire commercial viability. Early-eighteenth-century poetry praised the contraceptive attributes of "condums" or "machines" for sale at commercial outlets in London, and the frontispiece to The Machine—or Love's Preservative of 1744 depicts men and women seated at a warehouse table, making and testing "love's preservatives" by hand.[9] The abundance of raw materials from slaughterhouses in Europe made condoms a staple export in cities like London, where a 1783 handbill advertising the wholesale business of one Mrs. Philips boasted of thirty-five years' experience supplying "apothecaries, chymists, druggists . . . ambassadors, foreigners, gentlemen and captains of ships going abroad" with "the best goods in England on the shortest notice and at the lowest price."[10] But condom manufacture was not exclusive to England. The legendary Italian lover Casanova (1725–1798) bought some in a Marseilles brothel from a "tradeswoman [who] sold them only by the dozen."[11]

Before the 1850s, most condoms in the United States were skins imported from Europe, whose commercial slaughterhouses, catering to the dietary demands of the continent's urban populations, sustained a brisk trade. According to one investigator, skins were routinely "brought in from Europe . . . in small carefully-guarded packets that got by the customs officials without paying duty."[12] Smuggled or not, newly arrived condoms were openly advertised by American dealers. One New York dealer promised readers of the *Druggists' Circular and Chemical Gazette* the finest skins "from the best manufacturers in Paris."[13] Although the few slaughterhouses in the United States could not support the high-volume business that flourished in Europe, American manufacture was not out of the question. Directions in an 1844 guide published in Philadelphia offer a laborious but low-tech alternative to imported skins:

> Take the caecum of the sheep; soak it first in water, turn it on both sides, then repeat the operation in a weak ley of soda, which must be changed every four or five hours, for five or six successive times; then remove the mucous membrane with the nail; sulphur, wash in clean water, and then in soap and water; rinse, inflate and dry. Next cut it to the required length, and attach a piece of ribbon to the open end. Used to prevent infection or pregnancy. The different qualities consist in extra pains being taken in the above process, and in polishing, scenting, etc.[14]

The recipe was probably intended for farmers, but city dwellers would have benefited, too. Urban butchers specialized in custom-made orders, and buyers and barterers knew to ask for certain cuts by name. Given how common homemade sausage making was in the years before meat packaging became a centralized industry, a request for sheep intestine from the neighborhood butcher would not have seemed extraordinary. When it came to condoms, moreover, intestines from a single animal could go a long way. Depending on how much of the intestine one used (all of it or only the prized caecum, the pouch in the large intestine containing the appendix), and which species it came from (a sheep's small intestine provides twenty-seven meters of casing, a cow's even more), an efficient producer could create dozens of condoms with intestinal matter to spare. By 1868, moreover, American entrepreneurs were importing $14,741 worth of processed animal membranes, ready to be transformed into condoms on American soil.[15] When Julius Schmidt began operations in 1883, growing numbers of urban butchers and the increased volume of imported membranes ($35,979 worth in 1883) would have furnished him and like-minded individuals with raw ingredients with which to produce skins for sale.[16]

Not all skins were the same, however, as the 1844 recipe's reference to "different qualities" suggests. Bottom-of-the-line skins were usually pasted or hand stitched together from unprocessed intestines; better models were made by repeated soaking, stretching, and drying. Named after the art of beating solid gold into gold leaf, "goldbeaters' skins" were top-of-the-line condoms created by working intestinal matter into a delicate, supple mass. Gradations in quality derived from "extra pains" taken with the same technique, not the application of a new one. Until mechanization and mass production were applied to condom making, the technology of skin manufacture went largely unchanged.[17]

Making rubbers was different but not difficult. The American rubber condom business came of age in the 1850s, the by-product of the discovery of vulcanization technology by Charles Goodyear (1800–1860). Goodyear's feat was to make natural rubber, an elastic substance obtained by coagulating the milky juice of various tropical plants (such as those of the genus *Hevea* or *Castilloa*), commercially practical. The problem with natural rubber, also called India rubber, gum elastic, or caoutchouc, is its thermoplasticity. In cold weather, natural rubber gets stiff and brittle. In warm weather, it loses its shape, becomes sticky and soft, and emits a foul odor. The susceptibility of natural rubber to temperature change made it unsuitable for many products, especially condoms, which, to be effective, must not melt or crack.[18]

Goodyear, an inventor from Connecticut, began his experiments aware of findings by German and American chemists indicating that rubber mixed with sulfur (which acts as an accelerator) eliminated the tacky consistency of rubber goods.[19] One day in 1839, purely by accident, he dropped a spoonful of rubber-and-sulfur mixture onto a hot stove. Instead of melting, the rubber flattened into a malleable solid that was "charred like leather."[20] Goodyear quickly grasped the enormity of his results. The application of high-intensity heat, long regarded as inimical to rubber stability, made rubber stable. It "cured" natural rubber mixed with sulfur by divesting it of its adhesive properties, creating an air- and water-proof elastic substance unaffected by temperature change. Goodyear's discovery (soon dubbed "vulcanization," after Vulcan, the Roman god of fire) opened the floodgates to American rubber manufacture. Entrepreneurs scrambled to meet surging consumer demand with a mélange of rubber merchandise, from water beds and breast pumps to raincoats, hats, and shoes.[21] At least a handful began to make condoms. Rubber caps were first described in the United States in 1858, full-length condoms in 1869. Soon to follow were rubber pessaries: caps, diaphragms, and IUDs.[22] The rubber revolution in contraceptives had begun.

For all the hullabaloo surrounding the outpouring of rubber wares, making them was not necessarily costly or difficult, as the case of condoms proves. In 1892, a one-of-a-kind exposé published in *The India Rubber World*, an American trade journal, investigated the clandestine world of condom manufacture and explained the mechanics of rubber production. The author, T. J. B. Buckingham, harbored no love for condoms or those who made them, believing that their manufacture discredited the rubber industry as a whole. All the same, he felt duty-bound to discuss, if only to disparage, a sector of the rubber economy whose annual sales were estimated to be thirty thousand dollars. Aware of the laws that forbade open discussion of contraceptives and eager to cast himself in a respectable light, Buckingham diplomatically titled his article "The Trade in Questionable Rubber Goods."[23]

According to Buckingham, the typical condom firm "would mean very little to the uninitiated." Small, dark, and almost bare, it consisted of "a moderate-sized room, with windows so draped that the outside world may not peer in, small zinc-covered tables, [and] racks in which hang rolls of pure sheet rubber." Few pieces of equipment were needed to make condoms, so "very little money is expended on the plant." Indeed, Buckingham reported, "everything looks as if the proprietor was all ready to pull up stakes and hurry away." The sparse environment undoubtedly reflected entrepreneurial savvy, for discretion and portability were advantageous in a world where Comstock-inspired raids were infrequent but possible. But it also indexed the low-tech character of condom production. In the shop Buckingham described, a work crew of six made condoms using a "simple process." First, workers spread natural sheet rubber on tables in preparation for cutting. The next stage varied. In some firms, workers used cutting dies to excise appropriately sized pieces, each of which was molded around a form and dipped into a vulcanization solution for curing. In others, they doubled up the rubber, cut pieces to size, affixed the edges, and finally dipped inflated condoms into a vulcanization solution until they were cured.[24]

Whichever method was used, making condoms was so easy—and this was the disturbing point—anyone could do it. Natural rubber obtained from a distributor (purchasable without difficulty, Buckingham noted, if one claimed to need it to make dress shields), sulfur for vulcanization acquired from a druggist, a table, cutters, and a little know-how: these were the prerequisites for successful manufacture. There were no inspection costs. Because condoms were unregulated, the decision to test finished goods lay at the proprietor's discretion.[25]

So simple was the process of making condoms, Buckingham observed, that entrepreneurs lured by the promise of high profits in a business that required little capital investment had flooded the market. If the condom trade was to be subdued, Buckingham predicted, the cause would be too much competition rather than the feeble enforcement of contraceptive laws. But as of yet, there were no signs of collapse. "Since early in the 1850s," he asserted, the American condom business had positively "flourished."[26] Others agreed. In 1889, Henry Sumner, a publisher of fertility control tracts, had proclaimed that "the sale of [condoms] is now enormous both in America and Europe."[27] Notwithstanding their illegality, condoms remained staples of bedrooms, brothels, and drugstores. An 1879 edition of *The Druggist's Cost Book* (a workbook in which traveling salesmen could record prices and preferred brands) left ample room for condom shopping: three lines for goldbeaters, three for full-length rubbers, and two for rubber caps.[28]

The entrepreneurialism of condom manufacturing was also evident in the production of other "illegitimate" contraceptives, such as rubber diaphragms and cervical caps. In 1925, Margaret Sanger claimed that Holland-Rantos (the company funded by her husband) was the first American manufacturer of spring-type diaphragms. Her assertion ignored a long history of diaphragm manufacture in the United States. Half a century earlier, businesspeople such as Joseph Backrach had established a brisk trade in over-the-counter models sold directly to women.[29]

Sanger was right in one way: womb veil entrepreneurs took their cue from European initiatives, which were numerous. In a treatise written in 1838, the German inventor Friedrich Adolph Wilde boasted of a method more effective than condoms or withdrawal: a cervical cap.[30] Fashioned out of an elastic resinous material (probably natural rubber), each cap was custom-made according to a wax impression taken of the prospective wearer's cervix during what must have been a trying examination.[31] In 1842, the German gynecologist W. P. J. Mensinga invented the first modern diaphragm, a hard-rubber ring covered with sheet rubber. Mensinga later upgraded his design, replacing natural rubber with vulcanized, thereby eliminating what one inventor described as the unfortunate tendency of earlier models to collect "sediment and [to] emit an unpleasant odor." Mensinga also added rubber-covered springs, which retained the diaphragm behind the pubic bone after insertion.[32] Mensinga diaphragms were used at the first birth control clinic, opened in 1882 in Amsterdam. By 1900, a growing number of European clinics had made the Mensinga diaphragm their contraceptive of choice.[33]

Americans wasted no time inventing devices patterned after European technologies. In 1846, four years after Mensinga's invention, the Rochester native John B. Beers patented "the wife's protector," a device to "prevent conception." It consisted of a wire hoop covered with "oil-silk, or some other thin membranous substance." A handle protruding from the ring's periphery permitted the user to place the ring so that "the membrane on the hoop is made to completely cover the os uteri, thus entirely preventing the semen from entering the uterus."[34] Whether Beers sold his design is unknown, but if he did not, others did. In a rare obscenity prosecution predating the 1870s, the Boston physician Dr. Walter Scott Tarbox was arrested in 1847 for advertising "Dr. Cameron's Patent Family Regulator or Wife's Protector" to more than one hundred households in Massachusetts. The Cameron protector cost a hefty five dollars, but according to its promoters, it was worth every penny. Easily inserted, the protector, when withdrawn, "bring[s] with it every particle of semen, rendering its effects positive; and as it absorbs nothing, can be cleansed in a moment . . . [and] will last for life."[35]

If Boston prosecutors had assumed that Tarbox's arrest would discourage diaphragm entrepreneurship, they were wrong. The Massachusetts

Supreme Court overturned Tarbox's conviction, and decades later, even after the Comstock Act cemented its illegality, the diaphragm trade showed no signs of waning.

Edward Bliss Foote, a graduate of the Pennsylvania Medical College, made mail and clinic sales of his one-size-fits-all diaphragm his ticket to financial success. In his 1864 edition of *Medical Common Sense*, a guide for lay readers, Foote dismissed douching and coitus interruptus as injurious to body and mind and recommended his six-dollar womb veil instead. Praising the veil's simplicity, he also emphasized how it enabled women to control their reproductive destiny. The contrivance's "application is easy and accomplished in a moment," he wrote. "It places conception entirely under the control of the wife, to whom it naturally belongs: for it is for her to say at what time and under what circumstances she will become the mother and the moral, religious, and physical instructress of offspring."[36] Set against centuries of male condom use and an intellectual milieu that pronounced intercourse and reproduction inseparable, Foote's celebration of a contraceptive as a tool of female empowerment was radical indeed. Here was a device that gave women control over their procreative destiny. Of course, the price of control was responsibility. A century later, when the sexuality-reproduction nexus had become culturally uncoupled and there were many female contraceptives, such as the Pill, to prove it, many feminists would identify the feminization of birth control technology as sexist and burdensome, not liberating.

After 1873, Foote tried unsuccessfully to repeal the Comstock Act, a move grounded in both his political views and his economic aspirations. In 1874, he was arrested and fined for sending circulars advertising his popular womb veil. Undeterred, he continued his diaphragm business, only to be arrested again in 1876 by an irate Comstock for "mailing obscene pamphlets, and advertisement of obscene pamphlets, and articles to prevent conception."[37] Fined but not jailed, Foote persevered, founding in the 1880s a "Sanitary Bureau," which served as the headquarters for a mail-order business that ultimately included syringes, condoms, his ever-popular womb veil, and supplies "not to be found in every respectable drug-store."[38] His 1876 run-in with Comstock would be his last, notwithstanding his refusal to give up what credit reporters described as a lucrative business. When he retired, he did so a wealthy man.[39]

Foote kept no records describing how he made his womb veils, but patents from the period suggest how simple the process likely was. In the 1840s, Beers crafted his device from a wire stretched into a hoop shape and covered with a membranous substance. In 1877, the Boston inventor Rhodes Lockwood patented a similarly assembled device. Lockwood lapped a metallic spring core, "such as [that] commonly used for watch-springs," reinforced it with a strengthening strip (to prevent breakage), and then covered it with India rubber subjected to heat and "vulcanized [into] soft rubber."[40] As with condoms, creating diaphragms was easy and inexpensive, an ideal venture for those with little money and a penchant for risk.

Foote was well remunerated for his risk, as were others. Gustavas Farr, a homeopathic physician, resided in Indianapolis but counted as womb veil customers women from around the country. Farr founded his business in about 1873, advertising his devices in circulars, newspapers, and periodicals such as *Waverly Magazine*. He sent "hundreds" of his products by mail and "thousands" more by express. In 1872, his estimated worth was a respectable two to three hundred dollars; by 1876, he had amassed a debt-free fortune of twenty-five thousand dollars in cash.[41]

In the sexual economy of turn-of-the-century America, womb veils were illegitimate, but intrauterine devices (IUDs) were not. Both functioned as contraceptive pessaries. But although NYSSV agents harassed Foote and Farr and raided the shops of half a dozen New York druggists selling "closed-ring pessaries" in 1885, they let vendors of open-ring pessaries go about their business.[42]

One difference that law enforcers and polite society seized upon to distinguish between the two types of pessaries was the intent of those who used them. Womb veils and cervical caps came of age in the nineteenth century as articles designed, promoted, and used specifically for contraception. As long as official medical discourse recognized them first and foremost as articles of fertility control, womb veils would remain dangerous devices without redeeming therapeutic value. Government officials destroyed Joseph Backrach's 420 womb veils, his entire stock of female contraceptives, an act presumably intended to shield 420 women from their pernicious influence.[43] Only when Margaret Sanger medicalized womb veils by placing control of their distribution in doctors' hands did diaphragms and cervical caps become respectable. Before then they were scorned, seized, and destroyed.

But doctors felt differently about intrauterine and intra-cervical devices, which were medicalized much earlier. Intrauterine devices have been used since antiquity. For centuries, Arabs and Turks used hollow tubes to insert small stones into the uteri of camels before long desert trips. This technique was likely used to inhibit human procreation at about the same time.[44] In the United States, IUDs first became popular in the late nineteenth century as a medical treatment for a wide range of gynecological disorders, from asymmetrical and prolapsed uteri to painful or excessive menstruation. Intrauterine stem pessaries, as physicians called the devices, could span five inches. They consisted of a rubber, metal, or glass stem attached to a cup or button that held the stem upright and prevented it from becoming lost in the uterus. Doctors acknowledged but generally disapproved of the IUD's contraceptive attributes, and most refused to insert them into women unless there was a "legitimate" medical need.[45]

Physicians were leading players in the commercialization of IUDs. They invented, endorsed, and inserted the dozens of models available at mid-century; in 1864, the *Transactions of the National Medical Association* counted no fewer than 123 designs, "from a simple plug to a patent

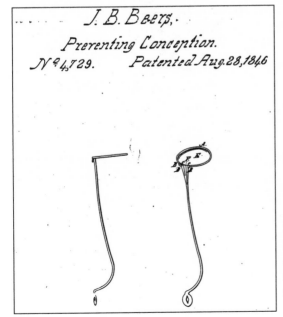

5. An example of an early IUD patented before the Comstock Act forced inventors and entrepreneurs to camouflage the use of birth control devices

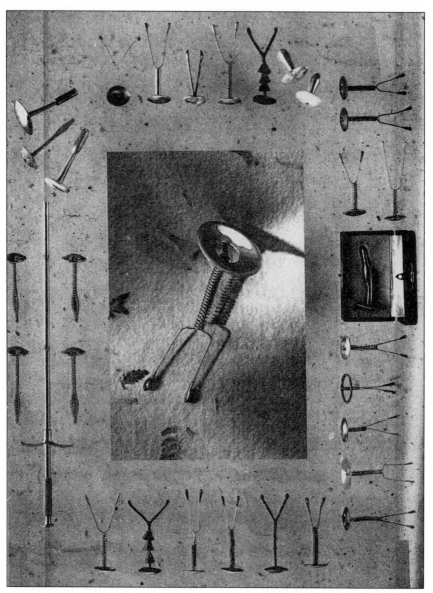

6. Late-nineteenth- and early-twentieth-century intra-cervical and intrauterine metal pessaries (Courtesy of the History of Contraception Museum, Janssen-Ortho Inc., Toronto, Canada)

threshing machine."[46] The IUD craze got so out of hand that one physician, in a playful parody of contraception published in 1867, warned that doctors' preoccupation with "filling . . . the vagina with such traps [was] making a Chinese toy-shop out of it."[47] Constructed from rubber, metal, ivory, and even wood, IUDs could be made by almost anyone, with little cost, knowledge, or equipment.[48] But as doctors knew, money and a professional identity—not to mention a battalion of female patients at one's disposal—did not hurt. In 1887, the president of the Illinois State Medical Society recalled the "craze [that] invaded our ranks a few years ago, [when] many of our over-zealous and enthusiastic brethren seemed to think that the surest and quickest way to reach a topmost round in the professional ladder would be to invent a pessary, and such a display of rings, oblongs, circles, semi-circles, curves, twists, turns, contortions and wind-bags was never witnessed before."[49]

Reputable manufacturers attempted to sustain this tradition of uterine intervention. The medical and legal credibility of IUDs and other therapeutic contraceptives (douching syringes, suppositories, medicated sponges, solutions, and the like) made them fair game for ethical firms who saw the cloak of legitimacy as an economic opportunity. In these companies' hands, contraceptives became a small, discreet, but omnipresent part of a diverse and lucrative product line offered to doctors and druggists nationwide. The B. F. Goodrich Company manufactured three soft-rubber IUDs—one pear- and two donut-shaped, each available in five sizes—and twelve hard-rubber models. Two of the latter models were one-size-fits-all rings encapsulating a spiral spring or copper wire, ten were hard-rubber designs of varying sizes and shapes that ranged from the standard Bow to the more menacing-looking Retroversion stem.[50] The U.S. Rubber Company and Goodyear also manufactured an assortment of IUDs, as did smaller concerns such as Davol and the Tyer Rubber Company.[51]

Rubber producers also made douching syringes. Syringes came in a variety of shapes and sizes and were frequently sold with screw-on pipe attachments. Those designed for the vagina were sold as "female" or "ladies'" or "married women's" syringes. Goodyear produced the Union Syringe (a possible reference to sexual union), Tyer the Ideal Safety Syringe.[52] Some syringes, like B. F. Goodrich's Summit Syringe, available in eight styles, were more versatile and included separate pipes for the rectum, ear, nose, urethra, and vagina.[53] All were designed to "clean" the targeted orifice by flooding it with liquids that eliminated discharges, including, if used vaginally, sperm. An 1883 ad for Dr. W. Molesworth's Vaginal Injecting and Suction Syringe promised to remove "by suction, without injury, all impurities or foreign matter that may be upon the walls and in the folds of the mucous membrane of the vagina, or within the mouth of the womb."[54]

Pharmaceutical producers supplemented the rubber component of the trade with chemical suppositories, powders, vaginal sponges, medicated tampons, and douching solutions, often called injections. Boston's George C. Goodwin sold twelve different injections in 1880, including one containing turpentine.[55] The Philadelphia-based manufacturing chemists John Wyeth & Brothers produced twenty-four types of vaginal suppositories in 1891. According to the printed formulas in the company's trade catalogue, many contained tannic acid, salicylic acid, and boric acid, substances considered potent spermicides in the late nineteenth century.[56] The Detroit Pharmacal Company, chemical manufacturers and jobbers, sold two-inch uterine bougies (thin gelatinous strips infused with medicine) containing two other popular spermicides: zinc sulfate and bichloride of mercury.[57] The H. K. Mulford Company, established in 1889 in Philadelphia, one of the nation's leading pharmaceutical centers, earned the distinction in 1895 of being the first firm to sell a commercial diphtheria antitoxin produced in the United States.[58] This success strengthened the company's commitment to vaccinology but did not deter it from producing contraceptives. Its 1899 *Price List of Pharmaceutical and Biological Products* lists ten kinds of antiseptic vaginal tampons containing boric acid, tannic acid, and alum.[59] As with other highly respected pharmaceutical firms involved in the manufacture of contraceptives at the turn of the twentieth century, Mulford did not specialize in birth control. Nor did it advertise its products as contraceptives. Instead, it offered antiseptic suppositories as part of a larger offering of established medical goods, including hundreds of tinctures, syrups, antiseptics, and powders.

Reluctant to make contraceptives exclusively, large manufacturers' halfway participation in birth control production kept the window of opportunity open to smaller players. One was William Halleck, who had established the Hygiene and Kalology Company in New York in 1897.

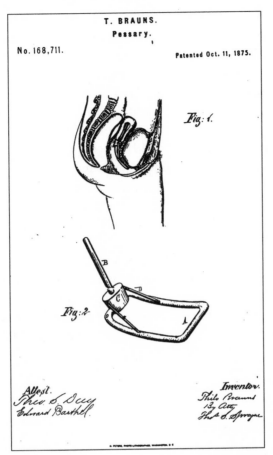

7. Patented to correct uterine displacement, this 1875 pessary doubled as a contraceptive

From the beginning, the company specialized in the manufacture and sale of rubber-stem pessaries, although it also sold douching syringes and abortifacients, which Halleck acquired from the Baltimore-based Sharp & Dohme, manufacturers and distributors of "ethical drugs" (later to merge with present-day pharmaceutical giant Merck). Halleck's hard-rubber IUD was called the Dilatare pessary. Its standard size was "that [which] will fit women who have given birth," but with twenty-three different molds at his disposal, Halleck was willing to supply the Dilatare pessary to customers on a "made-to-order" basis.[60]

Another seeking profit from the production of "legitimate contraceptives" was Antoinette Hon of South Bend, Indiana. Hon was a Polish immigrant who sold proprietary medicines to women under the name "Mrs. Hon." She founded her establishment in 1905 with the aid of her husband, Stanislaus J. Hon, who had received medical training in War- saw. Antoinette's business specialized in birth control, although she also sold stomach tablets and invigorating pills. Mrs. Hon's Healing Com- pound, an antiseptic douching powder containing boric acid, alum, and zinc sulfate, cost a dollar a box in 1917; her foil-wrapped vaginal Womb Suppositories, made from the same ingredients plus morphine in a cocoa- butter and lard-like base, cost $3.25 per order. Hon acquired the pills and tablets from a pharmaceutical supplier in Peoria, Illinois, but she and her staff made the contraceptive powder and suppositories in her Indiana of- fice.[61]

Like Sarah Chase before her, Hon found the contraceptive business accommodating to women. Many contemporaries denounced female entrepreneurship as a transgression of gender roles, but the contracep- tive business had already been branded illegitimate. This stigma served businesswomen well, creating an economic arena that tolerated, even

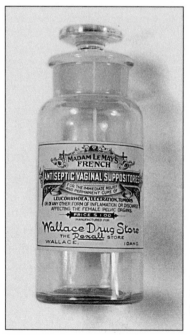

8. Used for a variety of purposes, including birth control, vaginal suppositories were a familiar part of the drugstore contraceptive trade

cultivated, women's commercial activity. Good credit and connections, essential tools for business success generally denied women, were less fundamental to the business of birth control than to others.[62]

In addition, many women would have already been familiar with the ingredients used in chemical contraceptives. Throughout American history, women had relied on homemade recipes for beauty enhancement, medical healing, and the relief of pain during childbirth. This tradition acquainted women with the principles of pharmaceutical practice and familiarized them with the potency and practicality of select herbs, food products, and chemicals. One woman's formula for suppositories found in papers dating to 1920 was precise and spermicidally sound, calling for a mixture of "acid citric—6 grains; acid boracic—1 dram; cocoa butter—90 grains."[63] Women could ask druggists to prepare suppositories and solutions from borax, carbolic acid, tannin, and salicylic acid, ingredients commonly found on the apothecary's shelf. Or they could prepare them themselves from recipes obtained from friends, family, and medical advice books.[64] For women with some knowledge of pharmaceutical science, the transition from creating birth control for home use to manufacturing it for sale would not necessarily have been difficult.

In selling products to female customers, moreover, women enjoyed a distinct advantage. At a time when almost all doctors, druggists, sales agents, and vendors were men, women contraceptive entrepreneurs made biological difference a marketing advantage, urging women to place their confidence in products designed by those with firsthand knowledge of childbearing and its prevention. Female experience, prospective customers were told, was the best mother of contraceptive invention. Hon's advertisements underscored this technique. "I am the woman that understands the sufferings of other women," she wrote passionately.[65]

Hon parlayed a culture that considered frank discussion of sexuality and intercourse taboo among mixed company into an asset. Her advertising asked: Could women feel comfortable broaching intimate matters with detached male doctors or druggists schooled in textbook ways? The answer was no. Hon's advertisements admonished the female reader not to "suffer in secret" or to become one of "thousands of women . . . ashamed to go to the man doctor."[66] Invoking the familial, she referred to prospective customers as "sister," linking buyer and proprietor through the common bonds of womanhood. Another layer to Hon's claims of sisterhood was shared ethnicity. Hon's primary customers were Polish, like herself. She advertised her products in Polish newspapers such as *Zgoda*, published in Chicago, home to 125,604 Poland-born immigrants in 1910 and 137,711 in 1920.[67]

In 1917, twelve years after she had begun operations, Antoinette Hon was still in business. Each day she received an average of thirty to forty letters ordering or asking about her wares. At a time when a middle-class, college-educated professional woman earning eighteen hundred dollars a year was thought to be doing well, Hon's annual salary was thirty-six hundred dollars.[68]

Hon's business capitalized on the medical endorsement of certain forms of birth control. But doctors did not appreciate contraceptive entrepreneurs like Halleck or Hon. In the eyes of the medical establishment, Halleck and Hon were dangerous quacks practicing gynecology without a degree. In 1917, Hon was charged with fraud for dispensing medicine without a license.[69]

Of course, doctors who refused to prescribe birth control were partly to blame for the proliferation of contraceptive entrepreneurs in the age of Comstockery. In the absence of medical leadership, women and men turned to the marketplace to acquire what doctors denied them. There they found men such as Julius Schmidt, with skins aplenty, and Joseph Backrach, with womb veils to spare. At the turn of the twentieth century, low production costs, high consumer demand, weakly enforced laws, and the reluctance of reputable manufacturers to specialize in controversial goods bequeathed ordinary folk such as Schmidt and Hon the freedom to participate in and profit from the bootleg birth control trade. From an entrepreneurial standpoint, these were the business's golden years.

FOUR

Black-Market Birth Control

Casanova wore the finest condoms money could buy, but he was hardly enthusiastic about them. It was emasculating and dispiriting, he complained, to have to "shut myself up in a piece of dead skin in order to prove that I am perfectly alive." Casanova's complaint, a familiar refrain among condom-wearing men then and now, did not prevent him from promoting condoms or wearing them during frequent visits to French brothels. The condom, he announced, was a "wonderful preventive" for "shelter[ing] the fair sex from all fear."[1]

Of course, no contraceptive was perfect. The savvy Italian knew that condom quality varied and that the *surest* way of sheltering sexual partners from fear was to inspect each one before use. Prior to intercourse, Casanova blew his condoms up, balloon-style, to see if they would burst or deflate.[2] In the days before condoms were subjected to mechanized air-burst tests, one did what one could.[3]

More than a century later, Americans had similar reactions to condoms and other birth control devices. They complained that rubbers and skins dulled sexual sensation and that postcoital douching was a chore. But they used these methods anyway, believing that to do so was better than doing nothing.

Although obscenity laws in late-nineteenth- and early-twentieth-century America were frequently violated and erratically enforced, they made contraceptives illicit goods to be confiscated, not merchandise to be regulated and inspected. Without government safeguards to protect consumers from unscrupulous merchants and shoddy wares, America's birth control buyers were on their own.

Refusing to let their procreative destinies be held hostage by absent safeguards, women and men invented strategies to shield themselves from quackery. They shared experiences with family and friends and sought advice from experienced contraceptors. To better the odds of pregnancy prevention, they used multiple contraceptives at once. They inflated condoms, Casanova-style, while yearning for superlative devices that felt and worked better. These precautions did not eliminate heartbreak, pain, or pregnancy. But they helped. National fertility rates dropped steadily after 1880, most sharply among African-Americans. In 1910, only France had a lower birthrate in the Western world.

It is difficult to gauge how safe, effective, and tolerable contraband contraceptives were before the advent of clinical testing in the 1920s and product standardization in the 1930s. Evidence from the period, however, sketches a scenario in which glaring incidents of quackery coexisted with a surprising degree of consumer confidence in bootleg birth control. If Americans stopped short of celebrating contraceptives as aesthetically pleasing or absolutely protective, neither did they denounce the devices as universally useless or prohibitively dangerous.

By modern standards, contraband contraceptives certainly seem to have been wanting. Take the ever-popular condom. Skins could be thick and smelly, especially if they were recycled, a cost-saving but odoriferous practice in which condoms were rinsed, dried, powdered, and then reused.[4] Hand-stitched low-grade skins sported protruding and uneven seams that could irritate genitals during high-friction sex. Chemicals used to create the finer goldbeaters' models left unsuspecting wearers vulnerable to chemically induced skin welts and lesions.[5] Making matters worse, the relative inelasticity of animal-based skins, no matter how well stretched or secured by ribbons or rings, rendered them less watertight and durable than today's formfitting models. By 1900, things had changed little since 1671, when one mother described skins to her daughter as both an "armor against enjoyment and a spider web against danger."[6]

Not the contraceptive panacea for which men and women yearned, the maligned skin was nonetheless bought and even praised, as it was in the anonymous 1744 poem *The Machine—or Love's Preservative*:

> By this Machine secure, the willing Maid
> Can taste Love's Joys, nor is she more afraid
> Her swelling Belly should, or squalling Brat,
> Betray the luscious Pastime she has been at.[7]

For all its drawbacks, the skin was most appealing for its potential to be, in Casanova's words, a "wonderful preventive." Lovers took precautions to minimize the risk of condom failure. They examined skins for cracks and structural weaknesses, moistened them to ensure a tight fit (Casanova purportedly dunked his in a canal before use), and incorporated such safety "rituals" into foreplay.

These strategies undoubtedly helped reassure skin users. But what probably eased their minds more was the arrival of rubber condoms in the 1860s. Historians have often discounted the significance of technological upgrades to birth control before the Pill, as if, in the long history of contraception, only a once-a-day oral contraceptive counts as new. In doing so, they have drawn attention to the ancient origins of many modern methods, an important point. But it is equally essential to recognize that technological modifications of traditional contraceptives that today might appear minor were regarded as revolutionary in their time. Such is the case with the invention of diaphragms that contained springs, and IUDs made of malleable plastic. And it was certainly the case with condoms created from rubber. In the nineteenth century, people viewed rubbers as a superior form of condom and contraceptive. George Bernard Shaw thought them the "greatest invention of the nineteenth century"—and this in a century that witnessed the birth of the internal combustion engine and the telephone.[8]

The American freethinker and publisher Gilbert Vale hailed India rubber sheaths as more durable than skins.[9] Rubbers reduced the risk of condom slippage or breakage. And because rubber as a substance is less porous than natural membrane, it is less likely to leak. (This is one reason why gynecologists today counsel against the use of skin sheaths as protection from sexually transmitted diseases such as AIDS.)[10]

Still, the quality of pre-latex rubbers varied. The hand-sewn rubbers described by T. J. B. Buckingham in his 1892 report were as seamed as many skins, making them both uncomfortable and poor retainers of fluid.[11] Seamless condoms were available, created either by working warmed natural rubber around a mold until its edges adhered or by dipping cylindrical molds into dissolved, masticated sheet rubber.[12] How successfully seamlessness fixed hand-stitched sheaths' tendency to leak is unknown, but as late as 1938, one birth control guide urged users of rubbers to inflate them to check for holes.[13] Seam or no seam, all pre-latex rubbers had a short shelf life. Rubbers deteriorated rapidly, especially when they came into contact with moisture. The magnitude of this problem is suggested by one advertisement for India-Rubber Capotes, which promised customers condoms "WARRANTED NOT TO DECAY."[14]

A more telling indicator of condom quality is the results of the first scientific investigations of condoms undertaken before inspections by the Food and Drug Administration (FDA) began in the late 1930s. A 1924 study by the physician and birth control advocate Robert Latou Dickinson found a 50 percent failure rate among couples using skin and rubber condoms at three birth control clinics in New York and London.[15] A contributing factor was likely the condoms themselves, first evaluated by the biochemist Cecil I. B. Voge, best known for his discovery in 1926 of a laboratory test for confirming pregnancy.[16] In 1934 and 1935, Voge assembled more than two thousand American sheaths representing twenty-one brands, a majority of which he purchased on "the open market." After inflating each sheath to a "moderate size . . . 8 inches long and 6 inches in diameter," he sealed the open end and suspended it for observation. Condoms that neither burst nor deflated after twenty minutes were placed against an illuminated background and visually examined for other defects: foreign matter, dirt, creases, thin spots, and weak tips. Only 41 percent of those tested—the strongest, cleanest, and most evenly textured sheaths—passed. Of those that did not, half burst upon inflation, a quarter were found to have pinholes, and the rest were declared otherwise unfit.[17]

Bursting condoms, holey sheaths, smelly skins: this is the material out of which modern sexual nightmares are made. Indeed, compared with today's sheer, odor-free, and resilient condoms—which are routinely subjected to a grueling twenty-five-liter air-burst test before being unleashed

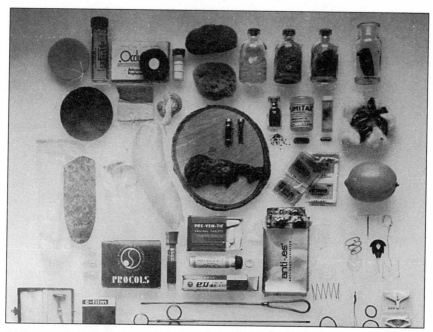

9. Contraceptives, past and present (Courtesy of the History of Contraception Museum, Janssen-Ortho Inc., Toronto, Canada)

on the public—early condoms do not measure up.[18] But that does not mean that men and women in turn-of-the-century America judged them ineffective. Evaluating contraceptive efficacy by the standards of a post-Pill world obscures the way Americans of an earlier era assessed birth control. Pregnancy is not a relative condition. But at the turn of the century, evaluations of contraceptives were informed by available options, which were more limited and less effective than they are today. Government regulation of contraceptives was unknown. Although being at the mercy of manufacturers and merchants was not ideal, it was an existence American consumers knew well. Until the FDA was established in 1906 to combat endemic quackery, most medical products—even legal ones—were sold without consumer protections. In a political and medical environment where the potential for health fraud was high and the unregulated market provided danger almost as often as relief, Americans could not help but evaluate contraband contraceptives for themselves.

Throughout the black-market era, moreover, contraceptives that would be almost 100 percent effective were unfathomable. The only reliable method was abstinence, something that has not always been in women's control. Male withdrawal, or coitus interruptus, was another popular technique. (Some physicians, referring to its grassroots practice, condescendingly termed it "the French peasant's withdrawal.") Free and easy to learn, withdrawal had a failure rate of about 20 percent. (Failure rates refer to the percentage of women who become pregnant after a year's use.)[19] Doctors' remonstrations against withdrawal, which linked it to insanity, impotence, blindness, and a host of other ailments, may have persuaded some men not to try it and others to "change their minds" at the last minute. Although modern science has invalidated such prophecies of doom, they may well have had a placebo effect on Americans in an earlier era. In 1895, one woman complained that her husband, a physician, had practiced withdrawal only to complain of being entirely "worn out [the] next day."[20]

The frequent failure of the so-called safe period, the point during the menstrual cycle when intercourse is least likely to cause pregnancy, was disheartening to Americans who practiced it, particularly because many physicians mistakenly insisted on its reliability. Doctors assumed that the reproductive cycles of lower mammals and humans were the same. Knowing from observation that animals ovulated during estrus, they reasoned that women must ovulate during menstruation and be least fertile midway through the menstrual cycle. As one Michigan doctor instructed in 1881, a woman trying to prevent pregnancy should avoid "having connection with her husband just before her menses," for "that is the time that nature evidently intended that conception should take place . . . it is then that all animals are in heat."[21] As early as the 1870s, postmortem examinations of women who died while menstruating without signs of a matured ovum had disputed this assumption. Most physicians nevertheless continued to insist on the simultaneity of menstruation and ovulation until the 1920s, when Japanese and Czechoslovakian studies of the laparotomic retrieval of ova from Fallopian tubes proved them incorrect.[22]

Many women, though, suspected that the doctors were wrong. Emily Fitzgerald had only to witness the world around her to know better. The wife of a western Army doctor, she began to suspect that the safe period was a myth. "I don't believe that there is a safe day in the month for me," she complained in 1875. "Indeed, I know there isn't—15th-16th-17th—

or any other." Emily and some women friends had discussed the problem at length. We have "meetings of horror over the subject," she wrote, "as we all . . . seem to be awfully prolific."[23]

The despair Emily and her contemporaries felt about a method that was supposed to be effective but was not probably shaped the criteria they used to evaluate other contraceptives. Compared with the safe period, condoms seemed a good bet. A failure rate of 50 percent also meant a 50 percent success rate, a significant measure of protection by the standards of an earlier age.

Although it is impossible to know how many couples used condoms in the late nineteenth and early twentieth centuries, a survey conducted by Dr. Clelia Duel Mosher provides clues. Mosher, born in 1863, first became interested in studying women's sexual practices in 1892, when she was a biology student at the University of Wisconsin. In preparation for a talk on marital relations she was to give at a local Mothers Club, she asked married women, most of whom were college educated and middle-class, to discuss their gynecological health. How often did they have intercourse? What contraceptives had they used?[24]

Mosher received an A.B. from Stanford University, and then went to the Johns Hopkins Medical School. After graduating from Hopkins in 1900, she moved to Palo Alto and eventually became assistant professor of personal hygiene at Stanford. Over the years, she continued the survey she had begun in 1892. By the time she completed it in 1920, the bound but never published questionnaires—discovered by accident in 1973—had chronicled the marital relations of forty-five women. Mosher's is the only known survey of its kind of Victorian women in the United States.[25]

Condoms were popular in Mosher's group, ranking second in frequency of use after the douche. Eleven of the twenty-eight contraceptive users had tried condoms, chiefly because they deemed them more trustworthy than other techniques. One woman, a former music teacher, turned to condoms after she and her husband, married in 1889, conceived by "accident" in 1891 during her "so-called 'safety week.' " Her pregnancy was physically and emotionally draining. When Mosher interviewed her in 1892, the new mother had regained her strength and vigor, but the couple had abandoned the safe period for the reliability of a "thin rubber covering for man." Another condom user, born in 1867, had conceived five times before switching to condoms. Two of the pregnancies had ended in miscarriage. When Mosher asked the woman what form of birth control she was currently using, her answer underscored her faith in condom technology: "Cundrum now," she replied. "Must not conceive again." Others shared her confidence. After one woman became pregnant using the safe period and a postcoital douche, her husband switched to condoms. The "French method of prevention," the relieved woman told Mosher, had been "perfectly successful."[26]

One of Mosher's respondents used a "woman's shield—pessary cap"— prescribed by a doctor because "she must not have more children."[27] Notwithstanding the doctor's confidence, it is unclear how effective womb veils were at the turn of the century. If the pessary was constructed to fit like a diaphragm, odds of its reliability were poor. Today diaphragms are prescribed only after the cervix has been measured, a technique that enables a medical practitioner to select the best-fitting size. Sizes are standardized—ranging from fifty to ninety-five millimeters—and manufacturers supply doctors with "fitting" models to ensure accuracy. Unfortunately, medical schools at the turn of the century did not train physicians to fit women with diaphragms or to rule out physiological contraindications such as cervical lacerations, erosion, or displaced uteri. In lieu of standardized sizing, womb veils were sold over the counter in ambiguous dimensions that varied by producer: "big" and "small," "one-size-fits-all," "mothers' size." Too large a shield could cause abdominal pain, cramping, vaginal ulceration, and recurrent urinary tract infections; too small, dislodgement and pregnancy. If the pessary had been designed to function as a cervical cap, the odds of pregnancy prevention were better. The cap works by forming around the cervix a seal whose suction prevents sperm from moving past its edges. (In contrast, the diaphragm works by suspending a spermicidal agent within the vagina.) Although today a doctor's fitting is recommended before a cervical cap is used, caps are currently manufactured in only four sizes (ranging from twenty-two to thirty-one millimeters). An exact match between the inner diameter of the cap rim and the base of the cervix is not required for the method to work. This made cervical caps usually more reliable than diaphragms at the turn of the century. Still, in a pre-latex age, even the best-fitting caps and diaphragms suffered from some of the same shortcomings as any contraceptive made of India rubber, including rapid deterioration. But if the fit was right and the material resilient, diaphragms and cervical caps had a high potential for success. Two early studies of the methods found failure rates ranging from 1 to 24 percent.[28]

Another of Mosher's respondents used an intrauterine device, a "Good-year rubber ring," as birth control. IUDs were the most painful and medically dangerous birth control method at the turn of the century. Compared with today's quarter-sized malleable plastic models, intrauterine stem pessaries were bulky and large, making them difficult and painful to insert. IUD use increased a woman's risk of cramping, dysmenorrhea, uterine perforation, and pelvic inflammatory disease—a potentially life-threatening infection of the Fallopian tubes, uterus, or ovaries, incurable in the days before antibiotics.[29] Still, women able to endure the discomfort of insertion and use often found them beneficial. Although the specific antifertility mechanism of IUDs is unknown, scientists agree that the presence of an object in the uterus prevents pregnancy most of the time. There are several theories on how IUDs work. One is that the IUD immobilizes sperm by interfering with its migration from the vagina. Another holds that IUDs expedite the transport of the ovum through the Fallopian tube, causing the egg to arrive at the uterus too soon. The most widely accepted theory is that the introduction of an IUD causes a local inflammation or chronic, low-grade infection that makes fertilization and egg implantation impossible.[30]

The douche was the most popular contraceptive in Mosher's study, although its failure rate was higher than that of the IUD. For excellent reasons, doctors today do not recommend douching. As a hygienic practice, it is unnecessary and potentially harmful, because the vagina is self-cleansing. Water and chemical solutions wash away beneficial bacteria, increasing chances of infection. In addition, forceful douching may remove the mucous plug protecting the cervix, uterus, and Fallopian tubes from disease, providing a biological expressway for pathogens. Studies have linked douching to a higher incidence of pelvic inflammatory disease, sexually transmitted diseases, and ectopic pregnancy.[31]

As a contraceptive, douching is equally unsound. Sperm move fast. By the time a douching solution is introduced, seminal fluid that has already penetrated the cervix and surrounding tissues is difficult, even impossible, to remove. In addition, douching, while flushing away some sperm, pushes others into the uterus, placing a woman on a fast track to pregnancy. Many douching solutions are either spermicidally benign or so toxic that they chemically inflame, irritate, or burn the vagina and cervix. Doctors and family planning counselors today consider douching the least effective contraceptive, and some refuse to classify it as birth control.[32]

Still, it would be a mistake to assume that couples who repeatedly used this method at the turn of the century were stupid. In an era when sperm motility and the spermicidal properties of chemicals were not well understood, douching seemed intellectually logical, presenting women with a technique to wash away sperm and devitalize persistent leftovers. Compared with the safe period, douching must have seemed particularly reliable. Before clinical investigations in the 1920s and 1930s revealed failure rates as high as 90 percent (about the same as using no birth control at all), many doctors endorsed its contraceptive efficacy in medical journals and to patients for these reasons.[33] One 1924 study found that, after condoms, douching was the form of birth control most frequently recommended by doctors, more popular among medical professionals than diaphragms and suppositories combined.[34]

Moreover, although douching failure rates could be alarmingly high, they varied enough (one study found a 42 percent failure rate) to suggest that the method provided some women with a modicum of protection. The shape of a woman's body, the solution she used, and when she douched were important variables. Dorothy Bocker, a physician at Margaret Sanger's Birth Control Clinical Research Bureau, found in her yearlong investigation of contraceptive methods that douching was less likely to work in women with wide cervical canals and prolapsed uteri.[35] The chemical makeup of douching solutions also influenced the method's success. An effective spermicide kills "very vigorous human sperms" within a minute without injury to the vagina. But many commercial preparations were too inert or caustic to qualify. Zinc sulfate douches, for instance, were frequently used to prevent pregnancy at this time. But because zinc sulfate acts slowly on sperm, it is not an effective spermicide. This might explain a comment made by one of Mosher's subjects: "Sulphate of zinc . . . is not infallible." Citric acid was a better bet, but only in the right concentration. At 1:1,000 parts, it immobilizes sperm instantly, but a more diluted concentration takes longer, increasing the likelihood of conception.[36]

Efficacy also depended on quick thinking and immediate action after intercourse, a disruption not all women would tolerate. As Bocker observed, douching is "psychologically bad because the woman, after normal intercourse, is relaxed and fatigued; and using a douche is an act of will as devastating to the woman as coitus interruptus to the man."[37] Moreover, only affluent women had access to running water, a bathroom, and the privacy that facilitated douching as a practice.[38]

Vaginal suppositories and tablets were easier to use, but their effectiveness varied. Many turn-of-the-century suppositories and tablets contained boric acid or quinine, ingredients not considered effective spermicides. Others contained lactic acid, so effective that in the 1940s some birth control advocates suggested that it be used alone for contraception. In theory, suppositories were double-acting: they mechanically paralyzed and chemically neutralized sperm. Usually based in cocoa butter or gelatin, they were intended to dissolve at room temperature. In practice, weather extremes in a pre-air-conditioning age and corresponding fluctuations in vaginal temperature made suppositories' diffusion, homogeneity, and contraceptive attributes unpredictable. Foaming tablets were also unreliable. Composed of an effervescent, moisture-activated mixture such as tartaric acid and sodium bicarbonate (which, when triggered, produced a protective foam), tablets often remained inert until *after* ejaculation.[39]

Without a doubt, black-market birth control carried significant risks, especially by today's standards. But these risks did not just victimize contraceptive consumers. They incited women and men to action. Inventing strategies to shield themselves from product failure and commercial exploitation, women and men at the turn of the century did their best to convert awareness of birth control hazards into techniques for self-protection.

One strategy was to employ several birth control methods at once. Today's contraceptives, used as directed, rarely have failure rates exceeding 9 percent, and most Americans feel confident employing one method at a time.[40] Sexually active Americans in a less certain world doubled, tripled, even quadrupled up. Amassing contraceptives as if they were battle weapons, they stocked their birth control arsenals well. To buck the odds, one woman in Mosher's survey used a vaginal suppository and a douche, another a four-pronged regimen of a suppository, pre- and post-coital douches, and the "mid month period." Yet another used "cundrums" and a diaphragm, reserving the safe period for when the couple "could afford chance."[41] A 1941 investigation of contraceptive practices revealed that 66 percent of those surveyed had "previously used various and often multiple contraceptive methods."[42]

Another way women and men limited their vulnerability to contraceptive failure was by sharing their experiences with different methods and brands. In an era when the only way of discerning an article's safety and efficacy was through trial and error, recommendations passed along from mother to daughter, friend to friend, and husband to wife guided worried birth control users through the turgid and sometimes treacherous waters of the contraceptive marketplace. Women in Mosher's study cited as sources of reproductive knowledge "some very frank talks" with mothers, physicians, friends, and relatives. One respondent appreciatively recalled, "[A] few months before my marriage a wise woman friend told me about the various ways of 'regulating conception.' "[43] Bocker's 1923 investigation of preclinical birth control practices identified a similar network of local and informal instruction, whereby women learned about contraceptives "from neighbors, relatives, and friends." Bocker spoke with one woman from a small Midwestern town whose determination led her to the doorsteps of the community member she believed possessed the most expertise: the "keeper of a brothel."[44]

So entrenched was this tradition of grassroots discussion that once birth control became legal, contraceptive manufacturers endeavored to discredit it through advertising campaigns designed to bolster consumer support of products that were "scientifically tested" instead of "just" recommended by friends. Convincing contraceptive users to forgo what manufacturers disparagingly labeled "back-fence gossip" was difficult, for during an era when scientific evaluation of commercial birth control was denied them, women and men had turned to each other for the very information manufacturers were now claiming to monopolize. Writing in 1888, the Boston physician H. S. Pomeroy found informal discussions of fertility control disdainful but common. "Many of those who have become adept in the art of avoiding parenthood," he railed, "have . . . learned their lessons of some kind friend or neighbor."[45]

Mindful of the dangers of contraband contraceptives, Americans used them anyway. Their potential benefits outweighed their risks. Frustrated by the high failure rate of "natural" methods such as the safe period, drawn to advertised assurances of reliability, turn-of-the-century Americans looked to the market for pregnancy prevention. In Mosher's study, a majority of women (70.3 percent) practicing contraception forsook natural methods for the "safety" of commercial contraception.[46]

How universal was birth control use? Measuring use of contraceptives is inherently difficult, especially for an age when birth control was criminal, few people recorded their experiences with contraceptives, and medical, marketing, and opinion surveys of national practices did not exist. The women interviewed in Mosher's study used black-market birth control frequently. But their affluence and education set them apart from American women as a whole.

Margaret Sanger was firmly convinced that elitism kept contraceptives out of the hands of those who needed them most: the working class. Sanger, the twentieth century's greatest champion of birth control, knew plenty about the sufferings of the poor. As a young bride in New York, she immersed herself in the world of radical politics, organizing strikes, pickets, and rallies for the Socialist Party and the Industrial Workers of the World. In 1912, she began work as a part-time visiting obstetrical nurse in Manhattan's Lower East Side, the poorest immigrant district of the city and home to New Israel and Little Italy. Tenements there were crowded, sanitation poor. The resilient spirit that triumphed within this urban squalor—captured in perpetuity by the photographer Jacob Riis— was lost on Sanger. What she saw was only misery, poverty, and degradation, a state of human suffering exacerbated by inadequate fertility control. Mothers exhausted by relentless childbearing, parents struggling to support families of ten, dozens of immigrant women "with their shawls over their heads waiting outside the office of the five-dollar abortionist": these were the images that haunted Sanger. When she launched *The Woman Rebel* in 1914, Sanger articulated the problem of birth control as a class issue:

> The woman of the upper middle class has all available knowledge and implements to prevent conception. The woman of the lower middle class tries various methods of

contraception and after a few years of experience plus medical advice succeeds in discovering some method suitable to
her individual self. The woman of the people is the only
one left in ignorance of this information. Her neighbors,
relatives and friends tell her stories of special devices and
the success of them all. . . . But the working woman's purse
is thin.[47]

What should we make of Sanger's insistence that trustworthy contraceptives were known only to the rich? Certainly, the poverty she observed was as genuine as her desire to alleviate it. But Sanger was prone
to exaggeration; even sympathetic biographers have noted her tendency
to overstate her case to bolster political support.[48] Her observations,
moreover, are frequently at odds with the conclusions she draws from
them. If income alone determined contraceptive access, why would a
woman able to afford a five-dollar abortion not be able to afford a
twenty-five-cent reusable condom? One of Sanger's most frequently recounted stories, that of Sadie Sachs, contains a similar inconsistency. As
Sanger told it, Sachs was the young immigrant wife of a truck driver
named Jake and the mother of three children. Struggling to raise a family in their overcrowded dwelling, Sachs consulted a doctor for effective
birth control. The doctor's reply was callous and succinct: "Tell Jake to
sleep on the roof." Soon after, Sachs became pregnant and died from septicemia following a self-induced abortion. Sanger repeated this tragic tale
often both to elucidate the special reproductive burdens of the poor and
to explain her decision to give up nursing for full-time birth control advocacy. If we set aside the possibility raised by one biographer that
Sanger embellished the story for dramatic effect, the tale illustrates less
the economic barriers to effective contraception than the medical profession's opposition to it.[49] Sadie Sachs lived in slum conditions, yet she
managed to see a doctor, which was more costly than buying condoms or
suppositories. Presumably, had the doctor recommended contraceptives,
Sachs would have been only too happy to buy them, though this would
have cost more money still. But all Sachs got for her efforts was bad medical advice. In the end, it was not poverty alone that condemned her to
a premature death but an unfeeling physician unwilling to help.

Not all doctors were as dismissive as Sachs's. Many approved of and recommended contraceptives to their patients. Medical journals of the era frequently published debates on contraception, indicating that professional discussion of the matter had not been foreclosed. Still, the prevailing attitude of the medical fraternity was one of opposition. Only a handful of late-nineteenth- and early-twentieth-century schools trained medical students in contraception, and until 1937 the American Medical Association (AMA) rejected birth control as a legitimate facet of medical practice. The weight of apathy and ignorance made it hard for even the most sympathetic doctor to practice good medicine. As late as 1930 (seven years after Sanger's first permanent birth control clinic opened under medical supervision), the *Journal of the American Medical Association* advised doctors seeking birth control information, "We do not know of any method of preventing conception that is absolutely dependable except total abstinence."[50] In the absence of medical leadership and scientific testing of contraceptives, physicians, like their patients, were on their own.

Doctors disagreed about the reliability of different techniques. Many endorsed the misnamed safe period. One proclaimed douching injections "an absolute protection," another, recalling a case where the syringe had failed, advocated the " 'skin covering' worn by the male." The condom, he insisted, was the only "absolute protection."[51] David Matteson, a doctor from Warsaw, New York, favored the sponge, "preferably a silk sponge . . . with a strong silk thread passed through it." Another doctor cautioned against such devices, warning attendees of an 1888 Washington Obstetrical and Gynecology Society meeting that articles that "occlu[de] the uterine orifice" had "failed too frequently to gain the stamp of certainty." Abstinence was the only method he could recommend with confidence.[52]

Diverse opinions reflected medical uncertainty about birth control in late-nineteenth- and early-twentieth-century America. Not only did doctors not have a monopoly of knowledge about effective birth control; in some cases, as with the safe period, they were wrong. In subsequent decades, as medical discussion, endorsement, and evaluation of contraceptives increased, the credibility of doctors' claims to expertise in this area grew. But at the turn of the century, it is unclear whether women and men were any worse off if they eschewed medical counsel. In any event, most did. Until the FDA approved prescription-only oral contraceptives in 1960, a majority of Americans, including the most affluent, acquired birth control over the counter, not from doctors.

A deterministic view of affordability such as Sanger's, moreover, masks the complexities of consumer behavior. Although household incomes may be fixed, perceptions of what constitutes a luxury and what a necessity are not.[53] The thousands of letters working-class Americans sent to Sanger and other birth control proponents reflect their view that contraceptives were not a prohibitively costly luxury but a commodity few working people could afford to be without. Not just a pregnancy preventive, contraceptives promised families barely making do a prophylactic against economic ruin. Ironically, poor Americans may have felt the lure of the contraceptive market most strongly of all.

This was certainly the case for one working-class man in Michigan who sought birth control advice from Sanger in 1923. He wrote that he and his wife had "a family of six children to provide for from a laborer's income." He asked Sanger to "impart to us that which will relieve the despair of our lives." Cost, to him, was irrelevant. "Price and money will not stand in the way," he told her, "as we both realize something has to be done."[54] Significantly, in the first large-scale clinical study of birth control methods in use in the United States, more of the predominantly working-class women and men surveyed had relied on purchased contraceptives—the condom, douche, cervical cap, or suppository—than on natural methods.[55]

In addition, the turn-of-the-century birth control trade was highly stratified, accommodating a broad spectrum of budgets. Contraceptive prices varied widely, from $.11 condoms to the $.35 generic one-ounce douching syringe to the $1.25 eight-ounce "Tyrian" Female Syringe.[56] A New York worker making, on average, $1.75 a day in 1890 would have spent a significant portion of a day's wages to acquire a fancy syringe. Yet he might have considered it a good investment, for, unlike cheaper suppositories, syringes were reusable.[57]

Cheap did not automatically mean less reliable. Almost all contraceptives in this era, including the doctor-endorsed safe period or the Vaseline method, had a high potential for failure. As the historian Linda Gordon has argued, class differentials in contraceptive practice at the turn of the century "were not so great as they are today, because the best available methods were not so good as they are today."[58] Before birth control production was standardized and devices were inspected for reliability, retailers were free to make outlandish claims and charge exorbitant prices. A high price could signify nothing more than one entrepreneur's scheme for getting rich. Although sites of birth control buying varied by class, the safety and efficacy of products typically did not. Whether they acquired bootleg condoms from doctors or "first-class druggists" or by mail order through the *National Police Gazette*, consumers assumed similar risks, for the production technologies, absence of regulation, and economics of patent medicine blurred class distinctions.

Significantly, non-elite Americans were most likely to encounter advertisements for birth control devices. Contraceptive advertisements appeared most consistently in "spicy periodicals" and "penny miscellanies," working-class and immigrant newspapers, "sensationalist tabloids specializing in sports, theatrical news, murders, police reports, and courtroom dramas," and "newspapers aimed at an urban class of stable boys, maids, day laborers, upwardly mobile young clerks and salespeople."[59] The *National Police Gazette* was the nation's largest repository of contraceptive ads. It promised its readers—mainly urban, working men and women—a good time, not a trenchant analysis of the day's political events. Stories on sex scandals, murders, dogfights, rat-killing contests, boxing matches, and other amusements filled its pages, interspersed with ads for impotence devices, gonorrhea cures, pornographic photos, and contraceptives.[60] In contrast, ads for birth control were conspicuously absent in highbrow publications. Editors and publishers, mindful of the law but also of the association of contraceptives with smut, excluded ads that might sully their publications' reputations. Literary respectability was partly defined by honoring the boundary between what was "fit" and "unfit" for print. The efforts of contraceptive peddlers to reach an elite audience through the periodical press usually failed. The E. C. Allen Company, a prominent publisher of literary and agricultural journals in the late nineteenth century, kept a scrapbook of medical advertisements it deemed "unfit" for print between 1880 and 1890. About a quarter of the 182 advertisements it rejected were for contraceptives, including ads for "Dr. Dix's Celebrated Female Powders," "gents' supplies," and the Eureka Medical Company's "vaginal tablets and pocket syringe."[61] The impact of exclusionary advertising practices was twofold. First, it underscored the unseemly nature of contraception. Second, it concentrated contraceptive advertising in publications most likely to be read by non-elites.

Identifying birth control as an issue that crossed class and ethnic lines, contraceptive entrepreneurs aggressively courted working-class and immigrant dollars. The success of Antoinette Hon is instructive. In an era when small-business failures were as common as the cold, Hon's lasted twelve years, sustained by immigrant women and closed only by government decree. Hon knew that working women had little money or time. She promised goods tailored for the budget-conscious that could be purchased "very cheap[ly]" and taken without having "to disturb your daily work." Her success attracted unwanted scrutiny, but it also demonstrated ongoing working-class and immigrant support of the contraceptive trade. Hon's dispensing medical advice without a license made her a "quack" in prosecutors' eyes, but in the 1917 case against her, chemists and doctors hired by the government begrudgingly conceded that the chemicals in her products were "very injurious to the spermatozoa."[62]

Whereas Hon found support from Poles, the Septigyn Company courted Czech immigrants. The Chicago-based firm sold Septigyn tablets, vaginal suppositories designed to "prevent conception" without "injury to the delicate tissues of the female generative tract." Septigyn advertised its tablets, a hundred of which cost five dollars, in circulars printed in Czech and English. Preferring a marketing scheme more personal than the anonymity of mail-order commerce, the company hired sales agents to distribute flyers and sell products door-to-door in targeted neighborhoods. How well the company did is unknown, but it was enough to irk the AMA, which launched a formal investigation of Septigyn in 1913.[63]

Demographic evidence supports the view that contraceptives were used successfully by Americans from different backgrounds. In the absence of other factors such as a higher incidence of abortion, malnutrition, or disease, low fertility rates suggest a conscious effort among a specified population to restrict childbearing through contraception (although they do not reveal which birth control methods people used). Because of the way information was collected, the U.S. Census (the data set demographers use to determine fertility rates) does not permit calculations of national fertility patterns by class in the late nineteenth and early twentieth centuries. What demographers *have* succeeded in doing is determining this information for individual communities and towns through household enumerations.[64] Although the local character of this approach makes demographers' findings specific to the communities studied,[65] the findings are nonetheless important, for they challenge claims made by Sanger and historians since that "the most reliable methods of contraception were known only spottily by working-class women in the late 19th and early 20th century."[66]

One study of marital fertility in five Massachusetts towns in 1880, for instance, found that married women in households with a high occupational status did not always have the fewest children. In three of the five towns they did, but in the remaining two, the smallest families belonged to either the lowest- or the middle-occupation group. Such findings should make us wary of generalizing about the class-specific nature of birth control, for as the authors of the study conclude, the "relationship between fertility and the occupational status of the husband may not be clear-cut."[67]

Demographic evidence also suggests that African-Americans used birth control at the turn of the century. National fertility rates for both white and black women declined after 1880, reaching an all-time low in 1940. Between 1880 and 1940, the average fertility rate of whites dropped from 4.4 children per woman to 2.1, for blacks from 7.5 children to 3. Whites were having fewer children on average, but the *rate* of decline was higher among African-Americans, dropping 53 percent between 1880 and 1940, compared with 47 percent among whites.[68]

Racist demographers in the early twentieth century ignored birth control as an explanation for rising black childlessness. Instead, they ascribed fertility decline to malnutrition, infection, tuberculosis, and infertility caused by venereal diseases resulting from sexual promiscuity. Foreclosing the possibility of black self-determination, demographers emphasized the "pathology" of African-American culture, characterizing blacks as morally deficient and medically diseased. One demographer went so far as to suggest that blacks' lack of self-control rendered them constitutionally unfit for the responsibility of contraception. "The negro," he asserted, "generally exercises less prudence and foresight than white people do in all sexual matters."[69]

But conscious use of birth control was definitely a factor. Far from being novices at contraception, African-Americans at the turn of the century had a long history of fertility control. Anthropologists have documented the use of coitus interruptus, periodic abstinence, botanical contraceptives, and intra-vaginal plugs made of crushed roots or grass among early Africans, and it is likely that they imported many of these traditions when they came to North America as slaves.[70] In the antebellum South, slaves proved extremely adept at using birth control and abortion to thwart their masters' plans to increase slave ranks through procreation. Slaveholders, in turn, accused black women of possessing "secret knowledge" that kept them childless. There is no reason to think that these traditions and this knowledge died with slavery. A black women's newspaper, The Woman's Era, seemed to support women's right to reproductive self-determination when it printed in 1894 that "not all women are intended for mothers. Some of us have not the temperament for family life."[71]

Birth control advertisements in black newspapers point to a mail-order and drugstore contraceptive trade within the African-American community. The June 6, 1896, edition of Omaha's Afro-American Sentinel, for example, a weekly journal "devoted to the elevation of Negro character in the United States," couched an ad for rubber condoms between one for binder twine and another for elixirs for opium addiction.[72] In 1904, the Atlanta Independent, boasting a circulation of fifty thousand blacks, advertised "Paxtine Toilet Antiseptic," a "vaginal wash" unrivaled "for thoroughness."[73] Cultivating an image of African-American propriety within a culture that portrayed black men as hypersexual and then punished them for it, black newspapers would not publish advertisements for sex devices. But they printed some contraceptive ads, and as birth control became more respectable, they printed more. From the mid-1920s on, ads for douching solutions, vaginal suppositories, and diaphragms in the black press were commonplace. So, too, were their purchase and use. In 1932, George Schuyler, editor of the National News, observed, "If anyone should doubt the desire on the part of Negro women and men to limit their families it is only necessary to note the large sale of preventive devices sold in every drug store in various Black Belts."[74]

African-American use of contraceptives did not erase demographic distinctions. Black families continued to be larger than white, but we cannot assume that ignorance about contraception "explains" this difference. Occupational and residential status also factored into decisions about contraception. Most African-Americans, working as tenant farmers, lived in the rural South, where the benefit of children to the household economy may have dissuaded parents from restricting family size. Among whites, those in rural areas also had higher fertility rates than those in urban areas, but because a higher proportion of the white population resided in cities, average white fertility rates were lower.[75]

Political considerations also affected African-American decisions. Just as fertility control had protected slaves from some of the cruelties of slavery, the growth of the African-American population after emancipation seemed to some leaders critical to black cultural autonomy. The separatist leader Marcus Garvey encouraged unfettered black reproduction, believing that racial solidarity came with strength in numbers. Birth control, he feared, would lead to the enfeeblement, if not outright extinction, of the black population. In 1934, Garvey's nationalist Universal Negro Improvement Association unanimously adopted a resolution condemning contraception.[76] The African-American historian, sociologist, and founder of the National Association for the Advancement of Colored People, W. E. B. DuBois, felt differently. He favored contraceptive use among African-Americans to promote the dignity and uplift of black womanhood but admitted that his was often a minority view in the African-American community. "They are quite led away by the fallacy of numbers," he lamented. "They want the black race to survive."[77]

The race consciousness DuBois identified hints at the complexities of contraceptive practice at the turn of the century. American attitudes toward and access to contraceptives were affected by a range of circumstances that frequently transgressed boundaries of color, ethnicity, and class. Above all, the decision to use contraceptives was personal, dictated not by legal codes but by individual wants and needs. Criminal statutes against birth control enabled quackery to thrive, and yet, despite the risks, Americans used birth control devices, relying on a range of strategies to maximize pregnancy prevention and health.

Long before Margaret Sanger made the fight for birth control a political movement, Americans from all walks of life had turned to the contraceptive market, seeking control over their fertility and their lives. And so it was that in the age of Comstockery the birth control business continued, changed but not subdued.

PART TWO

From Smut to Science

FIVE

Salute to Prophylaxis

Secretary of the Navy Josephus Daniels was on a mission. Daniels, a fundamentalist Christian, had been horrified to discover after his appointment in 1913 that chemical "preventive packets" were being sold on American vessels to protect men from venereal disease. Each packet contained an ointment that men smeared onto their penises after intercourse to ward off not pregnancy but the military's main microbial enemies, gonorrhea and syphilis. Equally disturbing, the previous Navy secretary, at the urging of the surgeon general, had sanctioned the sale. Like many Americans, Daniels feared that the availability of prophylactics would increase sexual immorality. "It is wicked," he wrote in 1915, "to encourage and approve placing in the hands of the men an appliance which will lead them to think that they may indulge in practices which are not sanctioned by moral, military or civil law, with impunity, and the use of which would tend to subvert and destroy the very foundations of our moral and Christian beliefs and teachings in regard to these sexual matters."[1]

Daniels vowed to return morality to America's ships. On February 27, 1915, he banned the sale of chemical prophylactics. The prevention of venereal disease would henceforth be a matter of willpower, not technology. Daniels pledged to augment Navy efforts to teach men self-control through talks and pamphlets, a strategy he called "moral prophylaxis." Abstinence protected men best. Had Anthony Comstock, who died that August, known of Daniels's initiative, he would have approved.[2]

Daniels's edict articulated a belief trumpeted by a large swath of the American population in 1915, two years before the country's entry into World War I. For many, VD remained the libertine's curse, and condoms illicit, not to mention illegal, gadgets of treachery. But Daniels's philosophy of personal restraint collided with the practicalities of war and the consequent support for public health measures. At the time of his death in 1948, the U.S. Navy had helped win two world wars. Only the first was fought without military-issued condoms. In 1917, when moralists such as Daniels held court, even the progressive Medical Corps refused to advocate condom use. By the 1940s, not only had condoms become an approved prophylactic, but military officials had complained that they could not get them to troops fast enough.[3]

Fear of controversy shaped the development of U.S. military policy on venereal disease prevention in the early twentieth century. Stigmatized as a problem afflicting the promiscuous, venereal diseases were distinguished from "serious" communicable diseases such as smallpox and the plague. Military and medical leaders were aware of a range of medical prophylactics—from condoms to genital ointments—but condoned only the least controversial. The result was a series of policy compromises that sacrificed the health of thousands of American men and women on the altar of public morals.

The U.S. Navy and Army established a comprehensive campaign of medical and moral venereal prophylaxis in 1909. Its targets were syphilis and gonorrhea, the two most debilitating sexually transmitted diseases in Western history prior to AIDS. Left untreated, syphilis, a disease caused by the bacterium *Treponema pallidum*, can lead to heart disease, paralysis, blindness, senility, or insanity. Gonorrhea, a highly contagious infection of the genitourinary tract, pharynx, or eyes caused by *Neisseria gonorrhoeae*, can lead to systemic ailments, including meningitis and pericarditis (inflammation of the tissue surrounding the heart); inflammation of the prostate, urethra, or scrotal tubes in men; and pelvic inflammatory disease and sterility in women. Although 95 percent of men with gonorrhea experience telltale medical problems (usually a pus-like urethral discharge or frequent and painful urination) within days or weeks of infection, women are typically asymptomatic until serious damage has occurred.[4]

Neither disease had been a stranger to the U.S. military. During the Civil War, as many as 20 percent of enlisted soldiers were infected. But despite the disease's prevalence among the rank and file, neither the Army nor the Navy maintained an official policy of prevention short of rejecting visibly infected men for duty. VD was treated as a character flaw rather than as a health problem. Enlisted soldiers were chronically underdiagnosed, and the afflicted were often treated punitively, as if their disease were secondary to their disgrace.[5]

Rising infection rates at the turn of the century and new medical treatments prompted the surgeon general to formulate a new approach that addressed the problem on scientific grounds. Between 1897 and 1910, hospital admission rates for VD in the Army rose from 84.59 to 196.99 per 1,000, with the sharpest increase occurring between 1908 and 1910.[6] Few doctors doubted that these admissions represented only the most advanced and severe cases.

As military leaders were expressing concern over a higher incidence of disease, medical advances were offering concrete solutions. Before 1900, doctors knew little about syphilis and gonorrhea. Indeed, until the early nineteenth century, many considered them different manifestations of the same principal illness. In 1837, the French venereologist Philippe Ricord established their distinctiveness, and then went on to plot the three stages of syphilis. By the 1870s, research had revealed the disease's long-term systemic dangers, linking syphilis to serious cardiovascular, neurological, and spinal disorders, problems previously thought unrelated. Charting the etiology of gonorrhea proved harder, partly because until the late nineteenth century physicians viewed it as a nonspecific and minor ailment, caused by controllable behavior such as excessive intercourse. Medical thinking changed after Albert Neisser, a German dermatologist, identified gonococcus, the causative agent of gonorrhea, under a microscope in 1879. By 1906, Neisser and his colleagues August von Wassermann and Carl Bruck had developed a diagnostic blood test for syphilis, the so-called Wassermann test. The test required laboratory facilities that many physicians did not have, but it freed disease diagnoses from centuries of medical subjectivity.[7]

Treatment breakthroughs were equally significant, spurred on by exciting innovations in biochemistry. Nineteenth-century therapies for venereal disease were ineffective and often harmful. Medical therapies for gonorrhea varied, but in the late nineteenth century most consisted of oral medications intended to have an antiseptic effect when excreted through the urethra. This was a more humane but hardly more reliable treatment than that proposed by the respected American physician Frederick Hollick in 1852 for chordee, a complication of gonorrhea that caused curvature of the penis and painful erections. Hollick recommended that the afflicted penis be positioned "with the curve upward on a table and struck a violent blow with a book."[8]

Syphilitic patients fared no better. Physicians treated syphilis with mercury, absorbed topically, orally, or in vapor baths. Mercury promoted salivation or profuse perspiration, which, according to the ancient humoral theory of medicine on which treatment was based, removed disease-causing humors. In practice, mercury poisoning was an unfortunate but not infrequent side effect, resulting in loss of teeth, bowel hemorrhaging, or even death.[9]

The first effective treatment for syphilis was salvarsan, an arsenic compound discovered in 1909 by the Nobel laureate immunologist Paul Ehrlich. Salvarsan was the 606th compound Ehrlich had tested on syphilitic rabbits, and it caused symptoms to disappear after injection. But the compound was expensive and dangerous, accounting for 109 deaths by 1914. By 1915, a less toxic but also less effective compound, Neosalvarsan, had become available. But routine use of the new treatment, which required intravenous injection (a technique still unfamiliar to many doctors), was far from universal. Physicians continued to use mercury into the 1920s, even in well-equipped American military hospitals, and an actual cure for syphilis and gonorrhea came only with the mass dissemination of sulfa drugs and penicillin after World War II.[10]

Chemical compounds were also the backbone of early-twentieth-century developments in disease prevention. These were among the most socially radical of the innovations to influence American venereology, for they assumed a human sexual desire that self-restraint could or should not contain. In seeking to minimize the medical consequences of sexual contact, disease prophylaxis, almost by definition, announced that the Victorian war for a morally regulated sexual order had been lost. This was anathema to moralists such as Josephus Daniels, and it was no accident that he objected more strenuously to the "prophylactic" part of the surgeon general's VD program than to any other.

By 1901, chemical prophylaxis for venereal disease had been widely used in Germany, then the world leader in pharmaceutical research. The U.S. Bureau of Medicine and Surgery described in 1903 a chemical prophylactic named Viro used by the German Navy. Each Viro packet contained two tubes, the smaller of which held Protargol, a silver protein salt and presumed anti-gonorrheal. Protargol was injected into the urethra after intercourse and "retained there from three-fourths of a minute to a minute." The larger tube held a formaldehyde-based cream to be rubbed onto the penis before and after intercourse. The cream created a chemical barrier, "a thin, dry protecting cover . . . [that] render[s] harmless the infected germs."[11]

Several U.S. Navy surgeons recommended the adoption of the two-pronged German system in the Asiatic Fleet, the Navy's largest. But the Fleet surgeon urged caution, warning that the availability of preventive tubes "might provoke harsh criticism against the service by moralists at home." The commander in chief of the Asiatic Fleet agreed. Calling attention to international differences in sexual mores, he noted that a "scheme of this sort might be possible in the German Navy, but would be impracticable with us."[12]

Lacking official support, American medical officers instituted a halfway chemical prophylaxis program aboard selected ships. To make the German system less morally objectionable, they confined chemical prophylaxis to postexposure treatment. This eliminated the German program's premeditated aspects, which, like condoms, readied men for sex and thus seemed to sanction it. Under the American system, men were protected from venereal disease only after intercourse, a compromise that reflected the nation's tug-of-war between science and prudery. Less prophylaxis than early treatment, the American variant denied sexually active men the same protections German men received. Yet for those who supported medical interventions to thwart the advance of VD, it was better than nothing.

The American system was first tried in 1905 aboard USS *Baltimore* in the Asiatic station. Men returning from furlough were required to report to the ship's sick bay. Each man was questioned. If he admitted to sexual contact, a medical officer examined his genitals and then washed them with a cotton sponge doused in a bichloride of mercury solution. Next, the man received an anti-gonorrheal urethral injection of 2 percent Protargol, which he retained for thirty seconds to a minute. Once the Protargol had been expelled, the medical officer rubbed 50 percent calomel ointment, a colorless antiseptic compound used today as an insecticide, "well into the glans penis, foreskin, and shank of penis." (Although Viro contained formaldehyde, studies had shown calomel ointment, made with calomel, lanolin, and Vaseline or lard, to be more effective.)[13]

In his 1906 medical report for USS *Baltimore*, the surgeon Raymond Spear reported favorable results. "Although the ship visited the ports of Sydney, Melbourne, and Auckland for a month each," he announced, "there was practically no venereal cases on board, and the crew was 'clean.' " By contrast, the "English ships which were in these ports at the same time as the *Baltimore* . . . had over 25 percent of their crews infected." Presuming levels of sexual activity to be the same among British and American soldiers, Spear concluded that low disease rates on *Baltimore* were "due to the preventive treatment entirely." The Navy Department and the Bureau of Medicine and Surgery soon received similar reports praising chemical prophylaxis from physicians on USS *Monadnock* and USS *Wilmington*. As evidence supporting the effectiveness of chemical prophylaxis mounted, the secretary of the Navy decided to act. He faced two competing realities: moral objections to prophylaxis and unacceptably high rates of venereal disease among soldiers. On January 9, 1909, he issued a discreet and confidential letter to "Commanders-in-Chief, Commanding Officers and Medical Officers" instituting chemical prophylaxis on all ships. The Army followed suit. By the end of 1909, the use of postexposure chemical prophylaxis had become standard military policy.[14]

The system had its drawbacks, including a lower efficacy rate than the 99.6 percent quoted in one Medical Department study. It required the honesty and cooperation of enlisted men, who upon admitting to sexual contact were subjected to humiliating examinations and painful treatments. One man who suffered through the procedure later recalled, "It burned like hell . . . we would rather have taken a pound—or maybe a ton—of cure than one hot ounce of prevention."[15] Understandably, soldiers wary of treatment often lied about their sexual experiences. Indeed, noncompliance became such a problem that in 1912 the Navy instituted a new policy, buttressed by federal legislation, denying pay to enlisted men who developed VD after declining treatment.[16]

Another problem with prophylaxis was its impracticality. The efficacy of the medicines depended on early treatment. As a result, men engaging in sex on overnight leave often went untreated. As early as 1910, the Navy and Army distributed on an experimental basis prophylactic packets, also called "pro-kits," containing calomel ointment, carbolic acid, and camphor for self-administration. Several manufacturers produced these kits for military and civilian use, but the most popular brand was Sanitubes, manufactured by the Sanitube Company of Newport, Rhode Island. In 1912, Surgeon General C. F. Stokes recommended their sale in ship canteens for the benefit of those going on extended liberty, a request the Navy Department approved. Sanitubes quickly became a staple on many ships.[17]

They also became the object of Josephus Daniels's wrath. The former newspaper editor from Raleigh, North Carolina, had supported the presidential bid of fellow Southerner Woodrow Wilson and was rewarded in 1913 with the Navy appointment, a post he held until 1921. A good evangelist, Daniels wanted to save sinners, not make them. He considered nonmarital sex a mortal sin and was baffled why his God-fearing colleagues would endorse a product that encouraged men to stray from the righteous path of abstinence. Couldn't they see the seduction of Sanitubes? The added temptation that came with the promise of worry-free sex? The grave decision to refrain from or succumb to illicit sex should be made unimpeded by technological trinkets, he argued. "The only absolute guarantee against venereal disease," he told one Navy chaplain, "and the only justifiable preventive measure, is continence" (which in the early twentieth century meant abstinence, not bladder control).[18] Sanitubes tilted the scales in the wrong direction. He saw their sale as tantamount to "the government advising these boys that it is right for them to indulge in an evil which perverts their morals."[19]

Intriguingly, Daniels supported the Navy's original postcoital chemical prophylaxis program. For him, this was not promiscuity but a sound public health measure to protect those who had already yielded to temptation. As he explained to one doctor in a private letter, men who willfully indulge in sin "are given opportunity at all naval stations and on board all vessels of the Navy to avail themselves immediately of the best preventive medical measures that can be devised. Such practice which seeks to save the guilty individual from the consequences of his act . . . is not inconsistent with the strong moral suasion which aims to prevent him from becoming guilty."[20]

It was a hairsplitting, even specious, argument. Although one was condemned and another sanctioned, Sanitubes and on-site prophylaxis had much in common. Both were postcoital measures. Both relied on the local application of chemicals to thwart the onset of disease. But Daniels's insistence that the mere availability of a prophylactic before intercourse (even one designed for use *after* sexual contact) promoted promiscuity set Sanitubes apart and struck a resonant chord in a country accustomed to such arguments. For decades, sexual purity reformers had invoked the same rationale to justify the continued criminalization of condoms. And only ten years earlier, Navy officials had made this very argument to rebuff overtures to establish the German system of precoital prophylaxis. It was not unexpected that such an old and persuasive logic would prompt the Navy to interdict the sale of all preventive or prophylactic packets in 1915. But in 1915, America had yet to experience the horrors of its first world war.

America's entrance into the Great War in April 1917 highlighted the social and economic costs of venereal infection and illuminated the extent to which sexuality was as much an issue of state policy as of private morality. By 1918, the financial, strategic, and human costs of a staggeringly high infection rate among America's doughboys had revealed the reality of a sexual appetite unsuppressed by moralists' warnings. Trouble on the venereal home front arose soon after Congress passed the Selective Service Act in May 1917, requiring all men between the ages of twenty-one and thirty (later, eighteen and forty-five) to report to local boards to determine eligibility for duty. Prior to the war, a man with VD was rejected for military service. But when draft examinations revealed infection rates as high as 25 percent among new recruits in some areas, the rule was discarded. Supplies of men were limited. As one Los Angeles physician observed, "If you were to attempt to get an army without having men who had gonorrhea, you would not have an army."[21] Altogether, about 5.6 percent of draftees entering the Army had a venereal disease. In public, government officials downplayed the domestic origins of disease. War propaganda liked to blame "French whores" and Europe's "laissez-faire attitude" for the corruption of American troops—just as early obscenity laws had sought to shield American virtue from Europe's bad influence.

All European forces operated brothels for their soldiers, relying on medical inspections to suppress VD rates.[22] But the surgeon general's statistics showed that five-sixths of all cases among U.S. soldiers were contracted on American soil.[23] Moreover, military leaders admitted that another reason for not barring men with VD was the possibility that large numbers would contract venereal disease at home to avoid service abroad.

Between April 1917 and December 1919, 380,000 soldiers—roughly one in eleven—were diagnosed with syphilis, gonorrhea, or chancroid. High infection rates among a segment of the male population previously believed healthy created a medical and economic problem of unprecedented magnitude. Diseased men had to be treated, but the financial costs were high. Physicians treated syphilitic patients, for example, with injections of Neosalvarsan and mercury over a period of weeks or months and monitored their progress with Wassermann tests. Severe cases required long-term hospitalization. The Army estimated that every case of venereal disease cost it approximately $231. By the end of the war, it had spent over $50 million on treatment.[24]

Military leaders also discussed venereal disease in terms of strategic cost and military efficiency. Infected soldiers drained the resources of the military, sapped its strength, and compromised its ability to fight. As General John J. Pershing, commander of the American Expeditionary Forces (AEF), explained, "A soldier who contracts a venereal disease not only suffers permanent injury, but renders himself inefficient as a soldier and becomes an encumbrance to the Army." Venereal disease was blamed for seven million days of lost active duty. Only the great influenza epidemic of 1918 ranked higher as a cause of "lost time."[25]

Influenza had triumphed over the best efforts of a galvanized public health community to halt the lethal virus in its tracks. Venereal disease, by contrast, was known to be preventable. Because the costs of treatment exceeded those of prevention, military commanders were able to marshal the efficiency argument to establish a far-reaching prophylaxis program once war was declared. A centralized VD program was in keeping with both a progressive ideology of rationality and social engineering and an acceptance of federal power to coordinate the war effort in Washington—the same power that led to conscription, price-fixing, and the first use of daylight saving time in the United States.

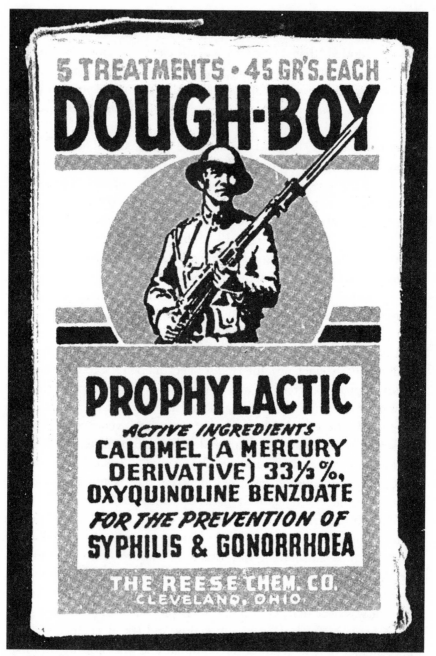

10. Chemical prophylaxis had two strikes against it. It did not prevent venereal disease, and it stung (Courtesy of Dennis O'Brien and George Goehring)

The twin objectives of the VD campaign were to contain the VD threat and to make America "fit to fight." The primary tool was education. On April 17, 1917, Secretary of War Newton Baker established the Commission on Training Camps Activities (CTCA) to teach doughboys about the benefits of abstinence and the wages of sin. Under the direction of Raymond Fosdick, CTCA leaders instructed battle-bound men in Army camps about social hygiene and venereal infection, often with the aid of stereoscopic slides depicting diseased genitals. CTCA propaganda warned that overindulgence led to impotence, a belief perpetuated in the marketplace, where scores of patent medicines for impotence were bought and sold. The soldier who stayed chaste protected his health in the short run and his virility in the long. "It used to be thought that [sexual] organs had to be used if they were to be kept healthy," one circular declared. "*This is a lie. . . .* The mere fact that famous boxers and wrestlers, explorers and athletes who want their bodies to be in perfect condition for a great struggle, keep away from women during the long period of training, proves that the use of the sex organs is not necessary to health."[26] CTCA training urged men to suppress sexual desire through sports such as boxing, prized for its ability to teach both discipline and timely bayonet-wielding skills. By the same token, the CTCA vilified as traitors men who had sex; they were soldiers who had "wasted" finite reserves of energy on pleasures of the flesh instead of battle.

Appeals to continence were supplemented by chemical prophylaxis, repackaged for the benefit of moralists as a treatment of "last resort." Having discontinued the sale of Sanitubes in 1915, the Navy maintained mandatory postexposure prophylaxis throughout the war. The Army embraced a similar strategy. Soon after American troops landed in France in June 1917, Pershing issued General Order No. 6, obligating soldiers to report to prophylactic stations within three hours of sexual contact. Pershing worried about the Army's ability to control the behavior of American soldiers in France, where prostitution was legal and regulated. But he was confident that postexposure prophylaxis would succeed whenever a doughboy's resolve failed. "The prophylaxis," he wrote to the surgeon general, "if properly used, is so surely a protection, that any venereal disease arising must be severely punished."[27] General Order No. 6 reflected this misplaced certitude and, for the first time, made the contraction of VD an offense punishable by court-martial.

The Medical Department also issued individual "pro-kits" to soldiers whose location made access to prophylactic stations impossible. Like Daniels, Pershing had opposed their general distribution during the war. But he changed his mind when venereal rates began to rise after the armistice was signed on November 11, 1918, and more American soldiers took leaves. Prophylactic packets began to be distributed in the Navy, too, although the policy change did not occur on Daniels's clock. Instead, Fosdick, having failed to convince the unwavering Daniels of their necessity, waited until Daniels was absent and then convinced his assistant secretary, the future president Franklin Delano Roosevelt, to sign the order.[28]

At no point during the war did military or medical leaders condone condoms as a suitable prophylaxis. Indeed, endeavoring to rationalize industrial rubber use, the government telegraphed at least one condom manufacturer and told him that he would soon "be unable to secure any further rubber because your business and article ha[ve] been declared a nonessential."[29] There is no question that the American military knew of their use by Allied forces; when it came to condoms, the United States was the odd ally out, the only country not to give its troops the benefit of full prophylactic protection. The British military distributed free condoms to its troops, and Dr. Hugh Hampton Young, one of the architects of the AEF's VD program, reported in 1917 that the New Zealand Expeditionary Forces used both condoms and chemical prophylaxis to prevent VD.[30]

American condom firms likely played a pivotal role in supplying Allied armies with what was forbidden at home. Before the war, Germany had been Europe's largest supplier of rubber sheaths made using the "cement" process, a technology pioneered by German chemists in the 1880s and adopted in Germany for the manufacture of a variety of seamless rubber articles. (Condoms were legal throughout Europe, even in Catholic countries such as Italy and Spain.) However, wartime hostilities forced England and other countries to look elsewhere for supplies. In 1915, L. A. Jackson founded the London Rubber Company as a vendor of barbers' sundries, including imported condoms. The company would go on to become the largest sheath manufacturer in England after it began the domestic manufacture of condoms in 1932 under the DUREX (DUrability, Reliability, EXcellence) trademark at its factory in Chingford. But before it exited the import business, London Rubber attempted to supplement the manufacture of several small English outfits with condoms imported from the United States and elsewhere.[31]

Evidence on the U.S. condom business during this era remains fragmentary, but it appears that several American condom firms that became industry leaders in the 1920s owed much of their initial success to wartime demands. Youngs Rubber, manufacturers of Trojans, started business in 1916, after war broke out in England but before condoms in America were legal. Merle Youngs, the company's founder, later credited his commercial success to overseas demand for American condoms: the war created a "tremendous demand . . . for these little articles."[32] Julius Schmidt—who recovered from arrest and renamed himself Julius Schmid, without the *t*—also saw his condom business increase during the war (and he would become the leading condom supplier to the U.S. military in World War II).[33]

Condom manufacturers weighed in in the prophylactic debate, hoping to profit from the new VD consciousness. A government resorting to far-reaching measures to suppress VD could presumably be convinced of the wisdom of quietly decriminalizing rubbers and issuing them to American troops. Julius Schmid and Youngs Rubber were both incorporated in New York, and one was likely the anonymous client referred to in the following letter sent by a New York attorney to the surgeon general in November 1916:

> I am desirous, for and on behalf of my clients, who are reputable manufacturers of rubber articles used by the medical profession, to get an expression of opinion from the highest source obtainable, upon the following facts:
>
> They manufacture large quantities of condoms, commonly called condrums, which are shipped to the war zones at the present time. The main point is, do you, as the Surgeon General of the United States Navy, recommend the use of this form as one of the preventives of disease?
>
> The purpose of this letter is that my clients are anxious to know whether they are within their rights to make this article, and if it is considered a benefit to mankind, by your Department. Your answer is *not* to be used for advertising purposes in any way.[34]

The endorsement was denied. But the letter, sent from the law firm of Alexander Rosenthal five months before the United States entered the war, indicates early American involvement in the overseas condom market. It also suggests the hopes American condom manufacturers harbored that support for prophylaxis in a country sensitized to venereal disease would enable them to sell their wares as legitimate medical devices in the United States. But high hopes did not blind them to the realities of the prevailing political and legal temperament in 1916. This anonymous client hired a lawyer to make discreet inquiries so that it could shield its name from scrutiny.

Discretion was an inevitable by-product of a political environment in which those who denounced prophylaxis were organized and had clout. Indeed, America's condom exceptionalism during World War I must be seen not only as a tragic chapter in the history of public health but also as a telling gauge of the obstacles faced by those who endorsed condoms and other forms of pre-exposure prophylaxis. Those supporting the abstinence-only cause were strange bedfellows: well-placed zealots such as Daniels; suffragettes and social purity reformers who condemned the tyranny of the sexual double standard; social hygiene advocates who feared women's carnal instincts and blamed them for the spread of venereal disease; and parents tormented by the prospect of young sons losing virginity and innocence. Add to this tempestuous mix the enduring appeal of abstinence as an idea in American culture and politics. It is tempting to dismiss America's wartime policy as a Victorian atavism—a prudish remnant of some long-forgotten past. But Nancy Reagan's "Just say no" approach to drug use and the vituperative opposition, even today, to proposals to distribute condoms in high schools compel us to reconsider.

There were other reasons why the U.S. military did not approve of condom use. The manufacture and interstate distribution of condoms were, thanks to Anthony Comstock, crimes under federal law. This point did not escape the attention of Daniels, who argued that prohibiting the sale of Sanitubes was the Navy's only legal option, for "articles which may be sold in ships' stores to officers and enlisted men are prescribed by law and do not include venereal prophylactic tubes, or their equivalents." There was also the issue of effectiveness, no small matter. The Bureau of Medicine and Surgery insisted until the early 1930s that postexposure treatment was close to 100 percent effective, a confidence that mitigated consideration of an alternative prophylactic.

But the military's stance on condoms was doomed to be short-lived, undermined during the war by the tolerance of renegade physicians and the everday defiance of troops. Immersed in an international environment that promoted condom use, American doughboys were quick learners. Those who had no experience with condoms learned about them from their compatriots or from lady friends: despite the CTCA's efforts, only about 30 percent of men who fought in France were abstinent.[35] Condoms were easily acquired in Europe and, according to the manufacturer Merle Youngs, were also sold "unofficially" in many government-operated American canteens. U.S. soldiers and sailors had special incentive to use them. Chemical prophylaxis could be painful and degrading, yet to forsake prophylaxis was to risk acquiring venereal disease, which was punishable by a loss of pay and a court-martial. Many rank-and-file troops dealt with the problem by circumventing official policy and using condoms on the sly, a trend widely commented on by contemporaries. One medical officer attributed the dwindling number of visits to the prophylaxis station to men's acquiring prophylactics "in the open market," where "some men purchase them by the dozen."[36]

More than four million men, many from working-class or immigrant backgrounds, served in the U.S. military during the war. What they learned they took home with them, infusing the civilian population with condom know-how at an unprecedented level. The impact of military experience on postwar contraceptive habits should not be discounted even if it cannot be precisely measured. Historians have attributed declining French fertility rates after the Napoleonic Wars to soldiers' sexual experimentation, and there's no reason to believe that the United States was immune to a parallel postwar education. Interviews with working-class women in Massachusetts and Rhode Island, for example, found that many first learned about condoms from husbands who had served in the war. Upon their return, moreover, veterans found a new reason to put knowledge into practice. By 1918, condoms had become legal.[37]

The decriminalization of condoms occurred in an intellectual milieu newly attentive to the links between medical science, private sexual behavior, and social welfare. As CTCA instructors lectured on the dangers of nonmarital intercourse, as politicians, doctors, and military leaders debated the best mechanisms for containing the VD threat, they pushed sex into a public arena and shattered the wall of secrecy that had made its discussion taboo. As one contemporary observed, prior to the war venereal disease had been "camouflaged under the name of the 'Social Evil' for fear of giving offense to the false modesty that existed." But the war had driven the subject "from darkness into light, compelling attention and focusing public opinion squarely upon a situation that had always been held too lightly and apathetically."[38]

The VD crisis freed Americans to reclassify sex as a legitimate subject of scientific and social research and made sexual behavior a matter of public welfare. Most important, it established a credible justification for contraception—public health—that placed the birth control debate on less incendiary grounds.

By 1918, the Victorian ethos of self-control had yielded to new ideas and institutions that took male sexual activity for granted and strove to subdue, even eliminate, its undesired consequences. In a nod to science, Congress passed in July 1918 a measure to create the Division of Venereal Diseases in the U.S. Public Health Service and allocated over $4 million for disease prevention and treatment.[39] The enactment followed an impassioned appeal from Congressman Julius Kahn of California that captured the scientific spirit of the new approach. "Cases of smallpox, bubonic plague, diphtheria and scarlet fever must be reported to the local health authorities," he noted. "But through prudery and mawkish sentimentality we have closed our eyes to the serious conditions that exist in our country by the prevalence of venereal diseases." The new initiative substituted science for sentiment. By 1921, the federal government had spent $4.5 million on its new public health campaign, including grants to promote research on "the discovery of medical methods in the prevention and treatment of venereal diseases."[40]

Against this backdrop, the 1918 ruling of Judge Frederick Crane of the court of appeals of New York was a timely acknowledgment of how contraceptives might promote public health. Crane ruled that physician-prescribed birth control acquired from a vendor used "for the cure or prevention of disease" was not "indecent or immoral." His ruling validated birth control as a public health measure, not a reproductive right. It was an important distinction that nevertheless endowed contraceptives with newfound legitimacy. Charges of smut and sin that had sustained objections to birth control devices under Comstockery lost their luster in the face of compelling evidence that contraceptives reduced disease.[41]

It was a mixed verdict for Margaret Sanger, the woman at the center of the controversy. The dispute stemmed from Sanger's illegal operation of the country's first birth control clinic, which she opened in Brownsville, a neighborhood in Brooklyn, New York, on October 16, 1916, with her sister, Ethel Byrne, also a nurse. For ten days, the two women tended to the birth control needs of 488 women. Police then raided and closed the clinic and arrested Sanger and Byrne for violating state law.[42]

Sanger's defense challenged the constitutionality of New York law, which made it a misdemeanor to give away or sell contraceptive information. Her lawyer argued that birth control was indispensable to efforts to reduce poverty, disease, infant mortality, abortion, and low intelligence. The Brooklyn trial judge John Freschi rejected the idea that birth control was sociologically practical or that "a woman has the right to copulate with a feeling of security that there will be no resulting conception." Sanger and Byrne spent a month in jail (a punishment Sanger would later use to great strategic advantage). But when the case was heard in the court of appeals before Judge Crane, the outcome was different. Crane acknowledged the social arguments for birth control but dismissed their consideration, insisting that they were "matters for the legislature and not for the Courts." Bypassing the question of woman's rights, he affirmed the legality of contraceptives as disease prophylaxis. Crane defined disease broadly as "an alteration in the state of the body, or of some of its organs, interrupting or disturbing the performance of vital functions, and causing or threatening pain and sickness, illness . . . [and] disorder." The definition, taken from the pages of *Webster's International Dictionary*, was subsequently interpreted to be general enough to cover the use of prophylactics against both venereal disease and dangerous pregnancies.[43]

Though not an endorsement of contraceptives as birth control, Crane's verdict provided Sanger with enough legal ammunition to open the first permanent birth control clinic in the United States in 1923. Under the auspices of protecting women from life-threatening pregnancies, a clinic doctor prescribed contraceptives, usually diaphragms. But the court's decision had its most immediate and conspicuous impact on the masculine side of the birth control business. Condom manufacturers seized the new opportunities afforded by Crane's ruling. After 1918, the condom industry flourished as skins and rubbers marked "for the prevention of disease only" became familiar sights in neighborhood drugstores and a host of male commercial venues: barbershops, newsstands, pool parlors, cigar stores, and, increasingly, gas stations. Crane's ruling legalized only doctor-prescribed condoms, a caveat consumers and druggists routinely ignored. As Merle Youngs, whose company boasted annual drugstore sales of twenty million Trojans in 1930, mused, no one needed a physician's prescription to purchase rubbers.[44]

Sold as disease prophylactics, condoms were used for birth control. Indeed, although the Crane decision broke new legal ground, it perpetuated in the ensuing decades an old pattern whereby consumers seeking contraception bought condoms disguised as something else. V. F. Calverton, a young radical critic interested in the problems of sex, characterized legal subterfuge as an "intelligent adaptation to an unintelligent morality" befitting a social order in flux. A journalist writing for *Fortune* magazine was less sympathetic but equally aware of the deception. The condom industry, she declared, is "based squarely upon the prevention of disease. The rubber (or skin) prophylactic . . . is never manufactured for any other declared purpose, although everybody in the industry knows perfectly well that it is otherwise used."[45]

For Sanger, the surging popularity of condoms was a bittersweet by-product of her struggle for legal recognition of contraceptives. Like her British counterpart, the contraceptive crusader Marie Stopes, Sanger viewed birth control as a woman's right and responsibility. "The question of bearing and rearing children," she would write in 1922, "is the concern of the mother and potential mother."[46] Female knowledge and control over contraception were preconditions of women's emancipation from the burdens of endless childbearing: "No woman can call herself free who does not own and control her own body."[47] Condoms compromised this objective by placing women's procreative destiny in men's hands. Like any enthusiast of family planning, Sanger recognized that condoms were better than nothing, if a woman could persuade a man to wear one. Sometimes, though, this was a big task. Until her death in 1966, Sanger championed the preferability of female birth control and promoted the manufacture of diaphragms and, later, the Pill, partly to re-

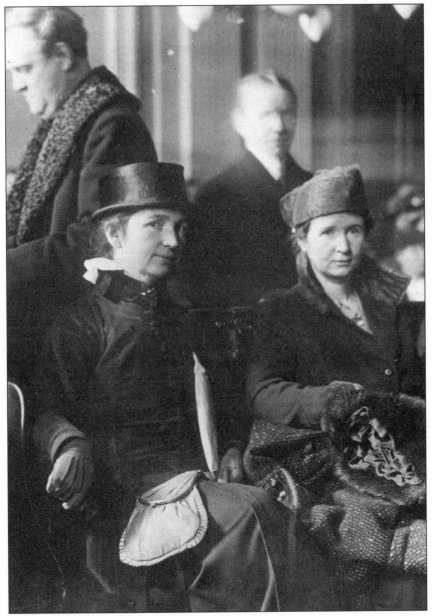

11. Margaret Sanger and her sister, Ethel Byrne, in court in 1917 (Courtesy of the Sophia Smith Collection, Smith College)

alize her dream of female empowerment through women-oriented technologies.[48]

The needs of women, which Sanger focused on, were not paramount in the minds of the various parties—public health advocates, military leaders, and politicians—who unwittingly helped propel condoms toward legitimacy. From the start, the campaign against venereal disease during World War I was hostile to women. A revised Progressive-era model of female sexuality, incorporating the new psychological theories of Sigmund Freud and Havelock Ellis, emphasized female desire rather than passivity but also made it easier to depict women as lustful predators. Military propaganda divided the female population into two camps: diseased prostitutes and mothers or virgins. "Live Straight If You Would Shoot Straight," a pamphlet distributed to sailors during the war, informed men that "all loose women are dirty." Men who resisted their allure "honored and protected the sisters, wives, and future mothers of the race we are fighting for."[49]

The war against improper womanhood went beyond barbed rhetoric. It also involved egregious violations of civil liberties. State and municipal laws passed at the behest of the CTCA's Law Enforcement Division empowered medical officers to arrest and detain without bail women suspected of carrying venereal disease. Prostitutes topped the list of suspects, but even a woman caught flirting with an officer could be arrested and examined without consent. Women testing positive for syphilis or gonorrhea were interned and quarantined. Attorney General T. W. Gregory justified these drastic measures as a valid exercise of the state's police power to protect "the interest of the public health."[50]

Not everyone agreed. In a January 1919 letter to several military and medical officers, one Civil War veteran from Iowa denounced the misogyny of government policy. Military propaganda blamed prostitutes for the woes of men when it was men who sustained prostitution. "A man who blames the woman, mother, sister, wife, daughter, has no manhood, is void in understanding, and is a damnable egotist and never should have been born," he wrote.[51]

It was a gutsy letter, for under federal law, the author, like the prostitutes he supported, was subject to arrest. Wartime suppression of civil liberties curbed both opposition to government practices and the prospects for a more radical vision of womanhood, disease, and prophylaxis. In a feverish attempt to mobilize public support for the war, the federal government denied Americans the right to voice their dissent. The Espionage Act in 1917 and the Sedition Act in 1918 outlawed open criticism of the government, the armed forces, and the war effort and gave the postmaster general the power to prevent unpatriotic materials from circulating through the mails. The new laws were enforced mercilessly against socialists and anarchists, who linked imperial aggression to class oppression. Among those arrested or harassed were birth control activists, including Sanger's inspiration, the anarchist agitator Emma Goldman, imprisoned as a traitor and deported in 1919. Goldman, Sanger, and hundreds of other women on the left had supplied the initial organizational impetus for the birth control movement, establishing birth control leagues across the country, lecturing on contraception, and demanding the sexual and class emancipation of women. As wartime hysteria and the ensuing Red Scare limited opportunities for political dissent, they also checked the momentum of a movement moored in a more progressive way of viewing women and prophylaxis.[52]

In a military climate in which women were depicted as diseased vixens, birth control and women's reproductive rights were not the War Department's primary concerns. The government distributed Sanitubes and urethral injections to protect men from women, not the other way around. But as a "legitimate" American condom industry grew and as skins and rubbers became increasingly visible on store shelves and in bedrooms, the U.S. military softened its stance on condoms.

Change occurred unevenly and cautiously. In the 1920s, some medical officers were openly advocating condom use in their hygiene instruction to enlisted men, much to the dismay of proponents of the old school. An angry commanding officer of USS *South Dakota* reported in May 1920 that his two medical officers favored chemical prophylaxis or "supplying the rubber 'French safe' as a means of prevention. Both of them apparently fail to appreciate the importance of trying to engender in the minds of the individual men a sense of their obligation . . . to make them understand the dangers and wrong of promiscuous sexual intercourse." The maligned officers, on the other hand, were probably just attempting to reverse what had become a major health disaster. In April,

8.84 percent of the crew had been put on the sick list because of venereal infection.[53]

USS *South Dakota* was not alone. Higher rates of venereal disease reported throughout the Army and Navy in the 1920s mustered support for the argument that abstinence, chemical prophylaxis, and Sanitubes were not enough. In 1927, the senior medical officer for the U.S. Asiatic Fleet declared postexposure prophylaxis "a practically useless expenditure of material and energy." Men needed instant protection. An "immediate means at hand is the use of a protector (condom)," he advised.[54] The same year, the Army's surgeon general endorsed in his annual report the suggestion of a medical inspector at Fort Benning, Georgia, that "gratuitous use of sheaths would help to reduce the rate. In addition, measures to inform all the men of the dangers from venereal disease should be emphasized, rather than wasting time advising continence!"[55]

References to the futility of abstinence surfaced often in medical reports in the late 1920s and the 1930s and indexed a newer, more indulgent perception of male sexuality. Hardly novel by international standards, the "men will be men" argument had prompted the dissemination of free condoms to British soldiers during World War I. By 1927, even Francisco Franco, the future Spanish dictator, had required cadets at the Zaragoza Army Academy, which he directed until 1931, to carry condoms at night. A ruthless disciplinarian, Franco would perform frequent spot checks and punish those unable to produce prophylactics. Franco was a Catholic moralist and self-described prude, but his military training in the early 1920s had compelled him to accept male lust as an irrepressible force.[56]

In the United States, this epiphany occurred later and was part and parcel of a larger cultural clamor against the emasculating effects of sexual prohibitions. In a society in which a growing proportion of men worked in offices and on assembly lines, references to men's "wild" and "raw" carnal nature were reassuring reminders of a forest-and-frontier manhood untrammeled by social and economic change. The cult of hyper-masculinity found enthusiasts in many places, including the Boy Scouts and intercollegiate football. But its most loyal following was in the military, where the prior policy of abstinence was mocked. Male "sexual aggressiveness cannot be stifled. . . . It cannot be sublimated by hard work or the soft whinings of Victorian minds," warned one captain.

"Armies and navies use *men*. Men of the very essence of masculinity." A colleague agreed: "We can preach, educate, scare, threaten and punish, but in the end men . . . become the arbiters of their own destinies." Whereas self-restraint once built character, it now depleted manhood and undercut military efficiency: "Imagine, if you can, an army of impotent men." It was unthinkable, or at least undesirable. Once cast as the inevitable outcome of promiscuous intercourse, impotence was now a threat used to win support for the military's revised vision of virility and, relatedly, condoms.[57]

Accepting the "reality" that "angels rightfully belong only in heaven," the Army and Navy quietly added condoms to their lists of approved prophylactics in the early 1930s. In 1934, one medical officer discussed the availability of "a great number of a reliable brand of condom" on the battleship on which he served.[58] There was no public announcement of the policy shift; the military rightly feared a religious backlash that came soon enough during World War II, when condom distribution was discussed in the general press. Nor was there discussion of birth control benefits for women, although one medical officer observed as an aside that condoms "serve a twofold purpose by obviating the unfortunate circumstance of illegitimate pregnancy." But even here, a woman's right to control her reproductive destiny was considered secondary (if it was considered at all) to the more important problem of illegitimate pregnancy.[59]

A report on venereal disease prevention at Fort Belvoir, Virginia, submitted to the surgeon general in 1936 contained what is likely the first accurate census of condom sales in the military. It showed that fifty-four hundred condoms had been purchased by soldiers at post exchanges in six months: an average of about five condoms per soldier. With condoms sold at the market price of three for ten cents, it was possible to conclude that rubbers "are not purchased for curios and . . . they cannot be bought as an investment for re-sale." Most promising about the volume of condom sales was the correspondingly low rate of disease. During the six months under investigation, "only 9 cases of venereal disease" had been reported, despite a "harvest of sexual experiences" and the application of only 262 chemical prophylactic treatments.[60]

The findings were encouraging and not confined to Virginia. In American stations and ships across the globe, the once-condemned con-

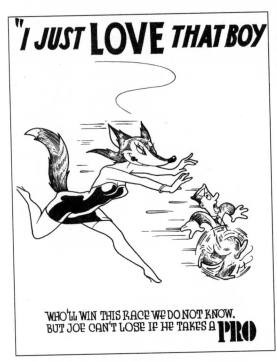

12. This World War II–era poster urged men to protect themselves from promiscuous, diseased women

dom became "the most widely used and safest prophylactic."[61] During World War II, soldiers could purchase ten-cent condom kits containing "three first-grade rubber condoms and a small tube of lubricating jelly" at prophylaxis stations and post exchanges and from vending machines strategically placed "so that easy access is the rule at all hours."[62] The training of enlisted men included detailed instructions on wearing a condom "with an inch or an inch and a half hanging at its tip, and not so snugly as the finger of a glove [or] the condom will tear. They are told to withdraw as soon as they have had their orgasm and then to remove the condom very carefully, trying not to contaminate the skin." And in a move that World War I moralists might have considered a shocking instance of "socialized immorality," military units were authorized to distribute, free of charge, condom kits purchased with company funds.[63]

Military demand for rubbers gave the American condom industry its biggest boost yet, doubling production capacity between 1939 and 1946. As in World War I, there was a nationwide rubber shortage, so severe that in 1942 President Roosevelt asked the public to donate household rubber products for recycling. But this time around, there was no government talk of suspending condom manufacturers' rubber supply. Indeed, some of that household rubber probably made its way into the 1.5 million gross of condoms American manufacturers produced in 1945.[64]

During World War II, condoms were government-inspected, thanks to a profound shift in Food and Drug Administration (FDA) policy. Although the 1918 Crane decision had declared condoms legal, sheaths were not required to be inspected for flaws before marketing. This state of affairs was disastrous for the causes of birth control and disease prevention. The biochemist Cecil I. B. Voge had discovered in his 1934–1935 tests on condoms that more than half were faulty. As the military began to adopt condoms en masse in the 1930s, it endeavored to offset the dangers of product variability by testing prophylactics itself. In late 1937, the FDA assumed that burden, standardizing condom inspection nationwide. The move was calculated to support the military and the Public Health Department's campaign to eradicate venereal disease, but the decision benefited all consumers of condoms, including those who used sheaths for birth control.[65]

With the FDA firmly on the side of condom consumers' health, a new chapter in contraceptive history began. Still, it would be years before condoms were safe, a point illustrated by a 1941 training film produced by the U.S. Public Health Service directing men to inflate condoms with water to inspect for leaks.[66]

By the 1940s, American condoms had come a long way. From a bootleg article to the darling of VD prophylaxis, the condom had reaped the benefits of changing views of sex, medicine, prophylaxis, and masculinity. With military legitimacy came added popularity and an overdue convergence of official policy and everyday practice. As one colonel in the Medical Corps remarked as early as 1936, "The soldier is now practicing what his civilian neighbor has been doing for years." Times had changed. "One has only to glance at the raw sewage output of a great city," he quipped, "to realize the part being played by rubber in our modern civilization."[67]

SIX

A Medical Fit

In a 1952 letter to the physician and fellow birth control proponent Clarence Gamble, Margaret Sanger reflected on her career. Her greatest achievement, she wrote, had been "to keep the movement strictly and sanely under medical auspices."[1]

Beginning in the 1920s, Sanger, Gamble, and a network of dedicated researchers, physicians, and activists made a once-radical movement middle-class and respectable. They established doctor-supervised clinics, promoted laboratory testing of contraceptives, encouraged the physician-fitted diaphragm-and-jelly method, and lobbied the American Medical Association (AMA) to reverse its long-standing ban on birth control. In public, Sanger refused to endorse specific brands or devices, fearing that the inevitable charges of impropriety would discredit the movement as a whole. Behind the scenes, however, her support of medicalized birth control shaped the course of contraceptive commercialization. By the 1930s, thanks largely to Sanger, the diaphragm and jelly had become the most frequently prescribed form of birth control in America, and Holland-Rantos its best-known manufacturer. Consciously distancing the birth control business from manufacturers who made contraceptives for the laity, Sanger helped inaugurate a regime of doctors, diaphragms, and corporate science.

When Sanger opened her first birth control clinic in 1916, she and her sister, Ethel, instructed eight women at a time on how to use over-the-counter contraceptives, including condoms, suppositories, and rubber pessaries. Although she later claimed that she referred women "to a druggist to purchase the necessary equipment," boxes of Mizpah pessaries she and her sister had dispensed were found by police when they raided the two-room clinic. The Mizpah (sometimes spelled Mispah) was a flexible, thimble-sized cervical cap made of corrugated rubber. Described in one 1900 advertisement as a "soft, light, and comfortable" uterine supporter, the Mizpah was inserted vaginally and positioned snugly to create an airtight seal around the cervical opening. Sold by druggists and mail-order vendors to treat the still commonly diagnosed condition of a prolapsed or distended uterus, the cervical cap was an effective over-the-counter contraceptive. Of all American-made contraceptives, the Mizpah, or "temporary French pessary," as it was sometimes called, was Sanger's favorite.[2]

Sanger's pessary education had occurred in Europe. At the urging of her then-husband, William, and her friend the labor leader Big Bill Haywood, she and her family sailed to France in 1913. In Paris, discussions with French radicals about contraceptive techniques nurtured her dreams of sexual emancipation and political revolution achieved through universal access to birth control. In March 1914, three months after her return to the United States, she began publishing *The Woman Rebel*, a feminist journal that demanded legal contraception and full woman's rights. Its June issue first used the term "birth control," a moniker coined by Sanger's friend Otto Bobsein as an alternative to the more awkward-sounding "voluntary motherhood" and "family limitation" then in vogue. After seven issues, the strident *Rebel* was deemed unmailable by the U.S. Post Office. Annoyed but undaunted, Sanger flouted the law again by writing *Family Limitation*, a home guide to contraception. This extraordinary pamphlet discussed douches, condoms, and cervical caps and recommended caps, whose use women could most easily and discreetly control. Sanger distributed 100,000 copies of her pamphlet, which implored women to learn how to insert caps into their own bodies and then to "teach each other" how to use them.[3] Sanger envisioned a world of grassroots birth control where women from all walks of life could use contraceptives without reliance on doctors, a populist approach she would soon abandon.

MOTHERS!

Can you afford to have a large family?

Do you want any more children?

If not, why do you have them?

DO NOT KILL, DO NOT TAKE LIFE, BUT PREVENT

Safe, Harmless Information can be obtained of trained

Nurses at

46 AMBOY STREET

NEAR PITKIN AVE. — BROOKLYN.

Tell Your Friends and Neighbors.   All Mothers Welcome

A registration fee of 10 cents entitles any mother to this information.

מוטערס!

זייט איהר פערמעגליך צו האבען א גרויסע פאמיליע?

ווילט איהר האבען נאך קינדער?

אויב ניט, װאַרום האָט איהר זײ?

מערדערט ניט, נעהמט ניט קיין לעבען, נור פערהיט זיך.

זיכערע, אונשעדליכע אויסקינפטען קענט איהר בעקומען פון ערפארענע נוירסעס אין

46 אמבאי סטרים ניער פיטקין עוועניו ברוקלין

זאגט דאס בעקאנט צו אייערע פריינד און שכנות.   יעדער מוטער איז ווילקאמען

פיר 10 סענט איינשרייב־געלד איהר בערעכטיגט צו דיעזע אינפארמיישאן.

MADRI!

Potete permettervi il lusso d'avere altri bambini?

Ne volete ancora?

Se non ne volete piu', perche' continuate a metterli al mondo?

NON UCCIDETE MA PREVENITE!

Informazioni sicure ed innocue saranno fornite da infermiere autorizzate a

46 AMBOY STREET   Near Pitkin Ave. Brooklyn

a cominciare dal 12 Ottobre. Avvertite le vostre amiche e vicine.

Tutte le madri sono ben accette. La tassa d'iscrizione di 10 cents da diritto a qualunque madre di ricevere consigli ed informazioni gratis.

Margaret H. Sanger.

13. Sanger's circular advertising the opening of America's first birth control clinic in Brownsville, Brooklyn, in 1916 (Courtesy of the Sophia Smith Collection, Smith College)

Family Limitation got Sanger into more trouble. In 1915, she found herself back in Europe dodging American law while continuing her contraceptive education. In London, she did research at the British Museum before embarking for the Netherlands, where she planned to tour the country's contraceptive clinics, learning "from personal observation."[4] The trip across the Atlantic was risky. War had broken out the previous year, and, as Sanger later recalled, crossing the Channel entailed "possible unwelcome encounters with . . . floating bombs [and] submarines."[5] She arrived safely, and immediately sought out the renowned physician and birth control advocate Dr. Aletta Jacobs.

Jacobs had an impressive résumé. One of eleven children, she was the first female physician in Holland. In 1882, four years after graduating from medical studies at Amsterdam University, she opened the first medical birth control clinic in the world, giving free contraceptive information and supplies to working-class women. Her initiative (and possibly

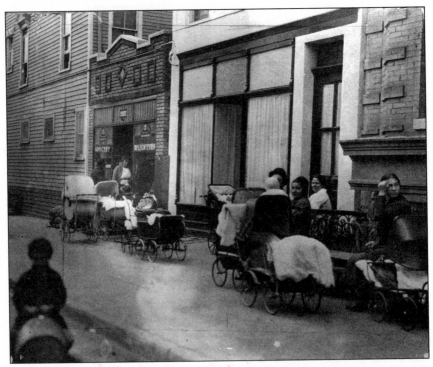

14. Mothers waiting in line to be seen at the Brownsville clinic (Courtesy of the Sophia Smith Collection, Smith College)

her well-known imperiousness) gave rise to a national system of contra-ceptive clinics, which helped reduce the country's maternal and infant mortality rates.

Jacobs clung fast to two principles. The first was the superiority of the physician-fitted Mensinga diaphragm, also referred to in medical litera-ture as the Dutch cup or Mensinga veil. Manufactured in Holland, the device had been invented in 1842 by the gynecologist W. P. J. Mensinga, Jacobs's friend and mentor and onetime professor of anatomy at the Uni-versity of Breslau. Jacobs loyally and actively promoted Mensinga's di-aphragm, helping to make it the most popular birth control method in clinics in Holland, Germany, and Russia. (The cervical cap, better suited to over-the-counter use, continued to be favored in England and France, where Sanger had first learned about it.)

Jacobs's second principle was the need for physician control over the distribution of contraceptive information and technology. Jacobs be-lieved, as Sanger would later, that birth control was strictly a medical matter. So adamant was she in her conviction that when Sanger re-quested a meeting with her, Jacobs refused. The American activist's po-litical credentials could not erase the fact that she was, in Jacobs's eyes, "only" a nurse and thus had no business involving herself in the dissemi-nation of birth control.[6]

Disappointed, Sanger made do. She learned about the Dutch system under the tutelage of Dr. Johannes Rutgers, Jacobs's second in command. Rutgers convinced Sanger of the need for medical clinics that favored the physician-fitted diaphragm rather than over-the-counter methods. The diaphragm's prescription and successful use entailed four distinct steps: a pelvic examination; measurement of the diameter of the vagina and assessment of its contours; selection of a corresponding diaphragm size; and, finally, instruction of the patient. Women were pronounced ready for "home" use only after they had successfully inserted and re-moved the device under a doctor's watchful eye. According to one physi-cian, the procedure required up to forty-five minutes of consultation and "depends on painstaking work with each patient." Even then, patient compliance was not guaranteed. Some doctors insisted on follow-up ap-pointments to double-check patients' technique.[7]

Sanger's acceptance of Rutgers's position on medical contraception and diaphragms shaped the future of the birth control movement. It encouraged her to give up her earlier vision of grassroots contraception, a laypersons' network in which women learned about birth control from each other and by reading educational pamphlets such as *Family Limitation*. Her acceptance also promoted a contraceptive technology that made access to physicians, a far from universal phenomenon in the United States, a precondition of effective use.

Returning to New York in the fall of 1915, Sanger was eager to start a clinic modeled on those she had visited in Holland, but she faced several formidable obstacles. First, U.S. law still regarded birth control as an obscenity. Indeed, while Sanger was away, Anthony Comstock had arrested her husband, William Sanger, for distributing *Family Limitation*. It would be one of his last arrests. During William Sanger's trial, Comstock caught a cold in the courtroom and died soon after of pneumonia.[8] Second, Sanger knew of no physicians like Jacobs and Rutgers ready to risk prosecution or AMA censure by operating contraceptive clinics on this side of the Atlantic. If she wanted a freestanding clinic, she would have to run it herself. Available supplies were a third problem. The Dutch Mensinga pessary was not available in the United States. When Sanger opened her clinic in the fall of 1916, she dispensed the Mizpah, the most frequently used American pessary, instead.[9]

Sanger's clinic did not remain open for long, but Judge Crane's 1918 ruling gave Sanger license to open a second clinic, this time under medical supervision. In 1921, Sanger established the American Birth Control League (ABCL), an advocacy group, which rented rooms for the new clinic. Recruiting a doctor to run it proved difficult. At the last minute, Dr. Lydia DeVilbiss backed out. Sanger persevered, and by late 1922 she had found her doctor: Dorothy Bocker, a public health advocate employed by the Division of Child Hygiene in Milledgeville, Georgia. Sanger warned Bocker that directing a freestanding birth control clinic was risky and that she might go to jail. But she also promised Bocker that the resulting notoriety would "get you such a good boost of publicity, that we can put you on the platform lecturing throughout the country for the next two years." Bocker knew little about birth control techniques. But she promised Sanger that she was "willing to learn."[10]

At about the same time, Sanger found another ally in James Noah Henry Slee. At first glance, Slee was an unlikely convert to the birth control movement. A widower with three grown children and twenty years Sanger's senior, Slee was a well-heeled member of Manhattan's business elite and its conservative Union Club. As president of New York's Three-in-One Oil Company, he was part of the same business establishment Sanger had vilified in her younger, more radical years. After meeting the incandescent woman rebel at a friend's house, Slee pursued Sanger with the ardor of a man deeply in love. Sanger had been separated from William for seven years, and they had recently divorced. Tracking her movements, placing full-page advertisements for his Three-in-One oils—suitable for typewriters, bicycles, guns, sewing machines, furniture, and razors—in the ABCL's *Birth Control Review*, and offering assistance at every turn, Slee coaxed Sanger to say "I do" once more. The two were married September 18, 1922, in Bloomsbury, London. The

MISPAH PESSARY OR SUPPORTER

Highly Recommended by Users

Shown with cap removed.

Reduced size of the MISPAH PESSARY

The attention of physicians, professional nurses and the interested public is invited to the above pessary or supporter. It possesses every decided advantage over any heretofore placed upon the market, whether of foreign or domestic manufacture. The need of an efficient device of this nature has long been recognized by the medical profession.

THE MISPAH PESSARY is sanitary, easily introduced by the patient, causes no pain or irritation.

No skill is required to adjust it.

A silk cord attachment permits its easy removal. Its collapsibility renders it easy of adjustment. The MISPAH is made of the purest and softest rubber, with silk cord attachment for convenient withdrawal.

Directions

Attach rubber cap and insert well up into the vagina.

Price complete with rubber cap $1.50.

Additional caps, 25c each.

15. The popular Mispah, or Mizpah, rubber cap was easy to purchase and to insert (Courtesy of the American Medical Association Archives, Chicago)

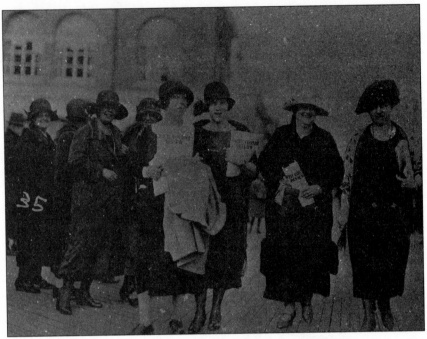

16. Volunteers distribute *The Birth Control Review* in Atlantic City in 1925 (Courtesy of the Sophia Smith Collection, Smith College)

marriage fulfilled a wish Sanger had confided to her sister from prison: that she "find a widower with money." Slee fitted the bill, and if it is crude to suggest that Sanger married him only for his money and connections, evidence indicates that, at the very least, she prized these assets greatly. At a time when prenuptial agreements were rare, Sanger insisted on most unusual terms. The two were to keep separate apartments, keys, and bank accounts. Slee was to pledge his unqualified support to her professional activities and personal autonomy. In professional circles, she would keep the name Sanger. Slee accepted her terms. Still, Sanger was ambivalent about the marriage. She kept it a secret for two years, during which time she stayed on close terms with several male suitors.[11]

With Slee's financial backing, Sanger embarked on a new chapter of her career, one that distanced the birth control movement from its radical origins and placed it on a more conservative path. Until his death in 1943, Slee honored their marriage contract with boundless generosity. More important, he contributed heavily to Sanger's cause. Between 1921 and 1926, his donations to the ABCL exceeded fifty thousand dollars, making him the league's single largest benefactor.[12] Spouse, fan, and friend, Slee was also Sanger's financier.

With Slee and Bocker on board, Sanger proceeded with her plans. On January 2, 1923, she opened her second clinic, the Birth Control Clinical Research Bureau (BCCRB), at 104 Fifth Avenue, across the hall from ABCL headquarters. Much had changed in the almost seven years since the Brooklyn clinic had opened, including Sanger's priorities. Rather than challenging obscenity laws, a course that might have made contraceptives universally safe and accessible, she set her sights on the passage of "doctors-only bills" to exempt physicians from criminal prosecution. In 1924, the ABCL made its first attempt to introduce a doctors-only bill into Congress (a strategy that sharply conflicted with that of the Voluntary Parenthood League, a rival organization established in 1919 that sought to repeal the Comstock Act altogether). The ABCL's mission failed when it could not get sponsors, but the attempt illustrated Sanger's new approach. Hoping to quell physician fears, she portrayed birth control not as a woman's right but as a medical prerogative.

Sanger's political transformation was partly a strategic accommodation to the culture of her times. In the 1920s, she remained committed to quality birth control for women, a goal few Americans and organizations openly endorsed. Not even the National Woman's Party, formed in 1921 by the militant Alice Paul, would support it. Sanger had learned through her failures the limits of sexual reform in early-twentieth-century America. She recognized too that medical science enjoyed increasing prestige and political clout. Narrowing her agenda, she sought birth control allies through an ideology that trumpeted women's health over their civil liberties and cast doctors, not patients, as agents of contraceptive choice.

By the end of 1923, the BCCRB, operating without a license (which the New York State Board of Charities had refused to grant), had supplied free contraceptive services to 1,558 patients. With a subsidy from Slee, Bocker published a study of patients' experiences in February 1924. It was the first clinical evaluation of contraceptives published in the United States and was distributed solely to doctors. Here was the BCCRB's chance to discredit quackery while shoring up the clinic's scientific reputation. Bocker made the most of the opportunity, railing against over-the-counter contraceptives, whose use bypassed physician expertise. She criticized condoms not only because they forced women to depend on men for fertility control but also because "devices break" and the "technique is rather difficult." Bocker was harsher with the Mizpah pessary, the diaphragm's chief rival. Sanger had praised the over-the-counter cervical cap in *Family Limitation*, but Bocker dismissed it. "Sold like a patent cure-all," Bocker complained, the Mizpah "is as likely to fail as any nostrum designed to remedy an undiagnosed disease." She cited a failure rate of "100 percent," although later clinical studies declared the Mizpah effective and safe.[13]

Bocker's report made much of the distinction between legitimate and fraudulent contraceptives—a distinction determined by the devices' retail status, not their efficacy. Over-the-counter birth control was inherently suspect. Contraceptives acquired from doctors were not. Hence, although it was the BCCRB's job to evaluate the safety and efficacy of *all* contraceptives, Bocker refused to test those she branded illegitimate. "Every effort was made [by clinic staff] to welcome new devices that were being developed by commercial interests," she reported. But "any device, method, or procedure that appeared irrational or fraudulent was dropped without trial." Hers was a curiously dismissive stance for a researcher. But Bocker's position reflected her eagerness to divide commercial contraception into two distinct realms: the ethical medical market and the fraudulent patent medicine market.[14]

Bocker gave high marks to the Mensinga diaphragm—used almost exclusively at the clinic—which Slee was smuggling into the country for Sanger.[15] Through international contacts, Slee had Mensinga diaphragms shipped from Europe to Montreal, where they were sneaked across the U.S. border in Three-in-One oil drums. Slee did not take lawbreaking lightly and resorted to it only after a customs collector pointedly told him that "there was no possible way of bringing them in lawfully."[16] The collector could not have been aware of how long this prohibition would last. Until 1971, the importation of contraceptives into the United States by laypersons remained illegal.

Slee's contraband operation was time-consuming, impractical, and risky, and Sanger knew she could not count on it indefinitely. To keep her clinic adequately stocked with Mensinga diaphragms, Sanger needed a domestic manufacturer. But who? On the one hand, there were plenty of manufacturers of Mizpah pessaries and rubber condoms around. A few blocks from the BCCRB, Youngs Rubber was manufacturing Trojans. Close, too, was Julius Schmid's company. Schmid was known mainly for its skins and rubbers, but by 1923 it had branched out into the diaphragm trade and was making a Ramses diaphragm in "a great many sizes" whose design was similar to the Mensinga's. Sanger was aware of Schmid's commercial activities and wrote about them later. Schmid might have welcomed a partnership with Sanger, producing diaphragms tailored to her specifications in the same way that the company would later manufacture condoms for the Navy. But Sanger was determined to dissociate her clinics from extant contraceptives and brand names associated with the over-the-counter trade. She wanted a company that would confine its sales to doctors. Rather than forging an alliance with Youngs Rubber or Schmid, Sanger turned to Slee, the man whose bounty and support she had come to know well.[17]

In 1925, Slee funded the establishment of the Holland-Rantos Company, the first all-birth-control firm to sell contraceptives exclusively to members of the medical profession. Established in May and incorporated in October under New York State law, it was headed by Herbert Simonds. Company letterhead described the firm's specialty as "Physicians' and Surgeons' Supplies."[18] Its objective was to make "available to American doctors the best possible contraceptive materials."[19] Slee's investment was bighearted, all the more so because Simonds had once been Sanger's suitor. An engineer, Simonds had courted Sanger during the war, when she was separated from William, taking the indomitable pacifist out dancing "almost every evening" while he waited to be shipped overseas. Still an admirer, Simonds began manufacturing diaphragms "fully expecting to be arrested."[20] But no one at Holland-Rantos was, although company officers used the mail to distribute Mensinga-type diaphragms and tubes of lactic acid jelly to druggists and doctors. Postal inspectors visited company headquarters but "were satisfied," Sanger wrote in May 1930, that "medical people only get supplies." A couple months later, in July 1930, a New York circuit court of appeals exempted from federal prosecution manufacturers who sold contraceptives exclusively to "ethical" vendors: licensed doctors and druggists. The ruling, *Youngs Rubber Corporation, Inc.* v. *C. I. Lee & Co., Inc.*, involved rival condom makers, but it established a shield of legitimacy that protected Holland-Rantos too.[21]

It was important for Holland-Rantos to promote the diaphragm directly to doctors without Sanger's involvement. Sanger's previous denunciations of medicalized birth control had alienated physicians. Moreover, though Bocker, a physician, supervised the clinic, Sanger's involvement and Bocker's sex did little to quell physicians' fears. Before 1915, the AMA did not admit women, and at a time when admission quotas of 5 percent for women were standard at coeducational medical schools, women remained a conspicuous minority in the profession. Promoting further opposition were the clinic's stand-alone status and its provision of free medical services to the poor. The AMA opposed socialized medicine, which it believed compromised doctors' professional independence and financial autonomy.[22] The physician and AMA heavyweight George Kosmak, a vociferous critic of extramural contraceptive clinics, railed, "If such clinics are needed for the medically indigent, they should be made an essential activity of an established hospital and removed from the domain of a doubtful sentimentality or misguided propaganda."[23]

The most organized opposition to Sanger's BCCRB came in the form of the Committee on Maternal Health (CMH), an association devoted to the scientific promotion and evaluation of fertility control that was founded in New York City in 1923 by the eminent gynecologist Robert Latou Dickinson, former president of the American Gynecological Society. Sanger's efforts on behalf of medical birth control would later earn Dickinson's support, but initially he considered her an adversary, an untrained presence in what ought to be an exclusively scientific domain. It did not help that Sanger was known to be outspoken and tendentious. In 1916, Dickinson advised a medical group in Chicago to seize control of contraception, "not let it go to the radicals, and not let it receive harm by being pushed in any undignified or improper manner."[24] From the outset, Dickinson conceived of the CMH as more likely, in its scientific and hence more objective moorings, to recruit doctors to the cause than Sanger.[25]

Sanger and Simonds suffered no illusions about how difficult it would be to change doctors' minds. They relied on James Cooper to win physicians' support. Cooper was a gynecologist who had worked as a missionary in China before entering private practice in Boston. His impeccable medical credentials, earnestness, and zeal, not to mention what Sanger thought were his "tall, blond, distinguished" good looks, made him a perfect choice for diaphragm crusader.[26] When Sanger decided in early 1925 that the time was ripe to launch a cross-country campaign to promote the Mensinga, she handpicked Cooper to be the ABCL's publicity agent. Cooper's participation would enable doctors to learn about diaphragms from a less threatening advocate. But a doctor of Cooper's stature needed a hefty salary to lure him from private practice, and Sanger implored Slee to help. She proposed a trade: Slee's financial assistance in exchange for her time and affection. On February 2, 1925, she pleaded:

> 1925 is to be the big year for the break in birth control. If Dr. Cooper's association with us is successful, I feel certain that the medical profession will take up the work. When the medical profession does this in the USA, I shall feel that I have made my contribution to the cause and shall feel that I can withdraw from full-time activity. . . .
>
> It is estimated that Dr. Cooper will cost about $10,000 salary and expenses for 1 year. His work will be to lecture before Medical Societies and Associations—getting their cooperation and influence to give contraceptive information in clinics, private and public. If I am able to accomplish this victory with Dr. Cooper's help, I shall bless my adorable husband, JNH Slee, and retire with him to the garden of love.[27]

With visions of retirement with "darling Margy" dancing in his head, Slee paid Cooper ten thousand dollars a year to spread the good word about medical birth control and the superiority of the Mensinga-diaphragm-and-jelly method. By the end of 1926, Sanger's tireless emissary had given more than seven hundred lectures in big cities and small towns in almost every state; sometimes he just rang doctors' doorbells and delivered an impromptu pitch.[28]

Sanger orchestrated Cooper's campaign, but the respected gynecologist was not simply her mouthpiece (although his salary, high even for a successful specialist, might have suggested otherwise). Cooper was a true convert to diaphragmatic birth control. He had even helped create a lactic-acid-and-glycerine-based jelly to be used with diaphragms.[29] Though she trusted Cooper's loyalty, Sanger kept careful tabs on him, demanding frequent reports. Cooper wrote to his boss regularly, detailing doctors' responses to his talks. Their sole concern, he assured her, was where they could acquire "ethical" supplies. Sanger broached this subject cautiously, fearful of the negative repercussions her open endorsement of Holland-Rantos might bring. In a letter to Cooper, she told him that the newly organized company was "getting supplies now and I believe will be able to take orders very shortly. However, I think your recommendations should be casual and not given unless urged to do so. . . . In this way it will look disinterested, as it must."[30]

Sanger was wise to be wary. Her detractors were plentiful and were constantly on the lookout for missteps that could discredit her and the movement. Sanger also had to cling to the trappings of commercial propriety to reassure doctors, who were forbidden by AMA guidelines and state laws to endorse publicly medical products for profit. Such behavior was condemned as quackery, the antithesis of the respectable image Sanger sought to cultivate. Sanger also had to think about the legal status of birth control organizations. The BCCRB and the ABCL and its successors—the Birth Control Federation of America, established in 1939, and Planned Parenthood of America, established in 1942—were nonprofit organizations whose tax and legal status hinged on commercial neutrality. To offset trouble on all these fronts, Sanger devised a code of business conduct. The BCCRB, operated by the ABCL until 1929, when it became independent, recommended methods but not individual brands, although, when asked, it provided a list of ethical manufacturers who sold only to doctors, which included Holland-Rantos. As the number of ABCL-affiliate clinics grew in the 1920s, Sanger made sure that their staffs understood that they were forbidden to be "affiliated with or subsidized by any commercial manufacturer of contraceptives" or to "derive any profit directly or indirectly from the manufacture, distribution or sale of contraceptives, either chemical or mechanical."[31] Sanger herself depended on fund-raising to bankroll her activism but turned down several lucrative endorsement deals, including one for a quarter of a million dollars to "speak on the radio for a chemical product."[32]

Sanger's dream of physician-controlled contraception thus depended, in part, on two competing principles: commercial disinterest and the success of a product manufactured by Holland-Rantos, a company she had helped create. Until the early 1930s, indigent patients were treated and

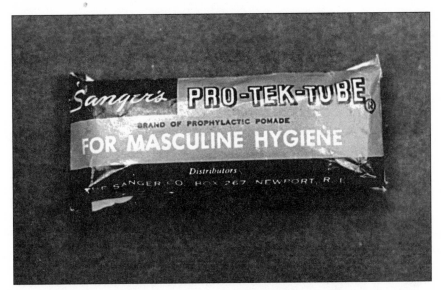

17. Sanger did not publicly endorse individual contraceptive brands, but that did not stop manufacturers from using her name to promote their wares

equipped with diaphragms for free at ABCL clinics, which numbered twenty-eight in 1929. To keep operating expenses down, Sanger counted on gratuitous or at-cost diaphragms from Holland-Rantos, which needed a wide profit margin to sustain its generosity. Holland-Rantos officers understood from the outset the company's mission to supply Sanger's clinics. That, after all, was the primary reason the company had been established. In a letter to Sanger dated February 1926, Herbert Simonds estimated that a sale of 5,000 diaphragms a month at $1.50 each "would show a good profit and still leave 15,000 to *give away*."[33]

Long after its products became popular with private practitioners, Holland-Rantos continued to offer discounted diaphragms to birth control clinics. The arrangement allowed thousands of women to acquire contraceptive supplies they might not have had otherwise, and it set up a model of corporate subsidization of clinics that other "ethical" manufacturers would soon match. But the two-tiered price policy angered surgical supply dealers and druggists, who accused Holland-Rantos of price-cutting at their expense. The company's response, outlined in a 1941 letter, was that it was "simply a matter of company policy to make materials available to birth control clinics serving the indigent . . . as a means of contributing something to the movement . . . so that the poor could be properly and adequately served."[34] The policy helps explain the above-average retail price of Holland-Rantos products. Clinic patients could get the company's Koromex diaphragm for under a dollar, but drugstore patrons and private patients in the late 1930s paid an average of three dollars—the highest price on the diaphragm market.[35] Medical prescriptions were Holland-Rantos's largest source of profit; the company made approximately one dollar in profits for every diaphragm it sold to doctors.[36]

Holland-Rantos enjoyed a lucrative partnership with physicians in private practice. The first manufacturer to sell clinic-approved Mensinga diaphragms exclusively to the medical profession, Holland-Rantos had had first crack at courting doctor loyalty.[37] After 1925, other American firms vied for but never caught up with Holland-Rantos's medical market share. The company also benefited from advance publicity. It introduced its version of the Mensinga diaphragm only after Cooper's advertising blitz and Bocker's (Slee-funded) report celebrated the device's efficacy in clinical trials and promised the medical profession at large that "it will probably be available soon."[38]

In addition, the profitable markup gave doctors a financial incentive to prescribe the company's Koromex brand. Although physicians were forbidden to endorse products, professional ethics did not stop them from benefiting from prescriptions filled in their offices. Because they were prescription-only products, Koromex diaphragms and jelly tubes guaranteed doctors a larger segment of retail-related profits than those sold over the counter. An investigation of the diaphragm industry in the late 1930s found that the average physician markup per device ranged from $.75 to $3.50, depending on design.[39] This could mean significant sales, even in a single practice. One study of contraception in a family practice in a Pennsylvania suburb from 1925 to 1936 found that 94 percent of the 884 white female patients were prescribed the vaginal diaphragm and jelly. Most—95 percent—were upper-middle-class women who could afford the device.[40]

Physicians also benefited from Holland-Rantos's promise of medical management of birth control. The company's prescription-only diaphragms underscored its commitment to the medical profession and boosted physicians' roles as supervisors of women's reproductive health.

In a laudatory and self-serving article on the history of Holland-Rantos published in *American Medicine*, a popular health journal read by doctors, Anne Kennedy, the ABCL's former secretary, Sanger's close friend, and the executive secretary and treasurer of Holland-Rantos, emphasized these themes. Kennedy neglected to inform readers that she worked for the company. She praised the Holland-Rantos diaphragm as "the modern professional method" and distinguished it from inferior "lay methods [such] as rubber prophylactics, douching preparations, tablets and liquids, suppositories, sponges, [contraceptive] tampons, and so on." The efficacy of these products was irrelevant to Kennedy. Their over-the-counter status made them inimical to medical interests, for they sought "to do away with the indispensable services of the physicians." Only the Holland-Rantos diaphragm, a scientific, doctor-controlled contraceptive, made the medical grade.[41]

A 1929 pamphlet sent to doctors by Holland-Rantos's Research Department raised similar concerns. It warned doctors "not to be confused with the cervical cap method." And it cautioned against prescribing suppositories (which destroy the vagina's "protective flora") and condoms (which break). "Here and abroad," the pamphlet insisted, "the weight of authority unquestionably favors the diaphragm."[42]

The message that Holland-Rantos was right for physicians was paralleled by studies concluding that Koromex diaphragms were right for patients. Bocker's was the first of many clinical investigations that endorsed the diaphragm-and-jelly method.[43] By the early 1930s, many such reports had been published in mainstream medical journals, increasing doctors' diaphragm consciousness. Most studies were based on medical data kept by clinics, which expanded in number from 357 in 1938 to 794 in 1942 and which were more likely to prescribe diaphragms than other methods. Even rubber shortages during World War II did not alter clinics' preferences. In 1943, Dr. Claude Pierce, the medical director of Planned Parenthood Federation of America, reported that the once-novel Holland pessary was prescribed in over 93.3 percent of all contraceptive clinic cases. The esteemed status of the diaphragm ensured more than a loyal following among public practitioners whose work provided data for study. It also guaranteed that most contraception studies read by private practitioners recommended the "Holland" diaphragm.[44]

Holland-Rantos couldn't have asked for better advertising. Six years earlier, when the AMA had finally endorsed contraceptives, the company inaugurated an aggressive advertising campaign targeting physicians in private practice. Presenting itself as the tried-and-true medical choice, the company reminded doctors of the long history of effective Holland-Rantos use. "Over 50,000 physicians, 234 clinics and 140 hospitals have already used the Koromex method," advertising copy declared. "Get in step with the AMA report."[45]

For physicians, the proven reliability of diaphragms was a real benefit. Many doctors had opposed birth control not on moral or religious grounds but for fear of endorsing a technique that did not work. There were good reasons for caution. Until the late 1930s, when the government started to enforce product standards, doctors were at the mercy of the market. Evidence of diaphragm efficacy thus reassured physicians and broadened their involvement in birth control even as it increased their reliance on a single method.

Like that of any medical technology, the effectiveness of the Holland-Rantos device was not preordained. Although the Mensinga diaphragm had been widely used in Europe, Holland-Rantos had struggled to engineer a version tailored to the idiosyncracies of the American market. The perfect diaphragm needed to be inexpensive to manufacture, effective after repeated use, aesthetically tolerable, and able to withstand variations of climate: "hot houses and cold winters, Florida dampness and Western dryness."[46] One company officer commented that "making a good diaphragm is like baking a cake. You have to put in the right ingredients in the correct amounts to get the best results."[47] There was also the issue of design, whose perfection necessitated three features:

1. Proper spring tension. The spring must be sufficiently stiff to hold the diaphragm without undue pressure or irritation against the pubic bone but not too stiff to interfere with its proper longitudinal position in the vaginal tract.
2. Dimensional accuracy. This includes diameter of spring, height of dome and size of coil.
3. Correct dome. This must be made of rubber that is soft, pliable and resistant to repeated sterilization.[48]

The company strove for product uniformity, but its goal was compromised by the fact that until the mid-1930s, most spring diaphragms were made by hand. "Molded" diaphragms were produced by rolling springs into cured Para sheet rubber, excising suitably sized pieces with molds, and affixing them to piano or watch wire bent to size. Workers making "dipped" diaphragms submerged spring rings into a liquid solution of natural rubber dissolved by naphtha, the same process used to manufacture rubber condoms. Holland-Rantos experimented with both techniques. Its first model was a dipped diaphragm, described as "attractive looking" but flawed. It had too many air bubbles, and insufficient spring tension made it unreliable. The second prototype was effective but ugly: a "heavy black article that was entirely unsatisfactory." The company finally settled on a handmade steam-cured model that was easily sterilized and durable. It "could be boiled almost indefinitely and well withstood deterioration in service." The company advertised its handmade production as a guarantor of product quality: "Cervical caps, like condoms, are turned out in large quantities by machines. But the vaginal diaphragm is strictly a hand-made article that requires an unusual degree of skill to fabricate." In 1932, Holland-Rantos manufactured the first latex diaphragm in the United States, substituting latex for Para rubber. But the basic design of its diaphragm remained the same. Modified over time, the Holland-Rantos diaphragm was given high marks by the Consumers Union of United States (the nonprofit group that today publishes *Consumer Reports*), which released its first evaluation of American contraceptives in 1937. Listing as "acceptable" only six brands of diaphragms, it described the Koromex model, one of the vaunted six, as possessing a "Dipped-rubber dome. Spring of moderate tension. Dated; guaranteed for two years." Consumers Union liked other diaphragms as much and noted that all of them were cheaper.[49]

Doctors also learned about the effectiveness of the diaphragm-and-jelly method in medical school. Course time devoted to contraceptive instruction increased dramatically in the interwar years as medical support of birth control grew. In a 1944 survey of 3,381 doctors—the first large-scale investigation of its kind—Dr. Alan Guttmacher, an obstetrics professor at the Johns Hopkins University, found that only 10 percent of graduates before 1920 had received training on contraception, but fully 73 percent of those who had graduated in 1935 or later had. Medical students benefiting from the more enlightened approach received a focused birth control education, one that relied on clinical data—which favored the diaphragm—to rank individual techniques. Not surprisingly, education influenced private practice. Guttmacher found a strong correlation between prescription practices and a physician's graduation year. Four-fifths (83.7 percent) of post-1935 graduates listed diaphragms as the method they prescribed most, whereas only a little more than half (57.4 percent) of pre-1910 graduates did.[50]

This medical reorientation was important for a number of reasons. It ensured the medical patronage and hence commercial viability of select birth control manufacturers, cultivating a relationship between doctors and business that the contraceptive industry would fortify in subsequent decades. In addition, as it fed the coffers of firms such as Holland-Rantos, this shift discredited companies that bypassed the medical profession, impeding the development of effective and cheap over-the-counter methods accessible to the laity. Moreover, in this new age of diaphragms and (primarily male) doctors, contraceptives meant birth control for women. When Bocker's study was published in 1924, condoms were doctors' most frequently recommended method of birth control, followed by the douche. Womb veils ranked a dismal fifth, even less popular with doctors than withdrawal or suppositories.[51] By the 1940s, however, diaphragms had become the No. 1 doctor-recommended contraceptive in the country. A 1941 survey by the Youngs Rubber Corporation (which acquired Holland-Rantos in 1947) found that 306 out of 453 doctors who recommended birth control prescribed "diaphragm pessaries." Only 26 recommended condoms.[52] Guttmacher's 1944 survey confirmed this reversal. He found that 69.6 percent of doctors ranked the diaphragm-and-jelly method their first choice for birth control. Condoms were a distant rival, accounting for only 9.5 percent of doctors' first recommendations. Significantly, the two surveys were completed *after* FDA regulations instituted in 1937 had radically improved the effectiveness of condoms, the method physicians had once preferred.[53]

It was not that doctors suddenly forgot about condoms. Condom sales boomed in the 1920s and 1930s, and medical reports touted the device's effectiveness at preventing VD. But even as men signaled their willingness to wear condoms by purchasing sheaths in unprecedented numbers, birth control advocates disparaged men's ability to be diligent users. If some medical reports were to be believed, American men were selfish, weak, and irresponsible, as ready to submit to condom use as they were to torture. In her pro-pessary report, Bocker had lambasted the condom as a technique that "places [the] wife at [the] mercy of unkind, careless, indifferent, or alcoholic husbands." Robert Dickinson of the CMH concurred. In a report published in the *American Journal of Obstetrics and Gynecology*, Dickinson warned that the sheath "is very commonly refused by the feebly virile and the selfish."[54] Although the medical malignment of male character was at odds with everyday practice, it marshaled support for female birth control and implicitly disputed the need for better or different male methods.

Also important to the popularity of female methods among doctors were changing attitudes within society and the profession that encouraged medical management of reproductive health. One concern was maternal mortality, death from pregnancy or childbirth. Although the likelihood that a woman would die from pregnancy declined during the interwar years, medical alarm about maternal mortality grew. The Chicago physician Joseph B. DeLee described childbirth in 1920 as a "pathologic process" few women escaped unscathed. "So frequent are these bad effects," he wrote, "that I have often wondered whether Nature did not deliberately intend women should be used up in the process of reproduction, in a manner analogous to that of salmon, which dies after spawning."[55]

Emphasizing the life-threatening risks of pregnancy enabled doctors to make a strong appeal for physician rather than layperson or midwife supervision of a woman's reproductive health. Writing at a time when most American women still gave birth at home, doctors such as DeLee hoped that the sterile conditions, trained staff, drugs, and equipment at physicians' disposal would encourage pregnant women to deliver in the hospital, the doctor's domain. Doctors also promoted medical birth control to prevent the development of pregnancy-related problems. In his 1933 address to the Section on Obstetrics, Gynecology, and Abdominal Surgery at the annual AMA meeting, Barton Cooke Hirst proclaimed pregnancy "incompatible with health or existence in some women." He ranked birth control one of the four most pressing gynecological issues of the day, along with death during childbirth, infertility, and cancer of the reproductive organs.[56]

By dissociating birth control from the morally charged issue of a woman's right to procreative self-determination and framing it as a valid form of disease prevention, the Crane decision of 1918 sanctioned physician involvement. In the new taxonomy of prophylaxis, contraception became therapeutically warranted. After 1918, doctors openly discussed and debated the conditions under which pregnancy was inadvisable and birth control indicated. "It is generally conceded," wrote one Philadelphia doctor in private practice, "that in the presence of tuberculosis, heart disease, chronic nephritis, previous cesarean section, and certain other subacute and chronic ailments, the occurrence of pregnancy is an additional menace to the patient's health."[57] Over time, the list of contraindications to pregnancy grew to include almost all recognized physical and psychological ailments and problems "sufficient to interfere with the discharge of ordinary duties of the earning of a living."[58]

As doctors came increasingly to regard birth control as therapy rather than smut, medical associations acknowledged, even endorsed, its place in preventive medicine. Like Catholic doctors who later prescribed oral contraceptives to treat menstrual disorders, doctors who opposed contraceptives for moral or religious reasons in the interwar years now had reason to accept their scientific benefits. By the mid-1920s, the American Gynecological Society and the Section on Obstetrics, Gynecology, and Abdominal Surgery of the AMA had endorsed therapeutic birth control. In 1937, one year after the Supreme Court upheld the right of a physician to receive by mail contraceptives "which might intelligently be employed by conscientious and competent physicians for the purpose of saving life or promoting the well-being of their patients," and after decades of characterizing contraceptives as immoral and dangerous, the AMA finally endorsed birth control—when prescribed by physicians.[59] Medical thinking had indeed shifted. As one doctor put it, "The large majority of the medical profession of this country has more and more to regard contraceptive practice in its true light; that is, not as a moral issue, but rather as a branch of preventive medicine." A sick woman "should be entitled to medical advice which will protect her from pregnancy just as much as citizens should be told to protect themselves from smallpox, diphtheria, or typhoid fever."[60]

The medical turn increased doctors' power over women's bodies. Only physicians could diagnose disease and determine the circumstances under which birth control was indicated. Then as today, there was a blurred line between what medical professionals considered best for the patient and what they thought benefited all of society. As the public health movement gained momentum in the early twentieth century, the rights and welfare of the individual were often subordinated to the needs of the community. The forced quarantining in 1907 of Mary Mallon, otherwise known as "Typhoid Mary," the first healthy carrier of typhoid in the country; the Supreme Court's ruling in *Jacobson v. Massachusetts* in 1905 that citizens could be vaccinated for smallpox against their will; and the Tuskegee experiments on syphilitic African-American males in the 1930s: all exemplify how arguments for public welfare and health triumphed over civil liberties in the early twentieth century.[61] They also hint at the nativist and racist character of public health policy. Mary Mallon was an Irish immigrant, the Tuskegee patients poor blacks. In both cases, defending public health meant singling out socially marginalized individuals less able to fight back and more likely to be stigmatized as diseased in the first place.

Similar intellectual currents affected public policies governing reproduction. As doctors in the 1920s claimed greater expertise in managing childbirth, venereal disease, and the entire spectrum of human sexuality—from everyday lust to sexual delinquency—eugenicist policy makers accepted biological explanations of and medical solutions for disease, poverty, crime, and "feeblemindedness." Arguing that these menaces to public welfare were inherited by individuals, they pathologized procreation as the source of social ills and called for the termination of the reproductive capabilities of unfit persons. For birth control advocates, the public welfare argument that anchored sterilization appeals was a double-edged sword. On the one hand, it gave contraceptives added respectability as tools of social engineering. On the other, it categorized them as instruments of social control, weapons in a eugenicist war against criminality and imbecility. Few doubted that these were serious problems. But the public welfare approach yielded a slippery slope toward state control once contraception became a public remedy rather than a private choice. The tension between the two would haunt the birth control movement for decades, victimizing those whom Sanger had initially tried hardest to protect, the underprivileged.

Eugenics was not a new concept in 1920s America. The Englishman Francis Galton first coined the term in 1883 to describe an applied science based on the supposition that intellectual, physical, and behavioral traits are inherited. Its objective was human perfection, its method, selective breeding. Galton, a cousin of Charles Darwin's, defined the term this way: "We greatly want a brief word to express the science of improving stock . . . which, especially in the case of man, takes cognizance of all influences that tend in however remote a degree to give to the more suitable races or strains of blood a chance of prevailing speedily over the less suitable than they otherwise would have had. The word *eugenics* would sufficiently express the idea." It derived from a Greek word meaning "good in birth."[62]

In the United States, the ideology of eugenics framed arguments for and against birth control in the late nineteenth and early twentieth centuries. Although the eugenics movement developed its largest following in the United States after 1910, scores of early enthusiasts linked contraception to recognizably eugenicist beliefs. The suffragist Elizabeth Cady Stanton and the popular birth control author Edward Bliss Foote, along with many free lovers and social purity advocates, supported female control of reproduction partly on the grounds that it would free women to select mates out of true love. Offspring would be healthier and morally stronger because of the purity of the sexual union from which they arose.[63]

The incorrigibly elitist Violet Blair Janin, the Washington, D.C., matron whose late-nineteenth-century letters and diary stand out for their detail and volume, subscribed to a more disdainful view. Five years before Galton coined the word "eugenics," she confided to her diary, "I wish a law could be passed to punish any man who has more than three children, unless one should die and he got another to replace it. Instead of pitying a man who has a large family when he cannot support them, I think public opinion should condemn him." Janin had recently read Thomas Malthus, the English economist and essayist who had argued that parents ought not to have more children than they could support. Janin fretted that the charity of the rich encouraged the excessive procreation of the poor. "It is wicked and contemptible for a man to bring unfortunate beings into the world," she wrote, only "to be provided for out of other people's charity."[64]

The distinction between "fit" and "weak" babies was central to early-twentieth-century eugenicist philosophy. There were two distinct intellectual camps in the United States. The first, known as positive eugenics, followed Galton's lead and called for the unfettered procreation of the fittest members of society to improve the American gene pool. Its rally-ing cry was virulently nativist and racist, premised on the assumption that Nordic-Teutonic Americans were genetically superior. Falling birthrates among the white, Protestant, and native born and the wide-spread emigration of foreigners from southern and eastern Europe (over twenty-three million arrived on America's shores between 1880 and 1920) prompted many Progressives, including Theodore Roosevelt, to condemn the use of birth control by "selfish" middle-class and upper-class women as "race suicide." Roosevelt argued that native-born middle-class women who practiced fertility control were forsaking their natural duties as women and citizens by purging America's stock of its finest ele-ments. Such behavior, Roosevelt warned in a 1911 article published in *The Outlook*, "means racial death."[65]

The second camp was known as negative eugenics, a still more insid-ious strain that sought to suppress, through coercion if necessary, the pro-creation of unfit groups. Its appeal mushroomed in the early years of the twentieth century, yielding myriad articles, pamphlets, and monographs, including Charles Davenport's widely read *Heredity in Relation to Eu-genics*, published in 1911. A Harvard-trained biologist, Davenport had tracked at his research center in Cold Spring Harbor, New York, the pedigrees of extended families believed to be transmitting "defective" genes. His study sought to prove that almost all undesirable attributes, including insanity, alcoholism, eroticism, pauperism, criminality, retarda-tion, and low intelligence, were inherited. It also associated fixed traits with specific ethnic groups. Americans of Anglo-Saxon or Scandinavian descent were the smartest and tidiest, Serbs "slovenly," Italians predis-posed to "crimes of personal violence."[66] Barton Cooke Hirst, chair of the AMA's Section on Obstetrics, Gynecology, and Abdominal Surgery, blamed "our loss of wealth, the venal government of cities and states, the ineptitude of Congress, the prevalence of crime, and the wave of dishon-esty that has swept the country" on the millions of immigrants who had "brought to this country some racial strains that were certainly not the best." Likening the causes of the country's woes to mishandled animal husbandry, he proclaimed: "If a breeder of live stock defied the laws of eugenics as we do, he would be ruined."[67] Eugenicists typically positioned

African-Americans at the bottom of the racial hierarchy. The professor and popular author Paul Popenoe and the petroleum scientist Roswell Johnson argued in their 1926 study, *Applied Eugenics*, that "if the number of original contributions which it has made to the world's civilization is any fair criterion of the relative value of a race, then the Negro race must be placed very near zero on the scale. . . . In comparison with some other races the Negro race is germinally lacking in the higher developments of intelligence."[68]

Cloaking their findings in the mantle of science, proponents of negative eugenics pressed for concrete measures to stem the racial degeneration of America. Like most Americans at the time, eugenicists supported segregation and antimiscegenation statutes. They lobbied successfully for national quota laws to restrict the immigration of southern and eastern Europeans. They criticized proposals to fund programs for retarded children and prenatal and obstetric care for the poor. These, they insisted, would encourage imbecility by increasing the life span and fecundity of defective citizens.[69]

Davenport and other eugenicists believed that the least intelligent members of the human species were, like lower animals, biologically programmed to be the most prolific. Hence it was especially important for society to halt the procreation of the unfit before they bred the human race into degeneracy. For many, the coerced surgical sterilization of unfit men and women was the only permanent, effective prophylaxis against racial decay. As one eugenics pamphlet proclaimed, "Eugenic sterilization, conservatively and sympathetically administered, is a practical, humane and necessary step to prevent race deterioration."[70] By the 1920s, scientists' reports of success with male and female sterilization had helped make the subject a mainstream political issue, with most Americans favoring its use on the institutionalized insane.[71]

Male sterilization referred to a vasectomy, the surgical tying of the seminal ducts. Dr. Harry C. Sharp performed the first male sterilization in Indiana in 1899 on a prisoner who complained of an uncontrollable urge to masturbate. Sharp published the results of the surgery, which he claimed had fixed the problem, in a 1902 article titled "The Severing of the Vasa Deferentia and Its Relation to the Neuropsychopathic Constitution." Sharp's insistence that the operation cured his patient's pathological desire illustrates how social views shaped ostensibly scientific conclusions. Subsequent research has shown that vasectomies do not affect sexual drive and that the desire to masturbate—by a man or woman—is neither a physiological nor a psychological problem. Yet Sharp was captive to the prejudices of his time and insisted that sexual deviance was of biological origin. Claiming victory in his crusade against neuropsychosis one surgery at a time, he went on to perform over 450 vasectomies on inmates and to lobby the Indiana legislature to pass the first eugenic law mandating the coerced sterilization of unfit persons, which it did in 1907.[72]

Sharp's medical involvement and political success encouraged other physicians to endorse compulsory sterilization to stem social degeneracy. Sexual surgery was also recommended for women, who had for decades been subjected to gynecological surgeries such as ovariectomies (the surgical removal of ovaries) to "cure" so-called nymphomania and hysteria.[73] It was not a huge surgical step from ovariectomies to salpingectomies. More complicated than a vasectomy, a salpingectomy (today called tubal ligation) involved incising the abdominal wall and tying the Fallopian tubes.[74] Eugenicists hailed vasectomies and salpingectomies as safe, effective, and simple. They rarely "failed," and no special training was required to perform them. Patient inconvenience and recovery time were purportedly minimal. One booklet circulated for general readership estimated that a vasectomy could be performed under a local anesthetic in fifteen or twenty minutes. The operation "is so simple and easily accomplished," gushed one pamphlet for men, "that the man need not remain away from his employment for a period longer than it takes to have the operation performed."[75] A New York judge promised in 1916 that it was "less serious than the extraction of a tooth."[76]

Sterilizations were also credited with saving taxpayers' money, an argument that increased support once the Great Depression arrived. The Human Betterment Foundation of Pasadena, California, the leading U.S. eugenics society at the time, estimated in 1930 that there were eighteen million Americans "burdened by mental disease or mental defect, and in one way or another a charge and tax upon the rest of the population." The economic burden to healthy Americans was considerable. "A billion dollars a year would be a low estimate of the cost of caring for these unfortunates," the foundation stated.[77]

In 1927, the Supreme Court upheld the constitutionality of state sterilization laws in its ruling in *Buck v. Bell*. The case involved a 1924 Virginia eugenics statute that legalized the coerced sterilization of "socially inadequate person[s]." Carrie Buck, the plaintiff, was single, white, pregnant, and only seventeen when she was brought to the Virginia Colony for Epileptics and Feeble Minded in Lynchburg. Although she insisted that her pregnancy was the result of rape, her condition and her status as the "daughter of an imbecile" and the mother of "an illegitimate feeble minded child" supplied the primary evidence substantiating the diagnosis of mental ineptitude. In his momentous ruling, Oliver Wendell Holmes, long admired for his heroic *defense* of civil liberties, declared coercive sterilization a valid exercise of the state's right to protect public health. "The principle that sustains compulsory vaccination," he declared, referring to the Court's 1905 ruling in *Jacobson v. Massachusetts*, is broad enough, "to cover cutting the Fallopian tubes. . . . Three generations of imbeciles are enough."[78]

The Court's decision licensed other states to pass similar eugenics legislation. By 1932, at least twenty-six states had enacted laws permitting the forced sterilization of individuals considered unfit. Although their provisions varied, most authorized sterilizations on men and women suffering from "feeblemindedness, insanity, epilepsy, idiocy, moral degeneracy, imbecility, habitual criminality, or sexual perversion." By 1937, almost twenty-eight thousand men and women had been forced to undergo eugenic surgery in the United States. Most—more than sixteen thousand—were women.[79] The Virginia act served as the model for Germany's Hereditary Health Law in 1933. During the Nuremberg trials following World War II, accused Nazi war criminals cited *Buck v. Bell* to justify the forced sterilization of some two million Germans.

Although eugenic theory began to be discredited as bad science in the 1940s, when the atrocities of the Holocaust were brought to light, it continued to shape policies affecting reproduction, birth control, and social equality. From the outset, support for eugenics and contraception overlapped, but not always as tidily as some have asserted.[80] Many eugenicists opposed birth control for the poor and persons of color. Convinced of the ineptitude of the unfit, they harbored doubts that blacks, immigrants, and the poor had the intellectual wherewithal or self-discipline to use birth control effectively—assuming, of course, that they could be convinced of its need. As one racist researcher callously observed, "The American negro may be supposed not to practice contraception largely. Some devices are expensive and intricate, others are expensive and distasteful to self-indulgent men."[81] Moreover, at a time when the efficacy of various contraceptives was still unclear, coerced sterilization seemed to many a surer bet than birth control. The Human Betterment Foundation had such a low regard for the self-control of the institutionalized insane that it rejected even abstinence "under lock and key" as a viable alternative to surgery. Aside from being expensive for the state, compulsory abstinence "is not 100% successful. Some childbearing occurs in any such institution. Some patients escape."[82]

At the same time, the scientific credibility of the birth control movement was enhanced by the search to limit the procreation of undesirable groups, and its leaders appropriated eugenic language to promote their goals. Like most Americans, Sanger supported sterilization for the incarcerated and considered birth control a necessary component of racial improvement. "Birth control," she stated emphatically in 1920, "is nothing more or less than the facilitation of the process of weeding out the unfit [and] of preventing the birth of defectives."[83] But Sanger also believed that socially structured inequality, especially differential access to contraceptives, caused inferiority. Poverty and criminality were made, not born: "Children who are underfed, undernourished, crowded into badly ventilated and unsanitary houses and chronically hungry cannot be expected to attain the mental development of children upon whom every advantage of intelligent and scientific care is bestowed."[84] This unshakable faith in the environmental rather than hereditary origins of human degradation was one Sanger carried over from her radical years. She earnestly believed that a desire to escape poverty (and its concomitant psychological degradation) would motivate women and men to use contraception. She endorsed the principle of reproductive autonomy and maintained that the establishment of public clinics promoting cross-class access to scientific birth control furthered that goal. But she was not above the paternalism intrinsic to eugenic thought, the conviction that sometimes people needed to be reeducated "for their own good."

This elitism was especially apparent in her dealings with African-Americans. In a joint effort between the Birth Control Clinical Research Bureau and the National Urban League, Sanger opened a second New York clinic in Harlem in February 1930. Like its sister clinic, the Harlem site aimed to bring birth control to the poor through the distribution of cheap diaphragm-and-jelly kits. But the all-white staff, and the storefront placard identifying the clinic as a research bureau, immediately raised suspicions within the black community that the clinic's goal was to experiment on and sterilize black people. Blacks' fears were not entirely unfounded. Sanger designated the Harlem clinic the official teaching site for physicians wanting diaphragm training. A fee of twenty-five dollars entitled trainees to "three sessions at the Harlem branch where they will not only be present, but will, under instruction, give examinations."[85] Naked, knees splayed, passive, and probed: being fitted for a diaphragm was not (and is not) what most women consider fun. But to be subjected to the procedure as an African-American woman by a novice, likely a white male, in the presence of others who watched and commented on his "work," could only have made a difficult situation worse.

Sanger also initially refused to cede control of the clinic to the Harlem Advisory Council, an autonomous board of black health professionals established to help run the clinic and to raise money. She insisted that the clinic met a need that "the race did not recognize" for itself.[86] When blacks continued to view the clinic suspiciously, she racially integrated its staff and reworded promotional pamphlets to emphasize the temporary and harmless nature of the contraception offered. It was not enough. In 1936, a year after the American Birth Control League took over as managers, the financially ailing clinic closed.

Unfortunately, unsuccessful efforts such as these did not motivate birth control leaders to rethink their racist and nativist assumptions. Before the clinic closed, Harlem Advisory Council member Mabel Staupers wrote Sanger: "If the Birth Control Association wishes the cooperation of Negroes . . . we should be treated with the proper courtesy that is due us and not with the usual childish procedures that are maintained with any work that is being done for Negroes."[87] But it was easier to chalk the clinic's failings up to black disinterest than to white racism.

By the 1930s, charges that public clinics and the diaphragms they dispensed were no match for the idiocy and fecundity of the urban poor had forced Sanger and her colleagues to defend the clinic-diaphragm formula as best for the medical profession *and* the masses. Few scientists and doctors questioned that the diaphragm-and-jelly method worked wonders in the laboratory and in the homes of the white middle class. But everyday use among African-Americans, immigrants, and the poor—the very groups whose fecundity American society was most intent on controlling—was an altogether separate matter. Was the method too complex for them? The question threatened to sabotage Sanger's work.

Robert Dickinson of the Committee on Maternal Health was among the doubters. Having described condoms in 1924 as too complicated for "the feebly virile . . . [and] the careless and the poor," he revised his assessment in 1931 in *Control of Conception*, a widely read medical book co-authored with fellow birth control proponent Louise Stevens Bryant.[88] Compared with diaphragms, condoms were easy. "Until some better device is perfected," the two chided, "the condom will rival the pessary [for] its use is much simpler to learn . . . [and its] cost to the worker and the white collar poor can be reasonable." Dickinson and Bryant warned that physicians' recommendations for birth control must take into account a patient's intelligence, living conditions, and character, keeping in mind that "all birth control is self control."[89] At a 1936 roundtable on contraceptive methods in New York City, Dickinson offered his most barbed criticism to date of the suitability of existing methods for the "impoverished and ignorant masses found in all parts of the world."[90] "There is no need to summarize how little we have provided for the people that have the greatest need," he asserted. "Consider the two and one-half million fertile couples that were on relief. How well can clinics, how well can doctors meet that particular need of the backwoods and the bayou, the requirements of the slum dweller or the distant mountaineer?" The perfect contraceptive for the masses had not yet been discovered. He concluded: "I propose three ways out. The first is research; the second is research; the third is research."[91]

Sanger struggled to devise a reassuring answer that validated current clinical methods without dismissing critics' concerns. She had painted herself into a corner. Having insisted that scientific birth control was too complex for anyone but doctors, she could not reverse course and claim that it was simple enough for the "ignorant slum dweller." Instead, the BCCRB touted positive results with patient compliance, including a 97 percent success rate with the diaphragm, "even" among women of "sub-normal intelligence."[92] Sanger continued to insist that poverty remained a compelling motivator: "their eagerness to prevent conception makes them very careful in following instructions."[93]

While refusing to relinquish her vision of medically fitted diaphragms for American women, Sanger conceded that meeting the contraceptive needs of developing nations might require a different and new technology. At the same 1936 roundtable at which Dickinson spoke, she discussed the backwardness of Indian and Chinese attitudes toward women's bodies and birth control:

> I found that it was going to be a very dismal thing to go to India, where the average wage of the Indian population is five cents a day, and advise there the use of a mechanical method, no matter how cheaply it could be made in this country. I knew that in advising a diaphragm it was not only a question of cheapness but the importance of being fitted by a qualified person. . . . The foam powder formula and method was one of the solutions; at least it offered a solution for the Oriental woman. In the first place, it probably can be made in the Orient with rice starch as a base. . . . It takes no particular knowledge of anatomy or physiology for the person to adjust it herself.[94]

For uneducated women in other countries, Sanger's original goal of simple, cheap, over-the-counter methods, outlined more than two decades earlier in *Family Limitation*, still applied. For American women, that time had passed.

In *Facts and Frauds in Woman's Hygiene*, a 1938 study of how women's health needs were shortchanged in American society, the consumer health advocates Rachel Lynn Palmer and Sarah Koslow Greenberg condemned the profits made by diaphragm-and-jelly manufacturers and demanded the "socialization of the birth control business." Palmer and Greenberg recognized what Sanger would not. A patchwork quilt of birth control clinics was no way of bringing contraceptives to the poor, at least not in a country where profits for manufacturers and medical professionals were more important than health care for the poor and where extramural clinics had to be funded by donations and defended against the argument that it would be cheaper for society to sterilize the indigent. In any society without universal health care, working-class people are systematically denied access to doctors and the services they monopolize. Of all people in the birth control movement, Sanger probably understood this best. To her credit, she never gave up her goal of quality birth control for all. She simply failed to achieve it. Throughout Sanger's life, most Americans got contraceptives where they always had, on the open market.

SEVEN

𝒥eminine ℋygiene

The contraception movement of the second and third decades of the twentieth century, spearheaded by Margaret Sanger, made "birth control" a household word. Sanger captured the media spotlight and provided the necessary cultural backdrop for the over-the-counter contraceptive revolution that followed.

The birth control business grew dramatically during the Great Depression. In 1938, with the industry's annual sales exceeding $250 million, *Fortune* magazine pronounced birth control one of the most prosperous businesses of the decade.[1] Yet soaring sales had little to do with doctors or the diaphragm, physicians' contraceptive of choice. In the late 1930s, diaphragm purchases accounted for less than 1 percent of total contraceptive sales.[2] Instead, the industry derived most of its profits from over-the-counter forms of birth control sold by pharmacies, five-and-dime stores, mail-order firms, and itinerant peddlers. Especially popular were feminine hygiene products. An innocuous term coined by advertisers in the 1920s, "feminine hygiene" was the euphemism manufacturers used for over-the-counter female contraceptives: vaginal jellies, liquids, suppositories, foaming tablets, and the ever-popular antiseptic douche.[3] (Advertising them as methods of birth control meant breaking the law.) Like the diaphragm, feminine hygiene products put women in charge of their procreative destiny. But they had advantages the diaphragm did not. They were bargain priced and could be purchased without a gynecological examination, in "the same matter-of-fact way as . . . toothpaste, aspirin, or sanitary napkins."[4] Condom sales also soared during the Depression, but it was sales of female contraceptives—which had outnumbered those of condoms five to one by the late 1930s—that fueled the industry's prodigious growth. By 1938, feminine hygiene accounted for 85 percent of annual contraceptive sales.[5] In the long run, the success of the feminine hygiene campaign was twofold: it encouraged more women to use birth control, and it ensured that the largest proportion of those who did used female-controlled, over-the-counter methods.

In 1936, the first survey of national attitudes toward contraception found that 70 percent of the 100,000 Americans contacted, and a majority in every state, favored medical birth control.[6] Yet as demand for birth control accelerated, the inability of medical institutions to satisfy the need for scientific methods became apparent. In the 1920s, birth control organizations in New York City received over ten thousand letters a year requesting information about safe methods. Because of chronic understaffing, most went unanswered.[7]

Officials who publicly promoted birth control also received a spate of inquiries. Judge Benjamin Lindsey of the Juvenile Court of Denver, Colorado, had no medical proficiency. But after he endorsed birth control in a series of articles in *Physical Culture* in 1925, hundreds of Americans sought his advice. One man implored Lindsey, "Give me the method of birth control taught by the lady in New York who has created such a stir."[8] Another, a recent college graduate, beseeched Lindsey to tell him the one true "secret" method "before the force of sexual instinct ruins my career and leave[s] me unprepared to meet the demands of its result."[9] A sixteen-year-old girl, the daughter of strict parents, asked: "This is embarrassing, but really where do babies come from? Do petting parties always turn out disastrously?" She promised to share Lindsey's contraceptive wisdom with "6 more girls like me . . . [whose] parents are like mine."[10]

Working-class women could get doctor-fitted diaphragms at urban birth control clinics, but there were not enough to go around. In 1932, only 145 public clinics operated to service the contraceptive needs of the nation; twenty-seven states had none. Rural residents were particularly disadvantaged. In states like Montana, Wyoming, Louisiana, and Mississippi, close by was not close enough because hundreds of miles separated clinics from prospective patients.[11] The number of clinics in the United States did grow from 357 in 1937 to 800 in 1943. But even in 1943, Planned Parenthood acknowledged that clinics were still "too recent" and "too few in number" to serve more than a "small proportion of the total population."[12]

Although Sanger had envisioned the doctor-fitted diaphragm as a contraceptive for the masses, at no point in American history was the device used by more than a minority of women, and among these, mainly affluent. A 1947 study of New York families, for instance, found that 27 percent of middle-class but only 2.6 percent of working-class couples used diaphragms with jelly.[13] Another study completed shortly before the release of the Pill in 1960 corroborated these findings, concluding that diaphragms remained the least popular contraceptive in the country.[14]

Affluent women also forsook the diaphragm for other contraceptives. Many consulted doctors who refused to prescribe birth control despite new AMA guidelines and legal exemptions. Women had also to consider a doctor's proficiency and experience when selecting a contraceptive provider, for even the most sympathetic physicians often had no training. Indeed, one gynecologist writing in the mid-1930s noted that until birth control education in medical schools became routine, "many women . . . could give most doctors pointers as to the contraceptive technique."[15]

In addition, an untold number of American women were uncomfortable discussing contraception with physicians. Some women may have felt that the birth control movement ushered in a new age of sexual candor, but there remained millions of Americans whose conduct was "rigidly governed by prudish customs and false modesty" and who preferred self-medication to a visit to the doctor.[16] Planned Parenthood believed that "it takes courage for a woman to go to a physician with such an intimate problem as that of contraception." In 1959, one woman admitted: "I have thought of going to a clinic for a diaphragm, but I'm real backward about doing that. I don't even go to the doctor to be examined when I'm pregnant. I never go until about a month before I have the baby." Her husband observed: "We have talked about the diaphragm. The nurse at the hospital where the babies were born wanted my wife to be fitted for one, but she won't go. She says she's afraid to go. She really isn't afraid, she's just embarrassed."[17]

Demographers and birth control proponents frequently branded suspicion of doctors a working-class fear, bred by "irrational" superstitions, but middle-class women shared similar inhibitions. Women who sought physicians' expertise for childbirth or infection did not find it contradictory to regard contraception as different and off-limits. One investigator discovered in the early 1940s that only 30.8 percent of middle-class families and 5.8 percent of working-class families got contraceptive information from doctors, including attending obstetricians. More astonishing was his finding that fully 60 percent of middle-class couples who used diaphragms "did so without medical advice and by a trial-and-error method," buying several sizes over the counter and fitting themselves. One couple "admitted having purchased four different-sized diaphragms before getting one that would stay in place."[18] Alarmed that "more contraceptives are distributed to the public through drug stores than through any other source," Planned Parenthood surveyed one thousand pharmacists from forty-one states in 1946. Every respondent stated that at least 30 percent of regular customers—often more—had sought out his birth control advice. In giving it, pharmacists tried to keep the business in-house. Although 63 percent of druggists recommended the diaphragm-and-jelly method, only 36 percent urged customers to see a physician first to be fitted. Most were happy to dispense the device without a prescription. A mere 1 percent suggested birth control clinics as a source of information or supplies.[19]

For consumers, the diaphragm's drawbacks went beyond the cost, discomfort, and other liabilities associated with its fitting. From the outset, the method was more flawed than Sanger liked to admit. In practice, the diaphragm was 80 percent effective after a year of use, making it safer than other methods but not, by any accounting, infallible.[20] It required planning, which deadened sexual spontaneity. Diaphragms were also messy and hard to clean in households without running water. Women uncomfortable or unused to touching their own bodies found proper placement difficult and incident-free withdrawal a challenge. One woman recalled the embarrassment of first-time use. After intercourse, she attempted to remove her diaphragm, only to have its spring action and her unfamiliarity with the device's mechanics land the diaphragm on the ceiling and splatter its contents—ejaculate, jelly, and all—around the room. A laughable but awkward moment for her and her partner, the incident motivated her to switch contraceptive methods. Permanently.[21]

Diaphragms were also expensive, especially for non-clinic patients. Excluding the costs of a medical consultation, the going rate for a diaphragm and a companion tube of jelly ranged from four to six dollars in the mid-1930s. In contrast, a dollar purchased a dozen suppositories, ten foaming tablets, a dozen condoms, or, most alluring of all, up to three two-ounce douching units (each of which typically made two gallons of douche-ready disinfectant), depending on the brand. With so many odds stacked against medical birth control, it is not surprising that its triumph came not with the diaphragm but with the Pill.

Until the 1960s, women got most of their contraceptive information and equipment from traditional nonmedical sources: neighbors, friends, advertisements, druggists and other commercial purveyors, and through the mails. Spurred on by public attention to birth control but unwilling or unable to secure medical guidance, women and men took contraception into their own hands, sometimes with tragic consequences. A Chicago physician noted with alarm in 1930 the growing number of doctors reporting the discovery of chewing gum, hairpins, needles, tallow candles, and pencils lodged in female patients' bladders. The doctor blamed these desperate attempts to restrict fertility on the "wave of publicity concerning contraceptive methods that has spread over the country."[22] But what this evidence really signaled was the failure of medically administered contraceptives to keep pace with demand.

People also turned to the market to purchase what they hoped were safe and reliable devices. The over-the-counter business thrived precisely because, while capitalizing on public discussions of birth control to which the medical community contributed, it operated outside customary medical channels. Pharmaceutical firms, rubber manufacturers, mail-order firms, and fly-by-night peddlers supplied women and men with something that clinics and private physicians did not: birth control that was conveniently located, discreetly obtained, and affordably priced.

Although the condom was the contraceptive most frequently purchased by men, most over-the-counter birth control was bought by and for women. The rise of the female birth control industry was an important episode in the advance of a consumer society in interwar America. Mass production, a predominantly urban population, and innovations in consumer credit supplied the underpinnings for the expansion of the consumer economy. The advertising industry, manufacturers, retailers, and political leaders provided a concomitant cultural ethos that celebrated the emancipating properties of consumption; the power to purchase was lauded as a desirable, deserved, and quintessentially American freedom.[23] Women became favored recipients of this self-congratulatory encomium.[24] In the 1920s, when advertising consultants agreed that purchases by women accounted for 80 percent of consumer spending (this in an economy increasingly dependent on consumer sales), the female orientation of advertising was readily apparent. Hoping to influence women's buying behavior, advertisers shrewdly cast women's timeworn role as consumers in a flattering light. Universally endorsing among themselves a psychological profile of the female shopper as mercurial and easily swayed by emotional appeals, advertisers attempted to convince women that consumption was inherently empowering. Advertising copy and images accentuated a common theme: that the freedom to choose between Maybelline and Elizabeth Arden lipsticks was the hallmark of women's newfound authority and liberation in the post-suffrage age.[25]

Just as consumption was trumpeted as a characteristically female freedom, reproduction was portrayed as a distinctively female task. On this latter point, women needed little convincing. By virtue of biology, pregnancy was an exclusively female experience; by virtue of convention, rearing children in the 1930s was principally a female responsibility. The birth control industry emphasized the naturalness of women's twin roles as consumers and reproducers. Conjoining these functions, manufacturers and retailers urged women to use their purchasing "power" to assume full responsibility for pregnancy prevention. The industry's sales pitch struck a resonant chord with American women in the 1930s. At a time when an unprecedented and increasing proportion of the laboring population was officially unemployed, and male desertion rates were at an all-time high, fertility control assumed added urgency. With advertisers' prodding, millions of women turned to the contraceptive market to achieve it.[26]

Contraceptive manufacturers did not create the desire to control fertility, but they preyed on and compounded women's fears of pregnancy to reap higher profits. Print and radio ads and commissioned door-to-door salespeople manipulated women's anxieties to hawk goods that were useless as contraceptives and dangerous to women's health. Under the guise of medical science, advertising promised women the latest advances in contraceptive technology. What women usually got instead were commercially prepared douches and suppositories less effective than conventional methods of birth control. "Although douching is relatively unreliable as a contraceptive," Planned Parenthood noted in 1943, "the power of the advertising and retail promotion put on these products under the banner of feminine or personal hygiene has built up a tremendous acceptance for them as contraceptives."[27] In addition, ads created new psychological anxieties by inflating the social significance of contraception. If pregnancy indexed impending financial hardship, its incorrect prevention could destroy a marriage or ruin a family. Birth control advertising in the 1930s implicitly asked the obvious: Could a woman in the "modern age" afford not to buy the newest contraceptives?

Aggressive advertising was instrumental to the industry's success. One 1947 study found that for both working- and middle-class women, advertising was a more frequent source of birth control information than medical clinics.[28] Appealing to women in the privacy of their homes, feminine hygiene companies sponsored advertisements on local radio stations. They blanketed women's magazines in the 1930s and 1940s with ads, many of full-page size. In 1933, contraceptive firms spent over $400,000 to promote products in romance, pulp, and movie magazines such as Love Story, Dime Detective, and Screen Book and in middle-class monthlies such as McCall's and Redbook.[29] Companies advertised to excess. One physician complained to the AMA that his "current issue of McCall's magazine is a veritable illustrated course in Gynecology and I am no prude."[30] Publishers' refusal to print advertisements explicitly for birth control exacerbated the problem. McCall's and Redbook would not accept "the advertising of any product which in the copy claims to be, directly or indirectly, a contraceptive" but were content to pocket the revenue from ads for less-effective feminine hygiene products, which their readers bought for the same purpose.[31]

The headlines of ads were designed to inculcate and inflate apprehensions in readers' minds. They conveyed the message that ineffective

NUMBER TEN IN A SERIES OF FRANK TALKS BY EMINENT WOMEN PHYSICIANS

"No wonder many Wives fade quickly

WITH THIS RECURRENT FEAR"

"I am a doctor. But I am also a woman — and a Latin. I cannot help but look at this whole problem with my feelings as well as my mind.

"As a woman, I think it tragic — and as a doctor, inexcusable! — when lovely young wives fade quickly after marriage. When fear disturbs their health, steals their beauty, turns their dispositions irritable. And, worst of all, when the unhappy husband wonders helplessly what has happened to the blithe young woman he married.

"You cannot blame a woman for her wretched fear of what *night* be . . . when a lapse in feminine regularity occurs. But you can deplore her ignorance of proper marriage hygiene, which permits that fear to exist.

"The proper technique of marriage hygiene is one of the blessings medical research has conferred upon womankind. It has alleviated woman's oldest fear. Antisepsis is a proved, familiar practice recommended by physicians in every land. The most important thing is your choice of an antiseptic. Some are good, some are not. My own preference is for "Lysol", in common with almost every other doctor I know.

"Lysol" combines the two most important qualities in a germicide. It is certain . . . yet safe. If instructions for its use are carefully followed, it will not irritate delicate feminine membranes, as other antiseptics may do which contain free caustic alkali. We even use "Lysol" in childbirth cases.

"Yet "Lysol" has the power to destroy the most active germ-life, which other compounds fail to do in the presence of organic matter. "Lysol's" extremely low surface tension lets it penetrate hidden folds, and that is vastly important in an antiseptic for feminine use.

"Its regular, unfailing use is the greatest precaution I, as a doctor, can suggest to guard against feminine irregularities — to allay the harassing fear that makes women old beyond their actual years."

(Signed)

PROF. DR. LINITA BERETTA

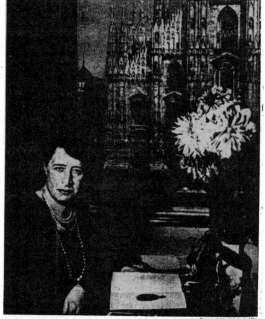

Photographed by Man Ray in Milan

Professor Doctor Linita Beretta, leading Italian gynecologist . . . Director of the Maternity Division of the State and Municipal Clinic of Quentiere Monforte, Milan.

© L. & F., Inc., 1933

LET "LYSOL" GUARD THE FAMILY'S HEALTH

Use it in your home as protection against colds, tonsilitis, sore throat, grippe, and to disinfect after these ailments. Use it for protecting and disinfecting in case of children's diseases — mumps, measles, etc. Excellent for athlete's foot. Helps to heal cuts, burns, etc. Protects mother and child in operations attending childbirth. Directions for every use on every bottle.

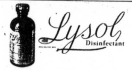

Lysol
Disinfectant

FACTS EVERY MARRIED WOMAN SHOULD KNOW

Mail coupon for a copy of our interesting brochure — "Marriage Hygiene." Contains the helpful advice of three world-famous women physicians. Check other booklets if desired.
☐ Preparation for Motherhood ☐ Keeping a Healthy Home
LEHN & FINK, Inc., Bloomfield, N. J. Dept. LH-N
Sole Distributors of "Lysol" disinfectant
Name_____
Street_____
City_____State____

18. Lehn & Fink's successful advertising campaign helped make the Lysol douche the best-selling female contraceptive in the country by the late 1930s

contraception led not only to unwanted pregnancies but also to illness, despair, and marital discord. Ads titled "Calendar Fear," "Can a Married Woman Ever Feel Safe?" "Young Wives Are Often Secretly Terrified," and "The Fear That 'Blights' Romance and Ages Women Prematurely" relied on standard negative advertising techniques to heighten the stakes of pregnancy prevention.[32] Women who ignored modern contraceptive methods were courting lifelong misery. "Almost before the honeymoon ends," one ad warned, "many a young bride is plagued by forebodings. She pictures the early departure of youth and charm . . . sacrificed on the altar of marriage responsibilities." Engulfed by fear, the newlywed's life only got worse—fear itself, women were told, engendered irreparable physical ailments. According to one douche advertisement, fear was a "dangerous toxin" because it "dries up valuable secretions, increases the acidity of the stomach, and sometimes disturbs the bodily functions generally. So it is that FEAR greys the hair . . . etches lines in the face, and hastens the toll of old age."[33]

As if these physical penalties were not disconcerting enough, feminine hygiene ads insisted that a woman's apprehensions and their attendant woes could ruin a marriage. On this point, the transcendent parable of ads was clear: the longevity of a marriage depended on the right commercial contraceptive. "She was a lovely creature before she married," one ad began, "beautiful, healthy, and happy. But since her marriage she seems forever worried, nervous and irritable . . . always dreading what seems inevitable. Her husband, too, seems to share her secret worry. Frankly, they are no longer happy. Poor girl, she doesn't know that she's headed for the divorce court."[34] And as ads—whose sole purpose was to convince women, not men, to buy contraceptives—hastened to remind readers, women alone shouldered the blame for divorce. After all, why should a man be held accountable for distancing himself from a wife made ugly and cantankerous by her own anxieties? "Many marriage failures," one advertisement asserted authoritatively, "can be traced directly to disquieting wifely fears." "Recurring again and again," marriage anxieties were "capable of changing the most angelic nature, of making it nervous, suspicious, irritable." "I leave it to you," the ad continued, "is it easy for even the kindliest husband to live with a wife like that?"[35]

Having divulged the ugly and myriad hazards of unwanted pregnancy while saddling women with the burden of its prevention, advertisements emphasized that peace of mind and marital happiness were conditions only the market could bestow. In the imagined world of contraceptive advertising, feminine hygiene was the commodity no modern woman could afford to be without. Fortunately, none had to. The path to unbridled happiness was only a store away.[36]

As advertisements reminded prospective customers, however, not all feminine hygiene products were the same. The contraceptive consumer had to be discriminating. Hoping both to increase general demand for hygiene products and to inculcate brand loyalty, manufacturers presented their product as the one most frequently endorsed for its efficacy and safety by medical professionals. Dispelling consumer doubts by invoking the approval of the scientific community was not a technique unique to contraceptive merchandising—the same strategy was used in the 1930s to sell women laxatives, breakfast cereal, and mouthwash. What was exceptional about contraceptive advertising, however, was that the experts endorsing feminine hygiene usually were not men. Rather, they were female physicians whose innate understanding of the female condition permitted them to share their birth control expertise "woman to woman."[37]

The Lehn & Fink corporation used this technique to make the Lysol disinfectant douche the leading feminine hygiene product in the country from the 1930s through the 1960s.[38] In a series of full-page advertisements titled "Frank Talks by Eminent Women Physicians," stern-looking European female gynecologists urged "smart-thinking" women to entrust their health only to doctor-recommended Lysol disinfectant douches. "It amazes me," wrote Dr. Madeleine Lion, a Parisian gynecologist, "in these modern days, to hear women confess their carelessness, their lack of positive information, in the so vital matter of feminine hygiene. They take almost anybody's word . . . a neighbor's, an afternoon bridge partner's . . . for the correct technique. . . . Surely in this question of correct marriage hygiene, the modern woman should accept only the facts of scientific research and medical experience. The woman who *does* demand such facts uses 'Lysol' faithfully in her ritual of personal antisepsis."[39] Another Lysol ad underscored the point. "It is not safe to accept the counsels of the tea table," explained Dr. Auguste Popper, a female gynecologist from Vienna, "or the advice of a well-meaning, but uninformed friend." Only the advice of scientific experts could be trusted.[40] The text was more

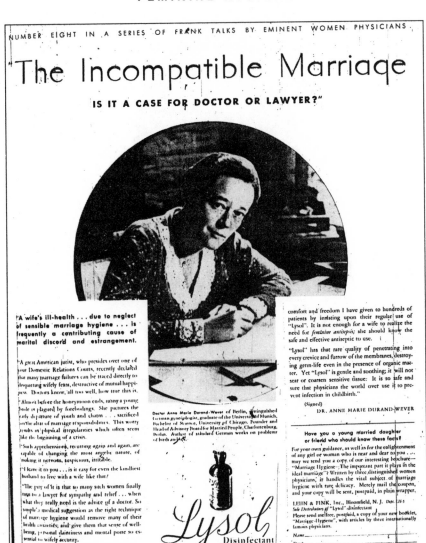

19. Although ads insisted otherwise, the stern-looking women who warned of the physical and psychological dangers of female fears of pregnancy were not physicians

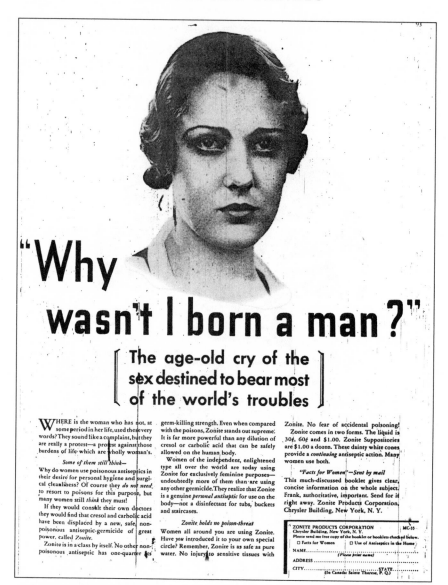

"Why wasn't I born a man?"

[The age-old cry of the sex destined to bear most of the world's troubles]

WHERE is the woman who has not, at some period in her life, used these very words? They sound like a complaint, but they are really a protest—a protest against those burdens of life which are wholly woman's.

Some of them still think—

Why do women use poisonous antiseptics in their desire for personal hygiene and surgical cleanliness? Of course they *do not need* to resort to poisons for this purpose, but many women still *think* they must!

If they would consult their own doctors they would find that cresol and carbolic acid have been displaced by a new, safe, non-poisonous antiseptic-germicide of great power, called *Zonite*.

Zonite is in a class by itself. No other non-poisonous antiseptic has one-quarter its germ-killing strength. Even when compared with the poisons, Zonite stands out supreme. It is far more powerful than any dilution of cresol or carbolic acid that can be safely allowed on the human body.

Women of the independent, enlightened type all over the world are today using Zonite for exclusively feminine purposes—undoubtedly more of them than are using any other germicide. They realize that Zonite is a genuine *personal antiseptic* for use on the body—not a disinfectant for tubs, buckets and staircases.

Zonite holds no poison-threat

Women all around you are using Zonite. Have *you* introduced it to your own special circle? Remember, Zonite is as safe as pure water. No injury to sensitive tissues with Zonite. No fear of accidental poisoning! Zonite comes in two forms. The liquid is 30¢, 60¢ and $1.00. Zonite Suppositories are $1.00 a dozen. These dainty white cones provide a *continuing* antiseptic action. Many women use both.

"Facts for Women"—Sent by mail

This much-discussed booklet gives clear, concise information on the whole subject. Frank, authoritative, important. Send for it right away. Zonite Products Corporation, Chrysler Building, New York, N. Y.

ZONITE PRODUCTS CORPORATION MC-55
Chrysler Building, New York, N. Y.
Please send me free copy of the booklet or booklets checked below.
□ Facts for Women   □ Use of Antiseptics in the Home
NAME..
(Please print name)
ADDRESS...
CITY.........................STATE.............
(In Canada: Sainte Therese, P. Q.)

---

20. Feminine hygiene advertisements portrayed antiseptic solutions and suppositories as the key to female liberation

than misleading. It was fraudulent. An AMA investigation found that none of the "eminent" gynecologists whose superlative words the ads quoted existed.

While insisting that women defer to medical opinion when choosing birth control, contraceptive ads simultaneously celebrated the tremendous "power" women wielded in the consumer market. Women who heeded physicians' advice and purchased "scientific" birth control were intelligently harnessing the advances of modern medicine to promote their own liberation. An ad by the Zonite Products Corporation claimed that birth control was not only a matter of pragmatism but also a "protest against those burdens of life which are wholly woman's." When it came to as important an issue as birth control, Zonite explained, the modern woman was not interested in the "timid thoughts of a past generation"; her goal was "to *find out* and *be sure*." It was no surprise, the company boasted, that Zonite hygiene products were favored by "women of the independent, enlightened type all over the world."[41]

Feminine hygiene manufacturers' creation of a mass market depended not only on effective advertising but also on the availability of advertised goods. Prospective customers needed quick, convenient, and multiple access to contraceptives. Manufacturers made sure they had it. Flooding a wide array of commercial outlets with their merchandise, companies guaranteed that contraceptives became a commodity within everyone's reach. Condoms were sold in locations where men were most likely to congregate; women were targeted in more conventional female settings—in stores and in the home.[42]

The five-and-dime store became the leading distributor of female contraceptives in the 1930s. By the mid-1930s, women could purchase feminine hygiene products at a number of national chains, including Woolworth, Kresge, McLellan, and W. T. Grant.[43] Already fashioned as a women's space, stores established sequestered "personal hygiene" departments where women could shop in a dignified and discreet manner for contraceptives and other products related to female reproduction such as sanitary napkins and tampons. Stores emphasized the exclusively female environment as the personal hygiene department's finest feature. The self-contained department was not only separated from the rest of the store, where "uncontrollable factors . . . might make for . . . embarrassment," but also staffed solely by saleswomen trained in the "delicate matter of giving confidential and intimate personal advice to their clients." As one store assured female readers in the local newspaper: "Our Personal Hygiene Department [Has] Lady Attendants On Duty at All Times." Female clerks, furthermore, were instructed to respect the private nature of the department's transactions; sensitive, knowledgeable, and tactful, they were "understanding wom[e]n with whom you may discuss your most personal and intimate problems."[44]

Contraceptive manufacturers actively promoted the creation of personal hygiene departments by emphasizing to store owners and managers the revenues their establishments would generate. Advertisements in retailing trade journals such as *Chain Store Age* recounted a plethora of feminine hygiene sales success stories; although the ads varied, they conveyed the same good news: selling feminine hygiene guaranteed a higher volume of customers and sales. The Zonite Products Corporation warned retailers not to miss out on the hygiene bonanza. "Did you know that feminine hygiene sales are six times greater than combined dentifrice sales?" one Zonite ad queried. "You'll be amazed [at] the way your sales and profits . . . will soar by simply establishing a feminine hygiene department. By this simple plan, many dealers have tripled volume almost overnight." Zonite offered free company consultations and sales training to encourage store managers to establish hygiene departments. Other firms with the same goal in mind sent complimentary counter displays, dispensing stands for "impulse sales and quick service," and window exhibits that could be strategically placed "where women predominate in numbers." The establishment of hygiene departments committed stores to the long-term retailing of feminine hygiene products, while the dignified decorum of departments lent an air of credibility and legitimacy to the products themselves.[45]

Manufacturers reasoned that many prospective female customers would not buy feminine hygiene products in a store. Many did not live close enough to one, and others, notwithstanding the store's discretion, might be uncomfortable with the public nature of the exchange. To eliminate regional and psychological obstacles to birth control buying, companies sold feminine hygiene to women directly in their homes. Selling contraceptives by mail was one such method. Mail-order catalogues, including those distributed by Sears, Roebuck and Montgomery Ward, continued to offer a full line of female contraceptives; each catalogue contained censored ads supplied by manufacturers. As a reward for bulk sales, mail-order houses received a discount from firms whose products they sold. Other manufacturers bypassed jobbers and encouraged women to send their orders directly to the company through conveniently supplied forms. To eliminate the possibility of embarrassment, ads typically promised that the order would be delivered in a "plain wrapper."[46]

To create urban and working-class markets, dozens of firms hired door-to-door sales representatives. All representatives were women, a deliberate attempt on manufacturers' part to profit from the notion that, as one company put it, "There are some problems so intimate that it is embarrassing to talk them over with a doctor."[47] The strategy also cashed in on public acceptance of itinerant nurses, who were the phalanx of the public health movement. At the Dilex Institute of Feminine Hygiene, for example, five female crews, each headed by a female manager, combed the streets of New York. The cornerstone of the company's marketing scheme was an aggressive sales pitch delivered by saleswomen dressed as nurses. As *Fortune* magazine discovered in an undercover investigation, however, the Dilex canvassers had no medical background. In fact, the only qualification required for employment was previous door-to-door sales experience. Despite their lack of credentials, however, newly hired saleswomen were instructed to assume the role of the medical professional, a tactic the institute reasoned would gain customers' trust, respect, and dollars. "You say you're a nurse, see?" one new recruit was told. "That always gets you in." Canvassers walked from house to house delivering by memory the standard Dilex sales speech:

> Good Morning. I am the Dilex Nurse, giving short talks on feminine hygiene. It will take only three minutes. Thank you—I will step in.
>
> Undoubtedly you have heard of many different methods of feminine hygiene, but I have come to tell you of THE DILEX METHOD, which is so much more simple and absolutely sure and harmless, and which EVERY woman is so eager to learn about and have without delay.

At one time this was a very delicate subject to discuss,
but today with all our modern ideas, we look at this vital
subject as one of the most important of all time, and for
that reason, we call to acquaint you with THIS GREAT
SECRET, a most practical, convenient way.

The Dilex Method meets every protective and hygienic
requirement. It is positive and safe and may be used with
the utmost confidence. Each item has been given the most
careful thought to fit the increasing strides in feminine hygiene. . . . ABSOLUTE FEMININE PROTECTION is assured.[48]

The saleswoman then attempted to peddle the company's top-of-the-line
contraceptive kit. For seven dollars, a woman could purchase jelly, a
douching outfit, an antiseptic douche capsule, and—most alarming of
all—a "one-size-fits-all" diaphragm. Poverty, women were told, was not
an impediment to the personal happiness the company was selling, for
the Dilex kit was available on the installment plan.[49]

Lanteen Laboratories of Chicago was bolder still. It double-dipped,
marketing fitted diaphragms to the medical profession and one-size cap
diaphragms to women directly through door-to-door and drugstore retailing and at company clinics that "prescribed" Lanteen products exclusively. Lanteen's clinics operated in Chicago, Detroit, and Milwaukee
and were modeled after Sanger's. They claimed to be nonprofit and to
prescribe "sure, safe, scientific methods," such as those used in European
clinics. Each bore the auspicious name Medical Bureau of Information
and employed an all-female staff who hosted weekly lectures on "plain
and complete medical information [about] the best scientific method of
birth control."[50] At the end of the talks, women were encouraged to try
Lanteen's color-coded products: the BLUE, a jelly for the young wife; the
RUSSET, a sanitary sponge; the YELLOW, "a particularly pleasant and
soothing douche solution" that doubled as a "general household antiseptic"; or the top-of-the-line BROWN, an "easily inserted and self-
locating" rubber-cap-diaphragm-jelly set purported to "fit all normal
anatomies."[51]

Medical Bureaus of Information also wooed customers through mailing schemes. In Chicago, for example, where the bureau was opened in

1929, Lanteen acquired lists of women who had recently given birth at county hospitals. The company sent each new mother a letter requesting her presence at the Medical Bureau of Information to discuss "the welfare of her baby." In one case, a twenty-two-year-old new mother complied. At the bureau, she was greeted by a woman dressed as a nurse who "entered into a lengthy discussion with her on birth control, its desirability and the various means of accomplishment." At a cost of six dollars (three for the device, three for printed instructions), the young woman received one of Lanteen's universally sized diaphragms—the only brand the clinics sold. Home insertion was painful. She complained to the bureau, but the baking soda and laxatives they recommended for relief did not help. The woman was eventually admitted to Cook County Hospital, where the 3.5-inch diaphragm was extracted with forceps from her urethra.[52]

For the "benefit" of those who could not reach company clinics, Lanteen sold a booklet, *Birth Control: Plain Medical Information*, instructing women how to prevent conception with Lanteen products. One pamphlet warned customers away from other brands. "The Medical Bu-

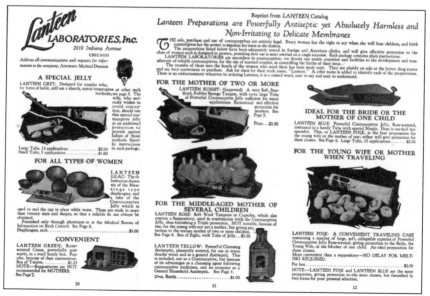

21. Lanteen's color-coded contraceptives promised formfitting birth control "for all types of women"

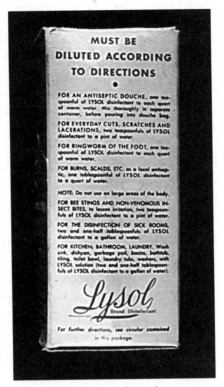

22. After disinfecting themselves, women could use Lysol to clean the garbage pail and toilet bowl

reau," it cautioned, "has found that nearly all of the many preparations on the American market which are offered, generally for some camouflaged purpose but presumably for the prevention of conception, are inadequate or worthless."[53]

Authorship of this best-selling pamphlet was attributed to Norman Carr of London, a medical doctor whose photograph on the front cover bore the requisite badges of scientific respectability: distinguished looking, gray-haired, middle-aged. A subsequent investigation found that Carr was a fictitious name. The man pictured on the cover was not a physician but a professional model whose photograph Lanteen obtained from the stock collection of an advertising agency. But American women had no way of knowing this. By the late 1930s, Lanteen Laboratories had sold, at a cost of ten cents each, more than fourteen million copies of the pamphlet in twenty-six editions. By 1942, Lanteen had become one of the two leading diaphragm-and-jelly firms in the country.[54]

Without lay guides or professional organizations to help them distinguish between reality and hyperbole, contraceptive consumers could hardly be blamed for embracing the over-the-counter trade. Among the many groups unwilling to expose the hucksterism and fraud of the feminine hygiene bonanza were the AMA and the federal government. The AMA established a propaganda department in 1913, which it renamed the Bureau of Investigation in 1925. Its goal was to disseminate information on nostrums and quackery. Only rarely, though, did the bureau address women's feminine hygiene inquiries. From the 1930s to the early 1960s, women who contacted the bureau about feminine hygiene were advised to "seek information on these products from your family physicians. As you perhaps know, the giving of information on contraceptives through the mails is an improper use thereof."[55] AMA inertia in this important area of public health was tied as much to concerns over professional neutrality as to the law. The medical organization, mindful of ongoing controversy regarding birth control, disavowed any responsibility for its distribution, sale, and use. The bureau told one woman who implored the AMA to denounce the feminine hygiene racket that the "American Medical Association is a scientific organization. It has no punitive power and wants none."[56]

The FDA was not in a strong position to rally to consumers' aid. Authorized to take action only against product mislabeling, it was powerless to suppress birth control manufacturers' rhetorically veiled claims. The FDA began to monitor condom quality in 1938, but its goal was to lower rates of VD transmission, not to protect the health of contraceptive consumers. Birth control fell outside the FDA's jurisdiction. As the chief of the agency's drug division informed one concerned consumer in 1938, the FDA "defines a drug . . . as any substance or mixture of substances intended to be used for the cure, mitigation or prevention of disease of either man or other animals." But pregnancy was not a disease; "articles intended solely for contraceptive use are not drugs as that term is used in the Act, and we have therefore had no occasion to make any investigation of their efficacies."[57]

The dangers and deficiencies of feminine hygiene products were well known in the health community. Concerned pharmacists, physicians, and birth control advocates routinely reviewed and condemned commercial preparations. Manufacturers' grandiose claims aside, not all contraceptives were created alike. For example, although safe and reliable spermicidal jellies, such as those made by Holland-Rantos and Ortho Products, were available and recommended by clinics and private physicians, ineffective jellies outnumbered them. Of the 189 contraceptive jellies on the American market in 1940, only a handful were found to be safe and spermicidal in laboratory tests.[58]

Critics reserved their harshest comments for the most popular, affordable, and least reliable female contraceptive, the antiseptic douche. By 1940, the commercial douche had become the most popular birth control method in the country, favored by women of all classes. It would remain the leading female contraceptive until 1960, when a breakthrough technology—oral contraceptives—knocked it off its lofty pedestal.[59] An inexpensive alternative to male and medical methods, the antiseptic douche was ineffective, even dangerous. Scores of douching preparations, though advertised as modern medical miracles, contained nothing more than water, cosmetic plant extracts, and table salt. On the other hand, many others, including the most popular brand, Lysol disinfectant, were soap solutions containing cresol (a constituent of crude carbolic acid, a distillate of coal and wood), which, when used in too high a concentration, caused severe inflammation, burning, and even death.[60] The Lysol douche did not prevent pregnancy; a 1933 study undertaken at Newark's Maternal Health Center, for instance, found that 250 out of 507 women who used Lysol for birth control became pregnant.[61]

Marketed under the proprietary name Lysol since the 1890s, the disinfectant, first used for medical antisepsis, was popularized in the second decade of the twentieth century by Lehn & Fink's advertising blitz, which targeted women and highlighted the product's versatile disinfectant properties.[62] Lysol was a caustic poison and in more concentrated form was retailed with a prominent skull-and-crossbones icon. Ingested, it could kill; applied externally, it irritated and burned. Lehn & Fink sold it for feminine hygiene anyway, ignoring a recommendation made by the 1912 Council on Pharmacy and Chemistry of the AMA that companies not advertise to the laity disinfectants, germicides, and antiseptics for application to the eye, gastrointestinal tract, or genitourinary tract. By

1911, doctors had recorded 193 Lysol poisonings, including 21 suicides, 1 homicide, and 5 deaths from uterine irrigation. In 1915, a Chicago man killed his wife, who had just given birth to their child, when, confusing Lysol with her regular medicine, he gave her the toxic substance to drink. As Lysol became more commercially widespread, injury and death rates grew. Coroners in New York City reported 40 suicidal and 4 accidental Lysol deaths in 1925 alone.[63]

Advertising downplayed the potential for injury by drawing attention to antiseptics' claimed gentleness and versatility. Ads praising Lysol's safety on "delicate female tissues" also encouraged the money-wise consumer to use the antiseptic as a gargle, nasal spray, household cleaner, and dressing for burns. Despite contradictory evidence, Lehn & Fink continued to insist that its best-selling douche was reliable, "convenient, and not poisonous or irritating." Similarly, the makers of PX, a lesser-known brand, sold liquid disinfectant that ads claimed could be used interchangeably for "successful womanhood" or athlete's foot.[64]

This strategy won sales by jeopardizing women's health. Even one-time douching was a potentially deleterious act, but women, guided by the logical assumption that "more was better," strove to beat the pregnancy odds by increasing the frequency of their douching and the concentration of the solution used. In one case, a nineteen-year-old married woman relied on regular douching with dissolved bichloride of mercury tablets for birth control. Eager to avoid pregnancy, she doubled the dose and douched "several times daily." Her determination landed her in a doctor's office, where she was diagnosed with acute vaginal and cervical burns. In what must have seemed a grave injustice, she also learned she was pregnant.[65]

Reports on douche-related deaths and injuries and the general ineffectiveness of popular commercial contraceptives failed to prod the medical profession to take a resolute stand against the contraceptive scandal. Nor, regrettably, did blistering indictments of manufacturing fraud trickle down to the lay press, where they might have enabled women to make informed contraceptive choices. In advertising text and in many women's minds, the euphemism "feminine hygiene" continued to signify reliable contraception. For unscrupulous manufacturers eager to profit from this identification, "feminine hygiene" continued to be a convenient term invoked to sell products devoid of contraceptive value.

Manufacturers absolved themselves of culpability by reminding critics that, by the letter of the law, their products were not being sold as contraceptives. If women incurred injuries or became pregnant while using feminine hygiene for birth control, it was not the fault of manufacturers. The Norwich Pharmacal Company, for example, manufacturers of Norforms, the most popular brand of vaginal suppositories in the country, deployed precisely such an argument to justify its advertising policy. Norform suppositories were advertised exclusively as "feminine hygiene," a term that the company's vice president Webster Stofer conceded had become synonymous with contraception in many women's minds. All the same, Stofer insisted, Norforms were not sold as birth control. Asked why the company did not then change its marketing slogan to avoid misunderstanding, Stofer expressed his regret that it was "too late" to advertise suppositories as anything else. "The term has become too closely associated with Norforms," he contended. "And anyway, we have our own definition of it."[66]

Women harmed by Lysol were doubly victimized by Lehn & Fink's refusal to take responsibility for the suffering its product inflicted. In 1935, the company defended itself in a lawsuit filed by one douche victim by arguing that the burns the woman had incurred could only have been triggered by "an allergy to Lysol." Lehn & Fink was blameless, for the company was "not under a duty to foresee that the particular individual would have an allergy."[67] In a 1941 case of vaginal scalding, the company hid behind weak government regulations to assert its innocence. Lehn & Fink regretted that a customer was hurt, but Lysol's packaging and directions were "in accordance with the requirements made of us by the Food and Drug Administration."[68]

As evidence about the hazards of its antiseptic douche mounted, Lehn & Fink continued to deny wrongdoing and to refuse to admit that it was in the contraceptive business. But it changed its formula in 1952 to substitute orthohydroxydiphenyl for cresol, which some researchers had come to believe was carcinogenic. FDA bacteriologists found the new solution to be "about one-fourth as toxic as the old" but still potentially lethal if swallowed by a young child.[69] The change left Lehn & Fink free to advertise Lysol as a germicide—a fact FDA scientists could not refute—"ideal" for the toilet bowl, ringworm, and sunburns and as an antiseptic douche for feminine hygiene. The new-and-improved solution did not shield women from injury or pregnancy. In 1961, a Lysol douche caused one woman's vagina to blister and bleed. Her husband, armed with her physician's report, complained to Lehn & Fink. The company's vice president admitted that feminine hygiene had long been one of Lysol's "major applications." He boasted that "millions of [Lysol] douches are being applied at regular intervals" across the country. What was astonishing was the company's defense. "Your report is the first of its kind on record," he informed the husband, in a striking example of corporate amnesia.[70]

Not every manufacturer of feminine hygiene products fared as well as Lehn & Fink. In the late 1930s, the Federal Trade Commission (FTC), which regulated product advertising to promote fair business practices, began to crack down on the feminine hygiene trade, issuing dozens of cease-and-desist orders to manufacturers. The FTC's actions did much to promote consumers' contraceptive health. But the regulatory assault occurred at the expense of small-business people, who had neither the financial muscle nor the political clout to repel it. Theirs was not always the best birth control available, but it was often no worse than what larger firms and "ethical" outfits made.

One businessperson adversely affected was Rosemarie Lewis, the founder and president of Certane Company, a Los Angeles feminine hygiene firm. Her tale is not the usual subject of business history, which has emphasized entrepreneurs who became captains of industry, not those who failed or just made do. Yet it is precisely Lewis's struggle, what she lost rather than what she gained, that reveals the dynamics of the birth control business in an era of flux. Understanding Lewis's commercial failure, we begin the long task of reclaiming a history of businesspeople—particularly women and minorities—who through prejudice and circumstance were unable to become titans of their trade.

History is about people, individuals who are agents of change and individuals who are powerless to stop it. The story of contraceptive corporatization involved both. Behind the seemingly faceless forces of regulation, technological innovation, and modernization, women and men fought to hold on to their livelihoods during an era of profound social and industrial transformation. Some succeeded, and others were ruined as the industry was transfigured. Like Rosemarie Lewis, all would learn that in history, timing is everything.

Lewis's story begins in Los Angeles. The city was home to 1.2 million people when Lewis founded Lewis Laboratories in November or December 1929 and began selling tubes of contraceptive jelly.[71] The move was bold and potentially risky. California law frowned on medical quackery, and its restrictions on birth control and abortion, passed in 1874 and not revised until 1931, were among the toughest in the country. Merely advertising contraceptives was a felony.

But paper laws were no match for the droves of lay practitioners who called L.A. home. Some said the climate was to blame. After ninety days of warmth and sunshine, the souls of "frozen folk of Vermont and Wisconsin" just melted, and they began to crave "something more exotic, if not more erotic, than the frigid stuff to which they have been accustomed."[72] L.A.'s streets teemed with chiropractors and more osteopaths than any other city in the country. According to one critic in 1933, "Any yeomancer, soothsayer, holy jumper, herbdoctor, whirling dervish, snake-charmer, medicater, tables turner, or Evil Eye—practicing any form of blackmagic, demonology, joint-jerking, witchcraft, thauma turgy, spirit-rapping, back-rubbing, physical torture, or dietetical novelty—any such will find assured success and prosperity in L.A. despite fierce competition."[73]

In this mecca of proselytism, Lewis set up shop, upholding a tradition of female contraceptive entrepreneurship that dated at least as far back as Sarah Chase, the single mother whose sale of contraceptive syringes in New York enraged Anthony Comstock. Like Chase, Lewis was her own breadwinner. Recently divorced from Max Lewis, she remained friends with her ex-husband and, in 1934, entrusted him with the management of a branch office she opened in Chicago. But the business was her doing, her initiative. She had never run one before. But in late 1929 she needed a job to survive.[74]

The Depression had just begun, but in the winter of 1929 many Americans remained optimistic. From the presidential pulpit, Republican Herbert Hoover dished out assurances of economic salvation the way mothers dished out morning porridge. "The crisis will be over in sixty days," he vowed in March 1930. In June, when it wasn't, he reassured voters that "the worst is over without a doubt." Hoover's words offered mainly false hopes to the growing contingent of unemployed, hungry, and homeless Americans, although a few people, like Lewis, initially experienced the Depression as a time of unparalleled prosperity.

By the time Americans elected Franklin Delano Roosevelt in 1932 and ended more than a decade of Republican rule, the great migration to California had begun. By 1940, it had increased the state's population by more than a million. With its bountiful land and resources, California became the final stop on a journey made by families from around the country, especially from the ravaged dust-bowl states of Texas, Arkansas, and Oklahoma.[75]

Los Angeles alone took in more than 100,000 migrants, although the city was not untouched by the Depression's cruelest blows. Between 1929 and 1933, the total amount of wages paid in the city was cut by almost half, the number of wage earners by 21 percent. Yet L.A. was more resilient than most cities. Its economy was young and diversified. Motion pictures, petroleum, rubber, meatpacking, auto assembly, women's garments—this diversity afforded the city a degree of protection, an ability to weather economic vicissitudes that devastated other towns.[76]

It was a city where a working woman was a familiar sight. This was true across the land, of course, as hundreds of thousands of women sustained family incomes by taking in laundry, dressmaking, and boarders and by opening up "household beauty parlors, cleaning and pressing enterprises, grocery stores, and the like."[77] Indeed, studies of women's work during the Depression have shown that the rigid sex typing of the 1920s, which funneled women's labor into nonmanufacturing occupations, cushioned the impact of the economic contraction that followed. But Los Angeles was more accommodating to women's occupational needs than most. In 1933, married women had a better chance of being gainfully employed in L.A. than in any of the twelve largest cities in the country.[78]

Rosemarie Lewis was among the city's army of women workers and one of hundreds of newcomers to the contraceptive business. The economics of austerity attracted small-business people to the industry, where, as *Fortune* magazine put it, they "discovered that birth control products could be produced at a quick and enormous profit with very little capital investment."[79] Of the four hundred known businesses making female contraceptives and feminine hygiene products in 1938, most were founded in the early Depression. Aided by a local chemist, Lewis began manufacturing antiseptic jellies and powders soon after the great crash. She had no formal schooling but was not uneducated. "I get a lot of different books and read up and try to be intelligent about it," she told the FTC.[80] In 1930, she renamed her business, of which she remained sole owner, the Certane Company—a good name for a firm that pledged to put women's minds at ease about pregnancy prevention.

By 1935, Certane had added suppositories, douching syringes, a one-size cervical cap, and diaphragms of varying sizes to its product list. The company made douching powder and jelly at its L.A. headquarters and diaphragms in its Chicago office. The Certane diaphragm—retailed as the Dia-Dome—came in sizes 47.5 to 100 millimeters. "We have a form and a mold for each," Charles Luntz, the company manager, explained, "and that form is dipped into liquid latex."[81] Other products were manufactured through outsourcing and then repackaged. Vaginal cones came from a local drug compounder, cervical caps from an L.A. rubber company. B. F. Goodrich made the rubber tubing on the douche shields, Kensington Glass Works the glass applicators used with the douching powders, and the Seamless Rubber Company of New Haven, Connecticut, the rubber bulb that attached to the glass applicators. With most products made off-site, Certane's labor force stayed small, comprising six employees and five traveling salesmen in 1938.[82]

By 1938, Lewis had carved out a birth control empire whose annual sales were between fifty-five thousand and sixty thousand dollars (at a time when few women earned over five thousand dollars).[83] Like other feminine hygiene manufacturers, she counted on advertising to familiarize women shoppers with the Certane name. Advertisements urging women to write for product information were published in numerous local newspapers such as *The Indianapolis News* and the Camden, New Jersey, *Courier-Post* and national periodicals such as *Motion Picture Magazine*. Lewis also circulated glossy pamphlets—*Women's Secrets, A Confidential Discussion of Feminine Hygiene*—brimming with customer testimonials "cheerfully written by satisfied users of Certane marriage hygiene products."[84] They were sent to druggists for store-counter promotion and to prospective women customers, identified by letters of inquiry and by engagement and "new mother" announcements in newspapers. The volume of promotional materials Certane mailed was considerable.

In one week in 1941, the Los Angeles postmaster counted 10,200 pieces.[85]

Lewis relied on the same phraseology employed by other feminine hygiene manufacturers to promote her wares. Certane diaphragms, cones, jellies, and powders were "preferred by doctors and thousands of women everywhere." They were "safe and dependable" and "easy to apply." "Endorsed by medical science," they gave women the "proper technique in modern feminine hygiene."[86]

By the time the FTC investigated the Certane Company in 1938, Lewis had climbed a long way up the industry ladder. Her company was not the leading distributor of feminine hygiene products and rubber pessaries, but it was probably among the top twenty. Lewis herself felt she had made it to the big leagues. She identified her primary competitors as Lanteen, Johnson & Johnson, and Holland-Rantos, not the smaller outfits that, according to one Planned Parenthood report, were plentiful and "buzzing [around] like bees."[87]

FTC records do not identify who filed a complaint against Certane, but at first glance, any of these large firms seem likely candidates. The FTC was established in 1914 by an act of Congress to promote competitive interstate commerce by investigating persons, partnerships, or corporations accused of practicing "unfair methods of competition," such as false or misleading advertising. Businesses the FTC determined to be in violation of the act were issued cease-and-desist orders, which a U.S. circuit court of appeals was empowered to enforce, set aside, or modify.[88] In theory, the FTC promoted fair play and restored competition to an economy increasingly marked by concentrated power. In practice, it often functioned as corporate capitalism's handmaiden, censoring the practices of smaller businesses that established firms considered threats.[89]

The FTC did not subject contraceptive companies to investigation until after the 1936 ruling *United States* v. *One Package* permitted doctors in every state (unless forbidden by local laws) to acquire contraceptive information and articles through the mails. The test case was arranged by Margaret Sanger, who had Dr. Hannah Stone, the director of the Birth Control Clinical Research Bureau, import 120 Japanese pessaries for medical use. Customs officials, prenotified of the shipment, seized the pessaries and charged Stone with violating the Tariff Act, an outgrowth of the Comstock Law that forbade the importation of "any article whatever for the prevention of conception by all persons." In his decision, Judge Grover Moscowitz of the District Court for the Southern District of New York read a distinction between legitimate and illegitimate use into the otherwise uncompromising wording of the Tariff Act. "From a medical standpoint," he ruled, "there are various types of cases in which it is necessary to prescribe a contraceptive to cure or prevent disease." To save lives, doctors must have the right to obtain contraceptives unfettered by government interference. Moscowitz declared the articles of contention—in this case, diaphragms—legally neutral rather than inherently obscene (as the Comstock Law had done). The test of criminality was intended use, evidenced by the character and class of distributors involved. One Package, affirmed on appeal by Judge Augustus Hand, exempted physicians from prosecution and asserted the legality of contraceptive commerce operated by and for doctors. The decision liberated the birth control business from its most oppressive legal shackles even as it excluded nonmedical professionals, like Lewis, from participation.[90]

The ruling was a coup d'état for Margaret Sanger, whose National Committee on Federal Legislation for Birth Control had lobbied since 1929 for federal laws to exempt doctors who prescribed contraceptives from criminal prosecution. Unsuccessful in the legislative arena, Sanger claimed victory in the courts and disbanded the committee in 1937. The court's decision was also a victory for "ethical" female contraceptive manufacturers such as Holland-Rantos and Julius Schmid, which sold diaphragms and jellies exclusively for use by medical prescription. But it was a blow to businesspeople such as Lewis, whose more liberal sales policy underlay Certane's success and violated the court's definition of commercial legitimacy. More obstacles were placed in Lewis's path in 1938, when Congress passed the Wheeler-Lea Act, making it a misdemeanor for any person, partnership, or corporation to disseminate false or misleading advertisements of a device that would injure a person's health when used as advertised.[91]

One can imagine why, in this new environment, where medical birth control was legal, over-the-counter sales frowned upon, and the female contraceptive industry recklessly competitive, Holland-Rantos or Julius Schmid might be tempted to ask the FTC to initiate an investigation of the Certane Company, an unwanted and increasingly successful competi-

tor run by a woman "quack." But the scant paper trail that survives suggests it was the American Birth Control League (ABCL), which Sanger
had left in 1929, that was to blame. Eric Matsner, the ABCL medical director, was irate that the Certane Company advertised its douche "as of
the type prescribed by Dr. James F. Cooper . . . medical director of the
American Birth Control League." Aside from the fact that Matsner, not
Cooper (who had died in 1931), was the organization's medical director,
the ABCL had its reputation and nonprofit status to protect. Matsner
contacted the Certane Company, informing Lewis that her advertisement "was misleading. . . . The American Birth Control League does not
permit the use of its name or that of its Medical Director in the sales promotion of any contraceptive." Matsner also issued a warning: if the "implied endorsement" was not withdrawn, "the matter will be brought
before the Federal Trade Commission."[92] Matsner wrote the letter on
March 8, 1938. A complaint against Rosemarie Lewis and the Certane
Company was filed with the FTC on July 12, four months later.

The complaint against Lewis charged her with circulating advertisements that "are false and misleading and in truth and in fact said products do not form or constitute safe and competent remedies against
conception and are not a guarantee against pregnancy." If Certane's
products were found to be ineffective, the company was competing un-
fairly against those who made reliable birth control.[93]

Lewis denied the charges. The FTC hearing began on November 18,
1938, in a hotel in downtown Los Angeles. The commission called to
testify three expert witnesses, "three of the most prominent gynecologists
and obstetricians on the West Coast," each of whom disputed the safety
and reliability of Lewis's products. One physician, discussing the Certane
douche, warned that "if not accompanied by proper instructions and
properly handled [it] would be a very dangerous instrument to place in
the hands of a woman." He condemned Certane's self-fitted diaphragms
and refuted its assurances of pregnancy prevention by insisting that
"there is no guarantee of any description against pregnancy except absolute continence from intercourse."[94] He failed to mention that doctor-
recommended douches and contraceptives were a common, albeit not
universally endorsed, facet of American medical practice.

Lewis's defense was a familiar one. Her advertising practices, she argued, were identical to those of other, more established firms—she men-

tioned Schmid and Holland-Rantos as examples—whose actions went unnoticed. "While I realize that the mere fact that my competitors use certain phrases is not in itself sufficient reason to permit me to use similar phrases or make similar statements," she pleaded, "if I am to remain in competition, you can appreciate how vital it is that I should be granted the same latitude as my competitors."[95]

Lewis was right, but the FTC dismissed her claims as "being entirely without merit" and issued an order against Lewis and Certane "to cease representing directly or indirectly that the Certane preparations or appliances will prevent conception or prevent pregnancy or that they are safe, competent, or effective preventatives against conception."[96] Lewis was not so easily deterred. Complying with the FTC order, she edited out references to birth control in Certane advertising. But she continued to sell her douches, solutions, and diaphragms to druggists, jobbers, and mail-order consumers.

It was not enough to save her. In a 1942 case initiated by the U.S. Post Office, she was charged with conducting an unlawful business through the mails. This prosecution was not business as usual. It was personal. By the 1940s, Post Office investigations of contraceptive purveyors had become extremely rare. Moreover, the new charge contradicted the FTC's own finding that Certane goods were too ineffective to be considered contraceptives. It was a lose-lose situation: reprimanded for selling products not good enough to be considered birth control, Lewis was now being charged for selling identical products that were. Because Lewis had revised Certane ads to comply with the FTC's order, Post Office inspectors resorted to cloak-and-dagger techniques to exact even moderately damning evidence. Posing as contraceptive consumers, they sent Lewis thirteen unsolicited letters, which, reflecting the Post Office's efforts to allay citizens' concerns, were now called test correspondence rather than decoy letters. They were just as slyly and graphically written, and their objective, after so many decades, remained entrapment. All masqueraded as letters from laypersons, signaled by the deliberate and condescending use of ungrammatical language. One letter, allegedly sent from a Van G. Okie, Dampton, Kentucky, read:

> Mom and I gest got back from a visit with our boy Fred what lives on Lawndale Ave. Mebe youse no where that is.

Fred married a city girl about 3 yr. ago & they ain't got no childs. Mom turns out one ever year and ever time she says that the last. We got 9 now and 7 at home. Fred is the oldest. So I asks Fred how they aint got no childs running around and he says Pop you and mom were borned 40 yrs too soon and shows me all that stuff he got from youse to keep from having children. I don't no offen I can get mom to where that thar rubber thing but I ken shoot that stuff up her. Youse let me no what it costs, so I can git sum. Mom says hes done having kids but she gets pregnent mighty easy I tells yuh.

Van sent Lewis a money order for a three-dollar Dia-Cap jelly kit and a request: "If that [kit is] what mom needs to keep her from gittin pregnent youse send it."[97] Lewis sent Van the kit.

But did that act make Lewis a lawbreaker? This was the question. Lewis had not called the kit birth control, and as she told those at her hearing, Certane Jelly, the Dia-Cap, and the Dia-Dome were retailed as "pharmaceutical[s] and not for contraception." When asked whether Certane products possessed contraceptive attributes, she referred to the testimony of the FTC's expert witnesses to assert her innocence. "According to the FTC [they do] not," she insisted, "and according to their physicians. They had the finest and best in Los Angeles, and they said no."[98]

The Post Office decided otherwise. It issued a fraud order, suspending Lewis's right to conduct Certane's business through the mails. It was a lethal blow. Although Certane products are listed in a 1945 Consumer Union report, no mention of Rosemarie Lewis or the Certane Company appears in contraceptive literature from 1950. Like so many other small entrepreneurs in this age of federal regulation and business consolidation, Lewis just disappeared from the corporate map.

The government continued its campaign against feminine hygiene manufacturers, but the results were mixed. The FDA's insistence that contraceptives were not drugs, and thus not subject to its jurisdiction, left the FTC in charge of regulating contraceptive commerce. But the FTC's authority was limited, confined to the elimination of false and misleading advertising. This regulatory vacuum encouraged companies to resurrect euphemistic language to obfuscate the intended contraceptive use of their products. Punished for daring to label its products birth control, Lewis's business was eclipsed by established firms such as Lehn & Fink, which profited from keeping women customers uninformed about just how bad a contraceptive the Lysol douche was.[99] For too many women, the freedom, pleasure, and security pledged by manufacturers such as Lehn & Fink amounted to nothing more than empty promises.

EIGHT

Condom Kings

While the FTC investigated feminine hygiene products, court rulings and the FDA unleashed a tidal wave of government regulations and guidelines designed to rein in the masculine side of the over-the-counter racket: the condom business. Stricter regulations and the adoption of new manufacturing technologies transformed the condom trade, improving merchandise quality and reducing the number of producers involved. By the late 1940s, the small-scale condom entrepreneurs who had made sheaths by hand in small shops had become a thing of the past. In their stead stood corporate Goliaths, automatic assembly lines, and name-brand condoms meeting industry specifications set by Washington.

War, disease, and the 1918 Crane ruling, which legalized doctor-prescribed contraceptives used for the prevention of disease, gave the condom industry newfound respectability and an economic boost in the second and third decades of the twentieth century. Condom production and retail statistics paint a picture of sustained expansion and profits. In Baltimore, for instance, the number of condoms sold more than doubled between 1914 and 1928, jumping from 3 million to 6.25 million.[1] V. F. Calverton studied the condom industry's growth. "At no time before had there been this immense expansion of the business of manufacturing, distributing, and selling [condoms] as is to be noted with the War," he wrote in 1928. "What before was merely a profitable business, now became a matter for large-scale production . . . [with] all of the paraphernalia of an enormous industry."[2] By 1931, the top fifteen U.S. manufacturers produced 1.44 million condoms daily, mainly buff-toned rubbers made from Ceylonese or Javanese rubber.[3]

Sales from the feminine hygiene business eclipsed those of condoms in the 1930s, but the number of condom users grew as more Americans turned to over-the-counter methods to meet their pregnancy-prevention needs. The streamlined look and sleeker feel of second-generation rubbers boosted condom popularity. Newer models were "thin and silky"—sheerer than the "surgeon's glove and of better quality rubber"—less clunky and more sensitive, certainly, than traditional condoms stitched out of sheet rubber. They were cheaper too. Consequently, for the first time, Americans embraced the practice of onetime condom use, a significant improvement in pregnancy prevention over the recycled condom of the past. A standard seven and a half inches long (a length considered one and a half inches longer than the "typical" erect penis), the new American rubber was suavely packaged. Tucked in small aluminum and tin boxes or fake cigarette cases, rubbers could be concealed in a man's pocket, undetectable and ready for use.[4] By 1938, the American condom business was a thirty-eight-million-dollar industry sustained by men who spent, on average, twice as much on sheaths each year as on shaving creams.[5]

Two men who profited from the condom boom were Julius Schmid and Merle Youngs. Schmid had come a long way since his 1890 arrest. He had married. His wife, the former Elizabeth Wolf, was also a German immigrant who had arrived in New York in 1892 with two small boys from a previous marriage. Elizabeth had two more sons with Julius: Carl, born in 1897, and Julius junior, born in 1898. Both would be instrumental to the family's success. The Schmids lived in a large house they owned in Queens, New York. Their residence doubled as a boardinghouse, which Elizabeth ran with the help of a female servant. In 1900, the Schmids shared a roof with nine boarders, all male laborers, whose world Julius knew well.[6]

Schmid told census takers in 1900 that he worked as a cap manufacturer. Likely this was a ruse to shield him and his brood from trouble.

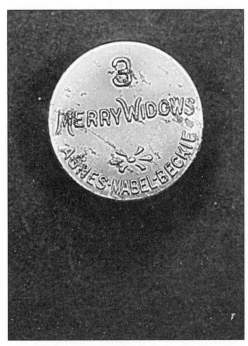

23. More than just a tin of rubbers, Merry Widows, popular in the 1920s, was an invitation to sexual play. "Proper" women waited until marriage to have intercourse, making widows Agnes, Mabel, and Beckie legitimately experienced and, better yet, available

Company letterhead would later boast that Schmid had been in the condom trade since 1883, a date consistent with surviving evidence.[7] Being a bootlegger, of course, necessitated deception. Lying about his job would have been commonplace for Schmid. As occupational aliases went, moreover, cap manufacturer was a good one, for the term "cap" had myriad meanings in turn-of-the-century America. In the vocabulary of prophylaxis, it referred to half-sized rubber or skin sheaths that sealed the tip of the penis. But it also referred to the capping skins that sealed perfume bottles, made out of caecum, the same material used for penis caps, full-length skins, and the sausage cases Julius had once prepared. Julius may have used caecum to make both kinds of merchandise. But if he did not, his self-identification as a cap manufacturer was linguistically shrewd, for it offered a convenient explanation for his unusual stash.

At the time of Comstock's death in 1915, Schmid had branched out into rubbers and launched what would become the company's signature Fourex line, soon to be supplemented by Paradise, Velveto, and the better-known Sheik and Ramses brands. Schmid made rubbers using the cold-cure cement technique, in which workers dipped glass formers into crepe rubber that had been milled and liquefied in a solvent, typically benzene, naphtha, or gasoline. Sheaths were then vulcanized at high temperatures. The technique had been widely used in condom manufacture in Germany since the 1880s, but Schmid was the first to popularize it in America.[8]

Whether manufacturing skins or rubbers, Schmid's guiding philosophy was the same. He believed that when it came to important issues such as contraception and disease prevention, consumers would be willing to pay more for merchandise that worked. Schmid's condoms were more expensive than most, but they were standardized, and tests performed in the 1930s found them to be safe and reliable. Early commitment to product quality helped Schmid cultivate a loyal consumer base and brand-name recognition, assets crucial to his long-term success.[9]

During World War I, Schmid's perseverance and business acumen paid off. Of all condom manufacturers in the United States, Schmid was

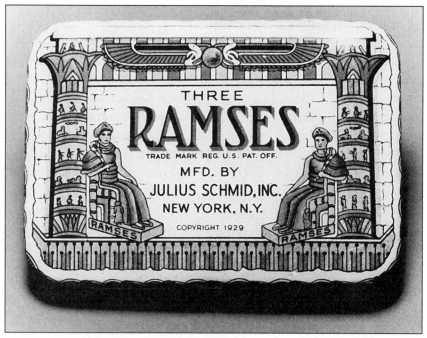

24. Ramses: Julius Schmid's flagship rubber condom, manufactured using the cold-cure cement technique (Courtesy of the Smithsonian Institution, NMAH/Science, Medicine, and Society)

best able to meet Allied needs, a demand for rubbers that the war had escalated and that Germany could no longer satisfy. In 1920, he was living the good life. He had moved his family to a house in Montgomery, New York, managed by a live-in staff of four: a secretary, cook, gardener, and servant.[10] Julius had incorporated his company in New York and bought a factory in Germany and another in Long Island City, Queens, where in 1927 a workforce of 150 made condoms. As prophylactic profits soared in the 1920s so, too, did Schmid's. He diversified production, branching out into the feminine side of the industry. He imported diaphragms from Germany for several years and then made arrangements in 1924 to begin their manufacture in New York.[11] Ramses diaphragms and jellies never became the cash cow condoms were. No one's diaphragms did. But in the prescription contraceptive market, they held their own against Holland-Rantos's Koromex brand. By 1932, Schmid had dismantled his German plant and reassembled it in Little Falls, New Jersey—a timely move that spared him the multiple misfortunes that would soon befall millions of German Jews.[12]

In 1938, in its first report on the birth control business, *Fortune* magazine pronounced Julius Schmid the undisputed king of the American condom empire. The formerly destitute German immigrant had achieved the American dream. A millionaire whose business earned him $900,000 per year, he had traded his wooden canes for the convenience of a mechanical wheelchair, which was loaded into his car, a Packard, whenever he traveled. Those travels had become increasingly infrequent. At age seventy-three, Julius retained his title as president and treasurer of Julius Schmid Inc. but depended increasingly on the administrative expertise of his sons, Carl and Julius junior. Both had been groomed in the contraceptive business from a young age and were up to the task. Indeed, after decades of innovation and expansion, the condom company remained strictly a family affair. Carl served as its vice president and treasurer, Julius junior as its secretary. Together, the three Schmids oversaw a business that spanned the globe and was one of the Depression's most profitable. The company imported lamb caeca from Australia and New Zealand to manufacture its XXXX, otherwise known as Fourex, skins. Branch offices in Chicago and San Francisco assisted with domestic sales and global distribution.[13]

Schmid's rags-to-riches ascent was an American success story, a bright and promising beacon in an otherwise enveloping fog of misery and economic despair. *Fortune* recounted only some of Julius's tale, neglecting, perhaps out of journalistic ignorance, perhaps out of deliberate calculation, to inform readers that Schmid the triumphant capitalist was also Schmidt the convicted criminal.

In 1938, the same year *Fortune* published its Schmid panegyric, the FDA began to inspect condoms. The move followed on the heels of a major court decision and the enactment of state statutes regulating the manufacture and sale of prophylactics preventing disease.

The regulatory ball began to roll in 1928, when Merle Youngs, president and treasurer of Youngs Rubber Corporation, makers of Trojans, sued C. I. Lee & Company, a jobber of medical supplies, for trademark infringement. Youngs, born in 1887, had entered the rubber-goods business as a young man but was a relative newcomer to the condom field. His company Fay & Youngs began to manufacture and sell Trojans, "prophylactic rubber articles for the prevention of contagious disease," in December 1916, ten years after Fay & Youngs had been founded. The war had treated Youngs well, as it had other condom makers. But once hostilities and the export trade were curtailed, he was stranded in a sea of competitors and saddled with surplus rubbers and renewed competition from Germany, whose companies wasted no time reclaiming their country's status as the Continent's leading condom producer.[14] In 1919, when he renamed the company Youngs Rubber, Merle Youngs was only one of dozens of condom entrepreneurs in the United States searching for a way of keeping their businesses afloat.[15]

Like other producers, Youngs's first response was to heighten domestic demand by making condoms more accessible to the common man. Legally protected by the 1918 Crane ruling, Youngs and other producers and jobbers sold their condoms, marked "for the prevention of disease only," in a cornucopia of male settings. Once whisper items typically acquired from a druggist or through the mails, condoms in the 1920s were sold by men of many trades: bellhops, elevator boys, street peddlers, barbers, bartenders, grocery clerks, razor-blade and tobacco merchants, waiters, tailors, filling-station attendants, bootblacks, students in fraternity houses, and operators of slot machines.[16] "Until 1915," Youngs later recalled, "I never heard of this class of goods being sold anywhere to the consumer, except in a drug store." After the Great War, however, con-

Look out for the Gift-bearing Pirate!

HE will offer you fat profits on Prophylactic Rubber Goods that are "sold only to drug stores." But he offers no protection; he does nothing to build up the druggist's business; he doesn't even give you a square deal. Instead, he sells the same goods he offers you, under another brand, to illegitimate people who steal away your profit, undermine your good will and ruin your reputation.

No druggist can compete against these illegitimate people . . . no self-respecting druggist will want to try . . . every druggist who wants his rightful part of this business must serve his customers with something the other people haven't got and cannot get. He must sell quality goods at a fair drug store price.

Shrewd druggists realize this; they concentrate on TROJAN BRAND. These goods provide exclusive advantages and superior quality features which are not even approached by any other brand offered to the drug stores of this country.

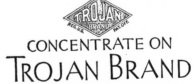

CONCENTRATE ON TROJAN BRAND

[ONE BRAND] [ONE QUALITY] [ONE POLICY]

We protect the druggist by selling only one brand; we have no other brands of these goods. Finest quality possible to manufacture; Guaranteed 100% Perfect. Sold to drug stores only, by responsible wholesale druggists and our own representatives.

Manufactured by

YOUNGS RUBBER CORPORATION, Inc.
145 Hudson Street, New York

25. After its court victory in 1930, Youngs Rubber promoted its Trojan trademark as an emblem of product superiority and commercial legitimacy

doms were "gypped around on street corners." Peddlers "would approach you on the street or in your office; barbers would approach you; you could get them in delicatessen stores, candy stores, tailor shops—every place, every conceivable place where a man might go to make a purchase, they would be offered to you."[17]

To distinguish himself from the competition, Youngs began in the mid-1920s to confine Trojan sales to the exclusive drugstore market. Trojans became the country's elite condom, a rubber available only from "ethical" druggists (who, ethics aside, turned a handsome profit on their sale). Youngs estimated in the thousands the number of "actual orders offered to us that had to be turned down on Trojan rubbers because [they came] from concerns not regarded as legitimate wholesale and retail druggists." Trojans cost about $1.50 per dozen and three for $.50, almost twice the price of bargain brands, such as Killian's Perma-Tex and Silvertex or Shunk's Texide, sold at non-drugstore outlets.[18] Triple-dipped and air-tested, Trojans cost more to make. But the primary reason for the high price was the druggist's add-on. Usually about 300 percent, price markups exceeding 2,000 percent were not unknown. "It is a common saying in the drug trade," noted the consumer economist Norman Himes in 1936, "that the sale of condoms pays the store rent."[19]

Youngs's exclusive retail policy sealed the loyalty of druggists, who touted the high price of Trojans as the consumer's guarantee of excellence. Of equal importance, the policy of exclusivity equipped Youngs with a marketing mechanism for distinguishing Trojans from generic "no-name" condoms. Merle Youngs wasted no time attacking his competition. Manufacturers and jobbers who sold condoms in bars and gas stations and on street corners had behaved "promiscuously," he complained. Because of their actions, the condom business "had been completely demoralized."[20]

In 1928, Merle Youngs filed suit against Clarence Lee in federal court, charging the New York jobber with infringing Youngs's Trojan trademark, awarded by the U.S. Patent Office the previous year. Youngs asked the court to issue an injunction to stop Lee's distribution of copycat Trojans. Lee had once enjoyed a business arrangement with Youngs as one of the company's jobbers, but Youngs had cut Lee off in 1924. Lee retaliated. He sold Trojans, stamping other companies' cheaper condoms with the Trojan label. This, then, was the crux of the dispute. Merle Youngs

cried piracy. Clarence Lee was a loathsome infringer, a "jobber of spuri-
ous Trojans." Lee called it tough luck; courts had never before upheld the
legitimacy of trademark protection for condoms. A lower court dismissed
the suit for lack of jurisdiction, the judge ruling that Youngs's business
was "contrary to public morals and an aid to and an encourager of lewdness and lechery" and hence was "sufficiently reprehensible to be outside
the field of equitable protection." The U.S. Court of Appeals for the Second Circuit, to which Youngs appealed, took a view more consistent
with newer ideas about disease prevention. Condoms were contraband
when they "promoted illicit sexual intercourse," but they were legal as
disease preventives. The test of legitimacy lay in the condoms' intended
use, not in their intrinsic nature. As such, the interstate trade, when
confined to *legitimate* medical and pharmaceutical outlets, was legal. Indeed, the court commended Merle Youngs's druggists-only distribution
policy, which it credited with uplifting an otherwise tawdry trade.[21]

The *Youngs* decision was significant for several reasons. First, by upholding the Trojan trademark, it legitimized the interstate condom business, providing manufacturers with an incentive to expand operations
and to adopt new production technologies to achieve economies of
scale. Second, mirroring larger efforts to eliminate medical quackery, the
court's decision delineated the parameters of dignified condom commerce. Replicating the class biases that had characterized criminal prosecutions against contraceptive purveyors since the 1870s, the court
distinguished members of established medical trades, namely physicians
and pharmacists, from over-the-counter vendors. Youngs Rubber's business was legal *only* because it confined Trojan sales to drugstores. Linking
legitimate use to retail venues, the court constructed an erroneous conception of the marketplace in which noble druggists sold condoms to
prevent disease whereas barbers, gas station attendants, and shoe shiners
sold them for illicit purposes such as birth control. The analysis was a
convenient fiction, but once it became the basis of the court's momentous decision, it helped reorganize the condom industry along these lines.

In addition, the *Youngs* decision encouraged companies such as
Youngs Rubber and Julius Schmid to treat brands as a basis for product
differentiation and consumer selection. Both Youngs Rubber and Schmid
hoped that the days of no-name rubbers would soon be behind them. In
1931, Julius Schmid applied to the U.S. Patent Office for trademark reg-

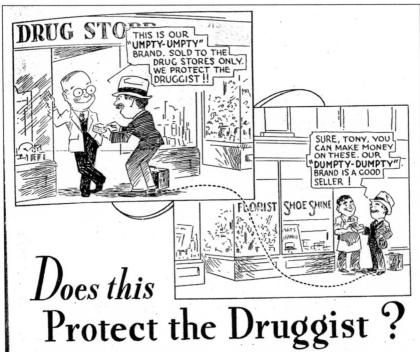

Does this
Protect the Druggist?

WHAT protection does "sold only to drug stores" offer on one brand of Prophylactic Rubber Goods when other brands, of like quality and from the same factory source, are supplied to illegitimate people who undersell the druggist and turn his customers against him?

The drug store should supply the largest part of the requirements of the neighborhood. But no druggist can hope to retain his customers' patronage if he supplies the same unsatisfactory quality that every peddler hands out. Shrewd druggists recognize this, and refuse to handle any goods that will not give absolute satisfaction and bring customers back. Every druggist's interest in this important part of his business should be far deeper than his immediate profit on the goods he offers his customers.

That is why thousands of druggists have concentrated their demands on Trojan Brand. The exclusive Trojan Brand advantages and superior Trojan Brand quality make these goods the safe, protected brand that will build legitimate business for any druggist; business which outside places cannot steal away.

ONE BRAND—ONE QUALITY—ONE POLICY —these are the Trojan Brand advantages which guarantee every druggist full protection, and freedom from undesirable competition. Concentrate on Trojan Brand — no other goods can rightfully offer you these Trojan Brand Advantages. Sold only by responsible wholesale Druggists and our own representatives. Ask your wholesale Salesman about the Trojan Plan for merchandising these goods.

Concentrate on

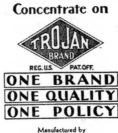

REG. U.S.   PAT.OFF.

ONE BRAND
ONE QUALITY
ONE POLICY

Manufactured by

**YOUNGS RUBBER
CORPORATION**

145 HUDSON STREET
NEW YORK CITY

26. Beginning in the late 1920s, Youngs Rubber allied itself with the drugstore trade. This policy paid off handsomely when subsequent government regulations restricted condom retailers to "ethical" vendors

istration of Fourex and Ramses, the company's most established brands.[22] Youngs Rubber, in turn, responded to its court victory by launching a yearlong advertising campaign in pharmaceutical trade journals celebrating Trojans' favored status and cautioning druggists to "beware the condom Pirate." In advertisements published in *Druggists' Circular* and *American Druggist*, the pirate was depicted as a man bearing "cheap, shoddy" merchandise who undermined druggists' authority by "offering customers unreliable sanitary rubber goods." Iconography highlighted the pirate's shady character, featuring him as either a lurking shadow or a businessman marked by a loudly patterned bandana, tooth decay, and oversize hoop earrings. His condom booty was stashed in a treasure chest that bore the telltale skull-and-crossbones insignia. This pirate meant trouble. "He sells the same goods he offers you," one ad warned, "under another brand to illegitimate people who steal away your profit, undermine your good will, and ruin your reputation."[23]

Even as the *Youngs* decision made brands more meaningful criteria for condom production and consumer purchase, technological innovations revolutionized how rubbers were made. Since Schmid had pioneered the cement-dipping technique in the United States, the chief problem condom manufacturers faced was fire hazard. Gasoline or benzene was required to break down and liquefy crude rubber, but both ingredients were highly flammable. To prevent a factory meltdown, condom makers had to avoid "fire, friction, of any kind, or a spark from a motor or a fan."[24] But even the best safety efforts could not ward off disaster. By 1930, Killian, Shunk, and Youngs Rubber had experienced devastating fires. One at Youngs Rubber in 1929 completely destroyed the factory's dipping room.[25]

Manufacturers earnestly searched for a technological way out of the problem. "We were very anxious to get away from the fire hazard," Merle Youngs recalled about the late 1920s. "The insurance was terrific, and you never knew when your plant was liable to go up in smoke."[26]

Latex and continuous assembly production offered solutions. By 1920, scientists had discovered a chemical formula that allowed latex—the milky liquid collected from rubber trees—to be transported uncoagulated in tin barrels from South America, India, and Indonesia. Latex was more expensive than crude rubber, but it was liquid in its natural state and not combustible. As companies such as U.S. Rubber began to distribute imported latex to American firms, condom companies experimented with techniques for transforming the substance into condoms. One man in the industry later recalled that from 1920 to 1930 "hundreds of the best brains in the country on latex and rubber were seeking to devise methods and apparatus" to allow the substitution of latex for rubber.[27]

Less flammable than crude rubber, latex was well suited to continuous assembly lines, which were already in use in the United States in the car, food, and textile industries. Manufacturers scrambled to be the first to apply this technology to latex condoms. Fred Killian of Akron, Ohio, reached the finish line first. Love showed him the way. In 1915, Killian married Elizabeth Terrell, who worked full-time rolling rings onto the open end of rubbers in a condom plant managed by her brother. After marriage, Killian worked for his brother-in-law, eventually striking out on his own. Killian had a flare for invention that was compounded by his wife's know-how. In 1926, he patented the first machine for the manufacture of a uniform condom ring. It went into immediate use throughout the industry and replaced the labor-intensive and time-consuming hand rolling. In 1930, after a relative died in a factory fire, Killian invented a condom assembly line that converted latex into finished condoms "automatically, rapidly, continuously and without the intervention of human hands."[28]

Killian's condom assembly line consisted of a five-hundred-foot-long conveyor belt that dipped glass molds into latex at the rate of one dip per second. After cylindrical brushes rolled a protective bead onto the open end of the condom, the condom was vulcanized in an overhead hot-air-and-water bath. Dried and dusted with talc, condoms were finally stripped with brushes from their formers and taken on continuous conveyor belts to an adjacent room where women workers manually unrolled and snapped the latex to remove wrinkles that might make the condom stick. This extraordinary machine, when operating around the clock, churned out eighteen hundred gross of condoms a day without danger to "life, limb, and property." It decreased production costs, and it generated rubbers that were thinner, more uniform, less susceptible to moisture, and longer lasting than cement-dipped condoms.[29]

It was a most marvelous machine—but only for those who could afford it. This excluded smaller outfits and prospective newcomers who could not pay the machine's hefty twenty-thousand-dollar price tag or Killian's leasing terms, which imposed a royalty fee of ten cents per gross. With the "patent situation," noted *Fortune* in 1938, "this industry has become concentrated in a few."[30] Flush with his court victory, Merle Youngs inspected Killian's machine in the early 1930s at Killian's Akron plant and "immediately entered into an arrangement to take one of those machines." He forked over the money, junked his old equipment, and watched the profits and output of Youngs Rubber soar. After installing Killian's machine in 1933, Youngs Rubber manufactured in a day what had previously taken a month.[31]

By the mid-1930s, the once volatile and competitive condom industry had been reduced to a handful of players. Leading the pack were Youngs Rubber, Julius Schmid, Killian, the Dean Rubber Manufacturing Company of North Kansas City, Missouri, and the Akron-based L. E. Shunk, headed by Louis Earl Shunk. By late 1937, when the FDA an-

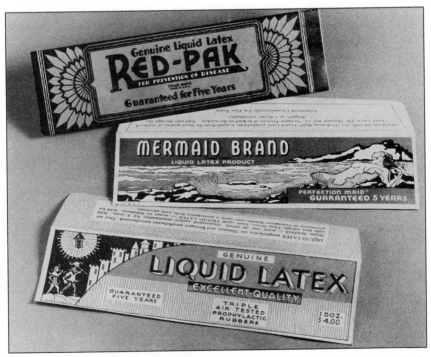

27. Latex rubbers, officially sold only for the prevention of disease (Courtesy of the Smithsonian Institution, NMAH/Science, Medicine, and Society)

nounced its plans to inspect condoms, these five stalwarts had taken control of over 90 percent of American condom production.[32]

Each firm succeeded by claiming different niches of what in 1937 remained a highly segmented market. Youngs Rubber stood behind the formula that had jetted Trojan to success: a reliable, premium-priced rubber sold exclusively to doctors and druggists, the ambassadors of reputable medical commerce. Julius Schmid also limited sales to licensed druggists and wholesalers. But whereas Youngs Rubber switched to latex, Schmid continued to produce skins and rubbers using the cold-cure cement technique. (Schmid's policy remained intact until 1963, when the company finally converted to latex because of ongoing fire hazard.) Skins were twice as expensive as rubbers, but many men considered them more stimulating. Cement-dipped rubbers, on the other hand, were thicker than their latex cousins and more dangerous and expensive to make, but they did not deteriorate when exposed to oil or grease, ingredients often used in sexual lubricants. By contrast, Dean, Killian, and Shunk covered the low end of the market, manufacturing single-dip latex sheaths for one-half or one-third the cost of Trojans. Their condoms sold for as little as three cents apiece at non-drugstore venues—including barbershops, rest rooms, and vending machines—sites where most Americans acquired sheaths.[33] As *Fortune* observed, years after the *Youngs* decision condom manufacturers were still drawn to the commercial potential of the non-drugstore market: "If he sells only to drugstores he cuts himself out of the mass market."[34] In 1938, bargain brands outsold top-grade Trojans, Sheiks, and Ramses by a margin of fifty to one.[35]

The regulatory trend favored product standardization, not differentiation. After the biochemist Cecil I. B. Voge's 1934–1935 widely publicized tests of more than two thousand American rubber sheaths purchased in the open market revealed that almost 60 percent of commercial condoms were flawed, state and federal agencies imposed standards to improve condom reliability. The root of the problem was inadequate testing. A 1938 study found that only 25 percent of prophylactics were tested by manufacturers before distribution.[36] One reason was cost. Although Killian's machine had mechanized dipping in 1930, testing in the mid-1930s remained "a skilled hand and eye operation infrequently supplemented by a compressed air jet for inflation."[37] Operators inflated each condom, either by blowing into it or by using a handheld jet, and then visually examined it for holes, weak spots, and creases. It was a labor-intensive task that added greatly to—indeed, more than doubled—total production costs.³⁸ The expense was imposed on consumers, not all of whom believed that manufacturers' assurances of condom infallibility justified the higher price. Used to self-testing condoms with air or water, many clung to tradition. "Some consumers seem to think that if they pay seventy-five cents for goods and test them themselves," Merle Youngs scoffed, "they are better off than if they paid a dollar or a dollar and a half and did not have to test them."³⁹ Youngs championed the manufacturer-tested Trojan but was not above selling defective condoms himself. Having adopted the air-jet "burst test" in 1928, Merle Youngs sold inferior condoms to jobbers as manufacturers' seconds, exacerbating low industry standards while profiting from them. Condoms that passed the burst test at Youngs Rubber were sold as Trojans. But "other grades or other goods are sold at different prices," he admitted in court. "If there is a flagrant hole or a flagrant defect . . . naturally they are sold too."⁴⁰

New state and federal statutes sought to put an end to manufacturers' indifference to reliability. In 1935, Oregon became the first state to enact a law regulating the safety and reliability of commercial prophylactics and contraceptives. Guided by the rationale outlined in *Youngs Rubber* v. *C. I. Lee*, the state limited the sale of birth control and condoms to druggists, jobbers, surgical supply houses, manufacturers, and retail drugstores licensed by the State Board of Pharmacy. Defining through omission the parameters of unrespectable commerce, it expressly forbade the sale of the same through vending machines and house-to-house solicitation. In addition, the law set up rudimentary inspection guidelines for condoms. Manufacturers and distributors of skin and rubber prophylactics who applied for a license had first to submit samples for evaluation and to sign an affidavit outlining the history and logistics of their operation. By September 1937, Iowa and Nebraska had passed similar laws.⁴¹

In 1937, the FDA hopped aboard the regulatory bandwagon. In October, FDA chief W. G. Campbell notified manufacturers of rubbers and skins that condoms would henceforth be subjected to FDA jurisdiction and inspection. "The Federal Food and Drug Act," wrote Campbell, "defines the word 'drug' as including 'any substance or mixture of substances intended to be used for the cure, mitigation, or prevention of disease.' "⁴²

Sold as disease prophylactics, condoms clearly fell within the FDA's jurisdiction. (Because pregnancy was not classified as a disease, contraceptives did not.)

When Campbell announced imminent FDA inspections, Youngs
Rubber spared no effort to seal Trojans' status as the country's leading
"no-fail" brand. Trojans' claim to fame, after all, was their "triple-tested"
safety. It would have been hugely embarrassing, and a blow to consumer
confidence and sales, for FDA inspections to prove Youngs Rubber
wrong. To promote compliance with "the test of the Federal inspection
people," the company took, as Merle Youngs remembered, "some of this
surplus money of ours and invest[ed] it in a more determined" testing effort.[43] Merle's brother, Arthur, was instructed to design the perfect testing machine.

Arthur delivered. On March 30, 1939, he applied for a patent for a
machine that tested condoms along a conveyor belt by immersing
sheaths stretched over a mold into a bath of liquid. His application specified that "the said liquid will pass through even the most minute hole or
perforation in the article and spread over the interior surface thereof between said article and mandrel producing a comparatively dark spot or
area which is readily perceptible to the human eye."[44] Youngs Rubber began using the machine in 1938. It was patented in 1940. The mechanization of testing benefited the company in two ways: it helped Youngs
Rubber meet the new FDA requirements, and it saved the company
money. Years later, Merle Youngs credited mechanized inspection with
cutting testing costs to one-seventh of what they had been when performed by hand.[45]

Youngs's quick technological response to new regulations, aided by its
formidable resources and marketing commitments, shielded the company
from the negative repercussions the FDA's new policy had on other firms.
Beginning in January 1938, FDA officers inflated sample rubbers from
the country's largest manufacturers and distributors with one cubic foot
of air and visually examined each for holes, dirt, spots, "putrid material,"
and other imperfections. They also inspected factories where condoms
were made to evaluate testing procedures. By June 1938, their spot
checks had resulted in the seizure of more than six thousand gross of substandard rubbers.[46]

In some FDA samples, defect rates ran as high as 93.7 percent. Most confiscated condoms—Texide, SilverPak, and Parisians—were made by Killian, Shunk, or Dean or by smaller rubber outfits such as Atlanta's Olympia Laboratory. The FDA charged makers and distributors with misbranding and adulteration because the strength of their prophylactics "fell below the professional standard or quality under which [they] were sold."[47] As a result of seizures, the Killian plant closed during early 1938, and the Shunk plant was closed for most of 1938. Dean was similarly affected. Between January 1938 and April 1941, the FDA seized sixty-nine shipments of the company's rubbers. Unable to withstand the regulatory onslaught, Dean discontinued condom making in its North Kansas City plant in 1941 and took up the distribution business, repackaging condoms purchased in bulk from other manufacturers.[48]

In 1938, Congress refined the scope of the FDA's authority in the Food, Drug, and Cosmetic Act, a comprehensive revision of the original Pure Food and Drug Act of 1906. The law, which went into effect on January 1, 1940, did not specify manufacturing standards for condoms but rather outlined requirements that all drugs had to meet: "freedom from defects which render them unsuitable for use; name and address of manufacturer, packer, or distributor on each package; no false or misleading statements, designs, or devices on labels."[49] The new law continued to allow the FDA to confiscate shipments of substandard condoms and authorized the fining (up to ten thousand dollars) and imprisonment (up to three years) of repeat offenders. Because quality-control measures did not apply to American-made condom exports, other countries quickly became the destination for manufacturers' seconds.

Youngs Rubber and Julius Schmid were uniquely positioned to benefit from the new regulations. Both companies had distinguished themselves in the 1920s by selling prophylactics that were standardized and extensively tested, the very qualities FDA inspectors in the late 1930s were looking for in a condom. Indeed, Youngs Rubber and Julius Schmid were the only condom companies to pass the FDA's comprehensive tests, and their chief brands—Ramses, Sheiks, and Trojans—were the only rubbers to make the Consumers Union's "recommended" list. As FDA standards increased the technological uniformity of condoms, brand recognition became more important to consumer selection, giving Trojans, Ramses, and Sheiks an advantage.[50]

In addition, by the time the new regulations went into effect, Schmid and Youngs Rubber had already identified pharmacies as the exclusive outlet for their merchandise. By the early 1940s, drugstores had become the single largest outlet for condom sales. Pharmacists and proprietors rewarded the condoms made by the two firms that had served, in the words of one industry analyst, as the "White Knights who helped them capture a lucrative product niche."[51] With pharmacists' support, the condom business became an oligopoly, with Schmid and Youngs Rubber holding court.

In 1940, Schmid's cement-dipped Ramses rubbers were the first condoms endorsed by the U.S. Army. The company prided itself on double testing all condoms destined for the American and Canadian markets, including the Dash and Lynx labels it manufactured exclusively for People's Drug Stores, a U.S. chain. In 1947, with established markets in North and South America and Europe, Schmid produced more than 133 million condoms annually—an extraordinary feat for a company whose founding father had once had nothing to spare but raw ambition.[52]

By 1950, Schmid and Youngs Rubber had gained control of more than 50 percent of the nation's $100 million condom trade.[53] In many respects, it was a good time to be an industry leader. By the mid-1950s, as the drawbacks of using the douche for contraception became more widely known and as consumer confidence in condoms increased, condoms had regained their former stature as the leading contraceptive in the country.[54]

Already, however, scientists were at work creating a new contraceptive that would put the tried-and-true condom on the back burner once more and restore consumer support for female methods.

PART THREE

The Medicalization of Contraceptives

NINE

Developing the Pill

It was one of the greatest inventions of the twentieth century, the capstone of decades of pharmaceutical research. It inspired songs, cartoons, political debate, and grateful letters from women around the world who flocked to their physicians' offices for prescriptions. The Catholic Church condemned it as immoral, and several African-American leaders denounced it as a technology of genocide. After reports of drug-related blood clots and strokes surfaced in 1962, scientists and journalists debated its safety, and many feminists openly worried that a generation of women had unwittingly become medical guinea pigs. But no matter how Americans felt about it, the object of excitement needed no special introduction. By the mid-1960s, Americans knew the wonder drug of the decade simply as "the Pill."

Approved by the Food and Drug Administration for contraception in May 1960, oral contraceptives ushered in a new era of birth control and medical practice in the United States. By 1965, the Pill had become the most popular form of birth control in the country, used by more than 6.5 million married women and an untold number of unmarried women, whose contraceptive habits were uncounted and (wistfully) ignored in official reports.[1] The Pill accomplished what the diaphragm had not. It created widespread doctor and patient acceptance of medical birth control. Its popularity cleared a path for subsequent prescription-only products such as intrauterine devices, Norplant, and Depo-Provera. The once-a-day contraceptive also revolutionized consumers' pharmaceutical practice. For the first time, millions of otherwise healthy women took a "medicine" unrelated to the prevention or treatment of disease.

The story of the Pill begins and ends with women: two who plotted its development, millions who dutifully swallowed it each day. In the middle, of course, there were men. A triad of brilliant scientists—Gregory Pincus, John Rock, and Min-Chueh Chang—conducted a barrage of tests of the drug on rabbits, rats, and eventually humans. The media singled out these men and hailed them as the Pill's "founding fathers," fueling suspicions later, once problems arose, that the men's scientific objectivity had been compromised by their sex.[2] Where, after all, was the Pill for men? But from the beginning, the Pill's lineage was more complicated, its implications for women more complex. Gregory Pincus, the Pill's chief researcher, had not thought to "invent" oral contraceptives until he was encouraged to do so by the proddings of Margaret Sanger and the boundless financial support of Katharine McCormick.

Sanger and McCormick first met in 1917, the year Sanger was tried and imprisoned for operating her Brooklyn clinic. Sanger had not yet converted to the political pragmatism that would come to characterize her leadership of the birth control movement. When the two met at a talk Sanger gave in Boston, Sanger was unabashedly angry and militant. McCormick was a philanthropist from a prominent Chicago family who, like Sanger, defied conventions when the cause was right. Born in 1875, McCormick was one of the first two women to earn a degree in science from the Massachusetts Institute of Technology. She majored in biology, acquiring expertise indispensable to her future collaboration with Pincus. After graduating from MIT, she married Stanley McCormick, the youngest son of Cyrus McCormick, founder of the International Harvester Company.[3]

In 1906, tragedy struck when Stanley was diagnosed with schizophrenia. His sufferings, combined with her fears that schizophrenia could be inherited, forged in Katharine a resolve to stay childless and made her an early convert to contraception. It also kindled in her a keen appreciation of the benefits of pharmaceutical research. Decades later, these two views encouraged her to fund, almost single-handedly, Pincus's work on the

Pill. But in the early part of the century, her priority was her ailing husband, who required constant care and attention. She built him a mansion in the hills near Santa Barbara and hired six musicians to play for him. She also participated in the search for a scientific treatment for schizophrenia. From 1927 to 1947, she funded Harvard's Neuroendocrine Research Foundation, where scientists were investigating the possibility of a biochemical basis for schizophrenia—a hormonal deficiency caused by a malfunctioning adrenal cortex. When Stanley died in 1947, she abruptly withdrew her support from the foundation but retained her faith in biochemistry as a tool for remedying serious medical and social problems.[4]

McCormick's wealth and stature did not blind her to the inequalities of her time, particularly those afflicting women. While Sanger was championing female emancipation through voluntary motherhood, McCormick took up the parallel cause of universal suffrage. She funded the suffragette *Woman's Journal* and served as treasurer and then vice president of the National American Woman Suffrage Association. After the Nineteenth Amendment was ratified in 1920, she helped Carrie Chapman Catt found the League of Women Voters, to which she was elected vice president.[5]

McCormick's interest in the birth control movement was a logical extension of her public activism and private vow of childlessness. She stayed in touch with Sanger and helped out when she could. She smuggled diaphragms into the United States for Sanger's clinics and entertained three hundred delegates to Sanger's World Population Conference in 1927 at her family's lavish Geneva château, originally built for Joseph Bonaparte.[6] But when Sanger asked McCormick to subsidize contraceptive research in the 1930s, she politely declined. Her resources and attention were already spoken for. She told Sanger: "[I am] deeply concerned over the research aspects of the birth control movement and wish very much I could enter that field in a definitely constructive way. Unfortunately, I cannot at present." Sanger understood. "The important thing is that you are with us in the struggle," she assured her ally. "There are times when goodwill and good wishes are stronger than money."[7]

By 1950, McCormick's circumstances had changed. Stanley's death in 1947 had left her with free time and a fortune exceeding fourteen million dollars. McCormick was "as rich as *Croesus*," John Rock would later ob-

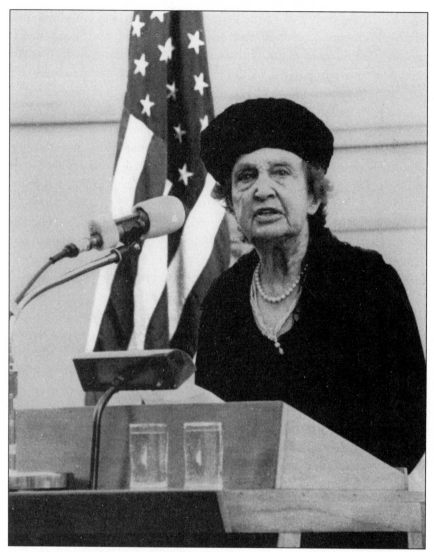

28. Katharine McCormick, woman of science, pictured here in 1963 at the Massachusetts Institute of Technology, her alma mater (Courtesy of the MIT Museum)

serve. "She couldn't even spend the interest on her interest."[8] In October 1950, at the age of seventy-five, she sent a letter to Sanger that would alter the course of contraceptive technology. There were, she wrote, "two questions that are much with me these days: a) Where do you think the greatest need of financial support is today for the National Birth Control Movement; and b) What the present prospects are for further birth control research, and by research I mean contraceptive research." For Sanger, it was a dream come true. She had been after McCormick for a sizable donation for years. She wrote a characteristically forceful reply, in which she discussed her hope that, with McCormick's help, a foolproof, simple method would one day be invented: "I consider that the world and almost our civilization for the next twenty-five years, is going to depend upon a simple, cheap, safe, contraceptive to be used in poverty stricken slums, jungles, and among the most ignorant people."[9]

Behind Sanger's response were several issues. One was the population crisis. From the beginning, the Pill was intended to supply critical ammunition in the war against unwanted population growth in developing nations. In the 1950s and 1960s, population control was not a fringe movement. Indeed, it was so enmeshed in the language and ideology of Cold War fertility control that Americans used the terms "family planning," "birth control," and "population control" interchangeably.[10] In addition to Sanger, its most outspoken proponents included John D. Rockefeller III; Dwight D. Eisenhower, one of the Population Council's charter members; and the British biologist Sir Julian Huxley, who articulated the fear of many when he warned in a November 1959 speech: "People do not exist to live all their undernourished lives in the illiterate ignorance of an Asian village. . . . Unless population increase is drastically cut . . . mankind will be reduced to the status of a swarm of maggots on the carcass of a dead cow."[11]

Although in 1958 it was estimated that the United States, with only 6 percent of the world's population, was consuming 50 percent of the world's resources, the crisis was attributed to the unchecked procreation of poor, uneducated persons in developing, and presumably unstable, nations. Without question, many advocates of population control had good intentions. They believed wider access to birth control would reduce hunger, poverty, and disease while fostering economic stability. But eugenicist sympathies frequently eclipsed honorable aims. Recasting the racism and class biases of the earlier eugenics movement onto an international stage, proponents of population control tethered predictions of global chaos, nuclear annihilation, and encroaching communism to the fertility of a teeming underclass. The expansion of undesirable groups in developing countries, advocates warned, would foment poverty, unrest, and the likelihood of war, creating an environment tailor-made for a communist takeover. Thus fear of self-annihilation through the depletion of natural resources meshed easily with Cold War concerns about the spread of communism and nuclear extinction. In his 1948 book, *Road to Survival*, William Vogt, the director of Planned Parenthood, portrayed a "cheaper dependable [contraceptive] method that can easily be used by women" as a precondition of global security. "If the United States had spent two billion dollars developing such a contraceptive, instead of the atomic bomb," he wrote, "it would have contributed far more to our national security while, at the same time, it promoted a rising standard for the entire world."[12]

Population control rhetoric made contraceptive research inseparable from the fate of international relations. But it also reflected its adherents' unequivocal faith that scientific research would eventually solve the population crisis. In a Cold War climate awed by technology, the gloom-and-doom predictions of Vogt and others were tempered by abiding hope in laboratory solutions to human problems. The early 1950s saw the peak of American enthusiasm for technological development. Americans had witnessed not only the atomic bomb, which had ended a terrible war, but also a batch of remarkable drugs: lifesaving antibiotics, tranquilizers, and cortisone, a steroid that enabled formerly bedridden arthritis patients to walk, even run. It was small wonder that Americans awaited news of the next engineered miracle with unbridled enthusiasm.

Sanger was one of many Americans who shared this Cold War optimism. As early as 1912, she had fantasized about finding a "magic pill" for contraception, and decades later, her mounting frustrations with the diaphragm method renewed that dream. In 1946, she confided to a friend that she was feeling "more and more despondent as I saw and realized more than ever the inadequacy of the diaphragm for reaching millions of women who need and should have something as simple as a birth control pill."[13] Sanger's health may also explain her preference for a pharmaceutical solution. She suffered from recurrent gallbladder attacks, which she treated with a variety of pills. After a heart attack in 1953, she added to her arsenal Demerol, a powerful, addictive narcotic that she continued to take after recovery. For much of her adult life, then, Sanger had first-hand experience with the ease with which drugs could be integrated into a person's daily regimen.

Sanger recruited Gregory Pincus to develop her "magic pill." Born in 1903 in Woodbine, New Jersey, Gregory "Goody" Pincus earned his B.S. in genetics at Cornell University in 1924. He went on to Harvard, which in 1927 awarded his M.S. and Sc.D. degrees simultaneously. By the early 1930s, as an assistant professor at Harvard, he had become a leading authority on mammalian sexual physiology and a lightning rod for debate when he engineered the first test-tube rabbit embryo. A triumph for scientific understanding of mammalian ovulation and fertilization, it triggered a media backlash that hurt Pincus's academic career. Critics saw in his work unsettling parallels to Aldous Huxley's *Brave New World*, the 1932 novel about a future dystopia where babies are born in test tubes and science has extinguished human error but also its spirit. An article in *Collier's* magazine titled "No Father to Guide Them" depicted a sinister Pincus, cigarette between his lips, holding up a sacrificed rabbit. Displeased at the notoriety, Harvard denied Pincus tenure.[14]

Harvard's loss was the birth control movement's gain. In 1944, the resourceful scientist moved from Cambridge to nearby Shrewsbury and set up the Worcester Foundation for Experimental Biology with Hudson Hoagland, a biology professor at nearby Clark University. The foundation's purpose was to strengthen ties between practical medicine and biology through pharmaceutical science. Hoagland remembered the glee the two scientists felt upon abandoning academia: "We welcomed the idea of freedom from bickering faculty meetings, futile committees, jealous colleagues, and teaching prescribed courses to often indifferent students."[15] But this independence left the research institute financially vulnerable. The foundation depended exclusively on grants. And even for eminent scientists such as Pincus, fund-raising took time. For a while, the foundation operated on a budget so tight that Pincus worked as a janitor and Hoagland mowed lawns. By the late 1940s, however, the two men had secured the financial backing of several granting agencies. One was the pharmaceutical house G. D. Searle.[16]

Headquartered in Skokie, Illinois, just outside Chicago, G. D. Searle was established in 1888 by Gideon Daniel Searle, a young druggist from Indiana. A small, family-run drug firm with a product line of traditional medicines, Searle was known in the trade as a specialty house. But like many pharmaceutical firms in postwar America, Searle was seeking to re-fashion its corporate identity by diversifying its product line. It wanted to embrace and to profit from consumer excitement surrounding "applied biology" and to make a name for itself as an innovative firm that brought the latest biochemical discoveries to consumers' homes. In the 1950s, Searle was looking for a proprietary "breakthrough" medicine and in-vested heavily in the field of steroidal chemistry to find it.[17]

When Searle hired Pincus, it had its sights set on the holy grail of pharmaceutical innovation: the steroidal hormone cortisone, whose ben-efit to arthritic patients had first been demonstrated in 1948. At the time, making cortisone was time-consuming and expensive, costing buy-ers nearly two hundred dollars per gram. In 1944, the Merck biochemist Lewis Sarett had used no fewer than thirty-six separate steps to synthe-size cortisone. In 1951, *Harper's Magazine* described the hunt for a cost-effective and efficient way of synthesizing cortisone as "an unrestrained, dramatic race involving a dozen of the largest American drug houses, several leading foreign pharmaceutical manufacturers, three govern-ments, and more research personnel than have worked on any medical problem since penicillin."[18]

Pincus persuaded Searle's director of research, the chemist Albert L. Raymond, that making cortisone by pumping serum through the adrenal gland of a sow might be the answer to Searle's quest. Pincus spent hun-dreds of thousands of Searle dollars exploring what turned out to be a dead end. In the meantime, Carl Djerassi, a chemist employed by the ri-val Mexican pharmaceutical firm Syntex, synthesized cortisone from diosgenin, a steroidal compound found in high concentration in the roots of Mexican yams.[19] The process would soon be outdated by a sim-ple and inexpensive microbiological method developed by scientists at Upjohn—but not before Djerassi's invention put Syntex on the steroidal map and his research team (standing next to a gigantic yam root) on the cover of *Life* magazine.[20]

Searle was furious. When Pincus contacted Raymond for additional funds for his next project, a proposed oral contraceptive, Raymond shot back a withering reply. "You haven't given us a thing to justify the half-million that we invested in you," he ranted. "To date your record as a contributor to the commerce of the Searle Company is a lamentable failure, replete with false leads, poor judgment, and assurances from you that were false. Yet you have the nerve to ask for more for research. You will get more only if a lucky chance gives us something originating from your group which will make us a profit."[21] Angered by Pincus's loss in the coveted cortisone race, Searle gave the scientist the supplies but not the funds to develop and test the Pill. Ironically, it would later consider the "Pincus pill" the most important drug it had ever brought to market.

Pincus's study of oral contraceptives began in 1951, after Sanger commissioned him to develop a simple but foolproof birth control method. The two met at a dinner in New York arranged by Dr. Abraham Stone, the director of the Margaret Sanger Research Bureau in New York. Pincus recalled that Sanger "was especially disappointed by the failure of conventional methods in India. She said 'Gregory, can't you devise some

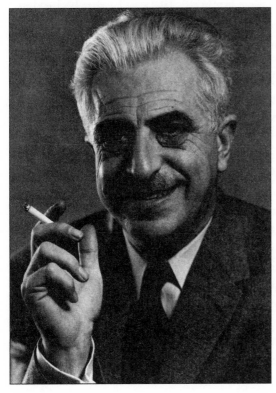

29. Gregory Pincus
(© Bettmann/CORBIS)

sort of pill for this purpose?' I said I'd try."[22] Sanger followed up with a two-thousand-dollar check. This was soon supplemented by a grant of thirty-one hundred dollars from Planned Parenthood Federation of America (PPFA), which, under William Vogt's leadership, had pledged as early as 1948 to finance research to develop a "simple, acceptable and reliable method cheap enough for use by poverty-ridden, illiterate and backward people who needed it most in all countries."[23] Between 1951 and 1953, the fund gave Pincus ten thousand dollars for his work on the Pill.[24] The allocation barely covered the salary of one member of his research team. But it got Pincus started.[25]

Pincus's work drew on the latest advances in endocrinology, the study of hormones. In 1905, the physiologist Ernest Starling had first identified glandular secretions in the body that, carried in the bloodstream from one tissue to another, stimulate the action of cells. Starling called these internal substances "hormones," after the Greek word meaning "to incite to activity."[26] Hormones regulate, among other things, metabolism, growth, and the reproductive cycle. By the 1940s, scientists had isolated and elucidated the chemical structure of two female sex hormones, progesterone and estrogen. Progesterone is secreted naturally in women by the corpus luteum, a mass of cells formed after the release of a ruptured egg. Once an egg is fertilized, the pregnant woman cannot conceive again because progesterone prevents the pituitary gland from secreting the hormones necessary to bring another egg to maturation within the ovary. Progesterone also checks conception by thickening the cervical mucus, which inhibits sperm penetrability, and by preventing the full development of the uterine lining, without which a fertilized egg cannot implant.[27]

Once physicians understood the role of progesterone in the female reproductive cycle, they began to use it to treat patients suffering from gynecological disorders such as painful and prolonged menstruation. The main obstacle to hormone production was cost. Scientists extracted sex hormones from natural sources, chiefly slaughtered animals—many of the first companies to supply hormones had close ties to the meat business. A minuscule amount of estrogen isolated by scientists in 1930, for instance, required the ovaries of eighty thousand sows.[28] Progesterone cost as much as one thousand dollars a gram in the 1930s, more than a standard automobile. Pincus's research associate Min-Chueh Chang later recalled that "you could only afford it then for thoroughbred horses, not humans."[29]

The progesterone price barrier was broken when Russell Marker, a maverick American chemist, discovered how to synthesize progesterone from diosgenin contained in the same yams that Djerassi would later use to synthesize cortisone. Marker's discovery reduced the cost of progesterone production and laid the foundation for hormonal birth control. Marker himself was unaware of the potential applications of his work. "I was never interested in the use of the hormone, only in making it available," he told one writer. "I didn't realize it could be used for birth control pills until I had quit."[30]

In Worcester, Pincus directed Min-Chueh Chang to inject laboratory animals with synthetic progesterone, called progestin, to test whether it inhibited ovulation. Chang's area of expertise was sperm. Born in China, he had met Pincus when he was a graduate student at Cambridge University in England, where Chang earned his Ph.D. in 1941 and where Pincus was a visiting professor in 1937 and 1938. Chang read Pincus's pathbreaking book, *The Eggs of Mammals*, in 1936. It made a huge impression. "*Everyone* in our field knew about him," Chang recalled. "You must remember that until then no one knew mammals had eggs."[31] When Pincus offered Chang a post at the Worcester Foundation, he readily accepted. Still, injecting female rabbits with progesterone, coordinating their copulation, and then slaughtering them to excise and examine their ovaries was uninspiring work for a scientist whose research interests and talents lay elsewhere.[32] Chang was a brooder. He worried about how experiments were progressing and about the motives of the drug companies his research would ultimately serve. He was wary of capitalism and companies bent on profiting from scientific discovery.[33] But with frequent reassurances from Pincus, Chang persevered and by late 1951 had graduated from rabbits to rats, whose ovulation cycle more closely approximated that of humans. Progesterone prevented pregnancy in both animals. In January 1952, Pincus sent a progress report to Planned Parenthood. He and Chang had "developed methods adequate for the possibly contraceptive activity of steroid substances in both rats and rabbits," he reported triumphantly. The "effective action of progesterone is indubitably demonstrated."[34]

Although Planned Parenthood announced Pincus's progress in its bulletin, the federation was having second thoughts about funding his work. Some PPFA officials considered it too risky—if Pincus failed, the organization and the birth control cause would suffer. But word of Pincus's progress gave Sanger just the impetus she needed to contact Katharine McCormick once more. "Have you had any information from the Federation as to what research is going on under their auspices?" she queried McCormick. "I am interested in what Dr. Pincus is doing on hormones, and if you have not heard from the Federation as to these projects that are in progress . . . I will be glad to send you copies and keep you informed." McCormick wrote back that she had "heard nothing regarding the research of Dr. Pincus." But she was intrigued. She had never met Pincus, but she knew his associate Hudson Hoagland, who had been active in research on schizophrenia before Stanley's death. In 1952, Sanger and McCormick met Pincus in Shrewsbury, toured his facility, and questioned him about his work. McCormick liked what she heard. By June 1953, she had pledged an annual contribution of ten thousand dollars. When Sanger told her that Planned Parenthood was threatening to cut Pincus's funding, McCormick promised more. She would foot Pincus's entire bill, including whatever funds he needed to conduct clinical trials—the final stage before FDA approval. McCormick was true to her word. Annoyed with what she saw as Planned Parenthood's mishandling of the project, she funneled funds directly to the Worcester Foundation: $150,000 to $180,000 a year during her lifetime and another $1 million as a bequest. All told, her contributions mounted to about $2 million.[35]

Not a single government dollar helped develop the Pill. Both the National Institutes of Health, the largest single source of funding for biomedical research in the 1950s, and the National Science Foundation refused to support reproductive research. So, too, did the World Health Organization, the central international agency addressing biomedical research.[36] Sargent Shriver, the future Democratic vice presidential candidate who would spearhead the government's war against poverty, recalled that in the 1950s birth control was "like syphilis—politically, you couldn't talk about it."[37] In 1959, President Dwight D. Eisenhower drove this point home, stating at a press conference: "I cannot imagine anything more emphatically a subject that is not a proper political or government activity or function or responsibility. . . . The government will not, so long as I am here, have a positive political doctrine in its program that has to do with the problem of birth control. That's not our business."[38] John F. Kennedy, the nation's first Catholic president, felt differently and endorsed a United Nations proposal to permit the United States to provide birth control assistance to countries requesting it. His successor, Lyndon Johnson, made contraception even more of a priority. In his January 1965 State of the Union Message, Johnson promised: "I will seek new ways to use our knowledge to help deal with the explosion in world population and the growing scarcity in world resources."[39] The government's about-face in the 1960s augmented efforts by philanthropic organizations, private citizens, and industry, which had long shouldered the financial burden of contraceptive development. In 1969, federal agencies invested $19.9 million in contraceptive research and development annually, making the U.S. government the single largest funder of contraceptive research and development in the world.[40]

The Population Council, a nonprofit organization, was more generous. Founded in 1952 by John D. Rockefeller III to "stimulate, encourage, promote, conduct, and support significant activities in the broad field of population," its biomedical division sponsored individual research projects on aspects of reproductive science—sex hormones, spermatogenesis, immunology—that might clear a path for new contraceptives. The Population Council granted ten thousand dollars to Pincus's Worcester Foundation for Experimental Biology in 1954 to study changes to sperm in the female reproductive tract. But it did not fund the oral contraceptive project, which Pincus had launched before the Population Council was established.[41] By 1954, however, Pincus had the full financial backing and personal support of McCormick, which was all his project needed.

Not content to be a silent philanthropist, McCormick involved herself with every stage of the project. She moved from Santa Barbara to Boston to monitor Pincus's activities. She visited Shrewsbury and entertained Pincus, his wife, Elizabeth, and their daughter, Laura, when they came to Boston. Although Sanger, the consummate networker, had first introduced McCormick to Pincus, McCormick would be the one to explain the technical details of the study to Sanger. With a scientific enthusiasm befitting her MIT training, McCormick tracked Pincus's progress, offering criticisms and commentary, asking a litany of questions. "Little old woman she was *not*," Pincus later recalled. "She was a grenadier."[42] Pincus admired her. In 1965, two years before she died, he dedicated his book, *The Control of Fertility*, to Katharine McCormick in recognition of her "steadfast faith in scientific inquiry."

The other important person who entered Pincus's life in 1952 was John Rock. The two met by chance at a conference. Rock was a Harvard-trained gynecologist and obstetrician who lived in Brookline, only forty miles from Worcester. As director of Brookline's Reproductive Study Center, Rock had been searching for ways of curing infertility. He believed that the temporary cessation of ovulation would give the womb a forced sabbatical, enabling it to be more effective once regular, unimpeded functions resumed. While Chang had been busy injecting laboratory animals with progesterone to induce sterility, Rock had been injecting women patients with progesterone and estrogen to help them get pregnant. The two men had opposite objectives, but their research began at the same starting point. By the time Rock and Pincus crossed paths, Rock had induced a state of "pseudo pregnancy" on eighty "frustrated but valiantly adventuresome" patients who had been unable to conceive for at least two years.[43] After being taken off the hormonal regimen, thirteen of the eighty patients became pregnant within four months. The breakthrough quickly became known among gynecologists as the "Rock rebound."

Rock was a devout Catholic. The father of five and grandfather of fourteen, he attended Mass daily and kept a crucifix on the wall above his office desk. He was, in many respects, a social conservative. He had opposed the admission of women to Harvard Medical School. He simply did not believe women were capable of being good doctors, he told his daughters.[44]

But Rock was also a man who valued conscience over conformity. Nowhere was this more apparent than in his views on birth control. He believed that there were times when contraception was medically necessary and in 1931 had publicly advocated the repeal of the Massachusetts contraceptive law on these grounds. As a professor of gynecology and obstetrics at Harvard Medical School in the 1940s, he taught students how to fit patients with contraceptives—this at a time when contraceptive instruction in medical school was still uncommon. That this training should come from a Catholic doctor in one of the least birth-control-friendly states in the country was nothing short of astounding. In 1943,

Rock published an article in the national medical journal *Clinics* titled "The Scientific Case against Rigid Legal Restrictions on Medical Birth-Control Advice." He listed poverty, genetic deficiencies, and maternal disease and disability as valid reasons for physician-prescribed contraception. But he also warned against recreational use: "I hold no brief for those young or even older husbands and wives who for no good reason refuse to bear as many children as they can properly rear and as society can profitably engross."[45]

Respected for his intellect, sincerity, and eagerness to engage life's most profound philosophical questions, Rock clashed with the Catholic hierarchy long before the Pill was introduced. He once performed a hysterectomy against the wishes of a priest who had told the patient that the operation violated Catholic precepts. "I tried to talk to him on the phone," Rock remembered, "but he was adamant. . . . I can't understand stuffed shirts like that priest who think they know everything."[46]

Pincus was eager to involve Rock in the study. Rock, the practicing physician, could bridge the chasm separating laboratory science and everyday medical practice. He was widely known and greatly admired. "If you went to doctors in New England in those days and asked who was the best obstetrician in the region," one man recalled, "you would almost surely be told that it was John Rock—he was a formidable figure."[47] Above all, he was Catholic. Pincus was Jewish. Pincus and PPFA backer Abraham Stone, also a Jew, feared the prospect of a Catholic backlash against the Pill or even anti-Semitic allegations of a Jewish plot to impede Catholic growth. Pincus's previous test-tube experiments had raised eyebrows. Rock's involvement might reassure the very constituency about whom Pincus worried most.

Rock was intrigued by Pincus's trials using progesterone alone and agreed to administer progestin to a new group of infertile women. His chief medical concern remained infertility, and he candidly told Pincus that long-term use of the hormone by women for contraception was "unthinkable."[48] His objective was to see if progesterone used without estrogen would trigger the Rock rebound. But a second goal, of particular interest to Pincus, was to determine whether progestin inhibited ovulation in humans. When Pincus contacted drug companies about securing supplies, he made an exhilarating discovery. Oral progesterones had already been synthesized, and they were purportedly more effective than the injected progesterone Rock and Pincus had been using. In effect, Pincus realized, the pill that Sanger had asked him to invent had already been made.

Credit for this important step in the development of oral contraceptives belonged to two chemists: Carl Djerassi and Searle's Frank Colton, a research chemist. Russell Marker's discovery had reduced the price of progesterone, but use of the drug was limited. Taken orally, progesterone was ineffective because of the way it was metabolized. Patients needing it received large doses, delivered in painful injections. Working separately, Djerassi and Colton strove to create a synthetic progesterone better than its predecessors, a progesterone so potent it could sustain activity when swallowed as a pill. After months of experimentation, Djerassi created a new molecule, norethindrone, with eight times the potency of natural progesterone. It remained active when *fed* to laboratory animals. Once he obtained positive results from animal and human trials, Djerassi applied for a patent on November 22, 1951. Unbeknownst to Djerassi, Colton had also succeeded in creating an orally effective synthetic progesterone—norethynodrel—using a slightly different process. Like Marker, neither scientist had birth control on his mind when he embarked on his progesterone journey. The idea was preposterous. "Not in our wildest dreams," Djerassi remarked later, "did we imagine [it]."[49]

But Pincus did, and he patiently awaited the results of Rock's 1954 experiments with administering various forms of progesterone—injections, progestin tablets, and vaginal suppositories—to fifty childless women at the Free Hospital for Women, where Rock worked in 1954 and 1955, and to nurse volunteers at the Worcester State Hospital. All participants were expected to comply with an elaborate protocol that included basal temperature readings in the morning, daily vaginal smears, urine collection, and monthly endometrial biopsies to ascertain if the drug inhibited conception.[50]

The first human trials of an oral contraceptive were encouraging. Rock was pleased when seven of the fifty infertile women tested became pregnant after he withdrew them from the progesterone. Pincus was ebullient, for the drug regimen had suppressed ovulation in most women. For the moment, however, he kept the news to himself. It was too early to draw sweeping conclusions or make public proclamations. Larger clinical trials would have to be done. But for the first time, Pincus's optimism overcame him, and he began to refer to the oral compound simply as "the Pill." He shared the news with his stunned wife. "My God, why didn't you tell me?" she asked. "Did you think you could ever get the pill?" Pincus was nonchalant. "In science," he replied, "everything is possible."[51]

But the first small-scale human studies also pointed to the many obstacles Pincus's team faced. Only half of the patients had complied with study protocol, and nurse volunteers—women *not* motivated by a desire to overcome infertility—had been particularly difficult to recruit and retain. As Pincus prepared to inaugurate broad field trials of the oral compound, he faced a battery of questions. Could enough women be recruited to participate in a birth control experiment? Could they be counted on to take the Pill daily? How many would drop out because of side effects or the medical indignities that came with being a study participant? "The headache of the tests," McCormick complained in 1954, "is the cooperation necessary from the women patients. I really do not know how it is obtained at all—for it *is* onerous—it really is—and requires intelligent, persistent attention for weeks. Rock says that he can get it only from women wishing to become fertile: those who wish to be sterile are not ready to take so much trouble."[52] Unlike laboratory animals, women could not be depended on to be obedient. In one of her more frustrated moments, McCormick wished for a "cage of ovulating females to experiment with" to hurry things along.[53] (In fact, even the laboratory animals at the Worcester Foundation were not always cooperative. When Chang first began administering progestin tablets to rabbits, many spit them out. He liquefied the drug and fed them through a plastic tube instead.)[54]

As Pincus was casting about for an appropriate site for long-term field trials, he set up another small-scale trial with fifteen psychiatric patients confined at the Worcester State Hospital. His objective was to determine the physiological impact of progestin on the reproductive cycle. This experiment, glossed over in subsequent media reports, was one of the more disturbing features of the Pill's development, a human trial that perilously approximated McCormick's imagined "cage of ovulating females." The trial forced hospitalized schizophrenics to participate in an experiment whose long-term side effects were unknown. Equally disturbing was the fact that the institutionalization of these women made birth control unnecessary. Denied sexual intimacies with men, they could not reap the contraceptive benefits of the drugs they swallowed. Pincus and his crew tested the Pill on other nonvoluntary populations, including sixteen psychotic men at the Worcester State Hospital. Pincus believed progestin might operate as an "anti-fertility agent in the male," a hypothesis tested with male prisoners at the Oregon State Penitentiary in 1957. Semen samples taken from prisoners given progestin showed lower sperm counts, leading the researchers to conclude that the drug was a male "desexing agent." In addition to impeding male fertility, the drugs "reduce sexual desire," causing Pincus to speculate that they might be used in conjunction with psychotherapy to "cure" homosexuality.[55]

What should we make of the use of institutionalized patients and inmates as human subjects? On the one hand, the ethical standards and expectations in the 1950s were very different from those today. In an era when the use of human subjects in medical experiments was poorly regulated, even the U.S. Public Health Service was conducting tests on syphilitic African-Americans until the early 1970s. On the other hand, we can explain Pincus's practices in the context of his times without condoning them. What made the Pill different from other experimental drugs, moreover, was its use on physically healthy women of reproductive age. The women on whom experiments were done were not afflicted with a disabling or life-threatening disease for which they sought a cure. Rather, these test subjects were physiologically healthy women intentionally subjected to the possibility of harm and a series of invasive procedures.

Pincus selected Puerto Rico as the site of the first large-scale clinical trial of oral contraceptives. The Caribbean island had been a U.S. territory since 1898. Its economy was predominantly rural and sustained by sugarcane cultivation. With over six hundred inhabitants, mostly Spanish-speaking Catholics, per square mile, Puerto Rico in the late 1940s was one of the most densely populated areas in the world.[56]

Overpopulation had contributed to overcrowding, poverty, malnourishment, and disease. High rates of tuberculosis, malaria, hookworm infestation, and syphilis had attracted the attention and medical interventions of the Rockefeller Foundation and the Public Health Service. But because of the steadfast opposition of the Catholic Church, birth control services had been slower to take root. Twice in the 1920s and

1930s, local birth control leagues had been forced to suspend their operations because of Catholic hostility. Federal programs had better luck. During its first term, the Roosevelt administration established the Puerto Rico Emergency Relief Administration (PRERA), which in 1935 sponsored a pilot program to offer free contraceptive instruction and supplies. The first PRERA clinic opened in San Juan in May under the supervision of Dr. José Belaval, the city's leading obstetrician. Encouraged by the popularity of Belaval's clinics, PRERA had launched an island-wide program by December. In 1936, another federal agency, the Puerto Rico Reconstruction Administration (PRRA), was established and took over the work of the now-defunct PRERA. The PRRA had an ambitious goal: a birth control clinic for every town. But by October, cuts in federal funding had terminated the PRRA's maternal health programs and the federal government's efforts to reduce the fertility rate of Puerto Ricans.[57]

Federal contraceptive programs may have been short-lived, but they proved that Puerto Rican women were eager for birth control. In December 1936, two months after PRRA programs were dismantled, a group of local philanthropists, public-minded citizens, and health advocates formed the Maternal and Child Health Association. With financial support from the American philanthropist, physician, and birth control proponent Clarence Gamble, the group opened a network of contraceptive clinics that provided birth control to thousands of women. The association also successfully lobbied the Insular Legislature to adopt Law 136, amending obscenity laws by legalizing the teaching and practice of contraception for medical indications, and Law 33, enabling the Commission of Health to organize contraceptive services through the Department of Public Health. In 1954, when Pincus decided on Puerto Rico as a testing site, there were sixty-seven birth control clinics on the island.[58]

Pincus's decision to conduct trials on Puerto Rico reflected several considerations. First, Puerto Rico had a well-established family planning movement spearheaded by a network of physicians Pincus knew and trusted. After delivering a series of lectures to medical personnel on the island, Pincus told McCormick in March 1954 that he found the physicians he had met "quite efficient and knowledgeable, and on reviewing the situation with them thoroughly, I came to the conclusion that work could be done in Puerto Rico on a relatively large scale."[59] The doctors were affiliated with the island's numerous birth control clinics, whose presence would support a "sufficiently large patient clientele" for the trial.[60] Second, there was the advantage of geographic isolation. Distant enough to keep away the probing American media, about which Pincus harbored suspicions because of his bruising Harvard experience, Puerto Rico was nevertheless close enough to facilitate frequent visits and regular communication. Puerto Rico's quasi-colonial status was a great attraction, for it made Puerto Rico both its own country and a territory under U.S. sovereignty and control. Should a crisis arise, the implied threat of American intervention might keep Puerto Ricans in line. And yet, as Pincus told McCormick, he could "attempt in Puerto Rico certain experiments which would be very difficult in this country."[61] Conducting large-scale trials in bluenose Massachusetts, where birth control was still illegal, was out of the question. In addition, because it is an island, Puerto Rico had a relatively stationary population that could be readily monitored.[62] Puerto Rico also had symbolic importance as one of the overcrowded and underdeveloped countries for which advocates of population control proposed contraception as a "cure." The field trial would determine "whether women without financial or education[al] advantages would find the drug acceptable and be able to follow conscientiously the necessarily complicated directions for its effective use."[63]

The Puerto Rican trial began in April 1956 under the supervision of Dr. Edris Rice-Wray, a faculty member of the Puerto Rico Medical School and the medical director of the Puerto Rico Family Planning Association. Volunteers lived in Rio Piedras, a new public housing project in a suburb of San Juan. Rice-Wray hired a female social worker who went door-to-door rounding up recruits. Rice-Wray recalled how easy it was for the social worker to find them: "[She] would say, 'I'm from the Family Planning Association'—like the Cancer Society or the infantile-paralysis campaign, so they could relate it to something they considered decent, you know. Then she said, 'We're very much interested in parents having the right to have the number of children they want when they want to have them. We have a pill that a woman can take twenty days a month and she doesn't get pregnant.' Well, they just couldn't get hold of it fast enough." Not every woman was eligible. Participants had to be under forty years of age and have at least two natural-born children as evidence of fertility. They also "had to be prepared to have another" child if oral contraception failed or if destiny placed them in the placebo-only control group.[64] Eligible women were given a medical examination to ensure that they were in good health. Women who met these criteria and were placed in the Pill group were given a bottle of Searle-supplied pills and instructed to take one a day from the fifth to the twenty-fourth day of their menstrual cycle. The pills were called Enovid, and each contained 10 milligrams of norethynodrel and .15 milligram of synthetic estrogen, which had first been added to a batch of norethynodrel in Searle's factory by mistake. When Rock and Pincus found that the "contaminated" pills reduced the incidence of breakthrough bleeding, they asked Searle to make the estrogen component permanent.[65]

Finding a steady supply of recruits for the Rio Piedras experiment and for a second, smaller trial established in Humacao in 1957 was not a problem. The difficulty was convincing women to stay on the Pill and to comply with study protocol. By June 1957, 295 women had enrolled in the two trials. But 162—more than half—had dropped out. Adverse publicity was one reason for high attrition rates. Within the first month of the Rio Piedras trial, El Imparcial, a local newspaper, published an article denouncing a "neomalthusian campaign" perpetrated by a "woman dressed as a nurse" who was distributing "sterilizers" that were "white and round and are contained in very small bottles."[66] Twenty-five women immediately dropped out. The Imparcial article was the first of many published in Puerto Rican newspapers to accuse investigators of racist motives. Articles made much of the fact that the Pill was not being tested on "continental" American women and accused "Nordic whites" of using "the coloured races as 'guinea pigs.' "[67] Ironically, Pincus had chosen Puerto Rico as the site for his experiment because he believed that clinical tests on women there could be carried out quietly. But this was a belief premised on assumptions about the indifference, docility, and ignorance of Puerto Ricans. The Puerto Rican press's interest in the ethical and racial issues posed by the drug trial proved Pincus's miscalculation.

Then, too, there were the medical side effects: nausea, dizziness, headache, stomach pain, and vomiting. By late 1956, 17 percent of participants had complained of them. So serious and sustained were these reactions that Rice-Wray wrote Pincus that a ten-milligram dose of Enovid "gives one hundred percent protection against pregnancy" but causes "too many side reactions to be acceptable."[68] Pincus disagreed. Be-

lieving these medical unpleasantries to be largely psychosomatic, he initially attributed them to the power of suggestion. "Most of them happen
because women expect them to happen," he told a journalist. Apparently, too, Puerto Ricans were more suggestible than Americans. "I very
much doubt that the nausea, etc. has anything to do with the tablets," he
told Rice-Wray. "We have never seen it in any of *our* patients."[69]

Although investigators reassured participants about their medical
problems while taking Enovid, Puerto Rican women evaluated the drug's
safety—as well as the pros and cons of being a medical "guinea pig"—
through personal experience. In July 1957, Adaline Satterthwaite, the
director of the Humacao trial, complained that the "great problem to
date has been the break-through bleeding." Doctors considered it a
normal phenomenon during the first month, but when "women see a
spot they immediately conclude that it is the menstrual period." Many
women, believing, erroneously, that the drug had failed, immediately
stopped taking Enovid instead of taking "two pills and going on as directed." Women were just as willing to learn from each other as they
were from trial personnel. When one woman under Satterthwaite's supervision was hospitalized with a severe headache, probably a migraine,
others immediately stopped taking the drug. Satterthwaite considered it
"unlikely that [the headache] was the result of the tablets" but lamented
that since the incident occurred, "it takes a lot of talking and revisiting
to keep the ladies taking the medicine." In fact, subsequent studies found
that headache-prone women taking oral contraceptives were particularly
susceptible to debilitating migraines.[70]

Nonmedical considerations also motivated Puerto Rican women to
abandon the trial. Disapproving husbands and priests talked several
women out of participation. One woman stopped under desperate circumstances when her husband, overwhelmed by his family's poverty,
hanged himself. Some women moved. Others separated from their husbands and stopped having sex.[71]

High attrition rates were offset by a steady stream of volunteers. In
1957, Pincus established a new trial in Port-au-Prince, Haiti, where
medical birth control clinics were unknown. By November 1958, 830
women, mostly Puerto Rican, had taken Enovid in one of the three trials. Their experiences constituted the backbone of the safety data Pincus
would soon submit to the FDA.[72]

Pincus shared the information he gathered with G. D. Searle, which supplied free Enovid for his trials. Initially, the company was cautious about its association with a contraceptive drug. Searle's president, John Searle, encouraged Pincus to publish his Puerto Rican results, because he was eager to ascertain public responses to the news. But he instructed Pincus "to avoid our being associated, even by implication."[73]

The company's change of heart, its decision to forge ahead with the marketing of the Pill, stemmed not from an epiphany but from a chain of reassuring events. Word of the Pill's success in clinical trials provoked much excitement. Pincus first broke the news in 1955 at the International Planned Parenthood Conference in Tokyo. Then, in November 1956, *Science* magazine published the first article on the Pill intended for a general readership. By 1958, other reports had appeared in *Time, Fortune, Reader's Digest, Ladies' Home Journal,* and *True Story.* The public relations pundits at Searle expected a flurry of public protest. None came. Searle's public relations director, James W. Irwin, remembered the anxiety surrounding those days:

> We were going into absolutely unexplored ground in terms of public opinion. My fear was that this would provoke an avalanche of letters. So I went to see various people. I sat down with a lot of my friends at the *Saturday Evening Post.* They decided to do two major pieces about the pill. I said "look, I want to warn you. This is controversial. You may get a sizeable protest." But there was none. I told the same thing to *Reader's Digest.* And there was none. We were overly cautious. All my experiences told me that you could not do this without getting your teeth knocked out—or some of them. And we didn't lose any teeth. We had underestimated the receptivity of the product. We got quite a surprise.[74]

There were letters. But most were written not by social or religious critics but by women eager, even desperate, to try the new anti-ovulant. A married couple from Oklahoma volunteered to be test subjects. They were both college students and anxious not to have children "at present." They had read about the Pill in a magazine and wanted Pincus to know that they were willing "to enter into any testing program which you may know of to study drug effects."[75] In a similar vein, one California man chastised Pincus about his selection of study sites. "Puerto Rico and Haiti are fine," he wrote, "but I would much rather you tried the pill in my own household." Perhaps, he prodded, "you would conduct your experiment closer to home in the near future?"[76] Rarely did correspondents question the need for a better contraceptive or fault the ethics of the human trials integral to the drug's development. Typical, rather, was the request of one thirty-year-old Indianapolis mother. She had six children, all under age eight. She was tired and fearful of marital intimacy. "We have tried to be careful," she confided, "but I get pregnant anyway." Could Pincus help? "As of yet can these anti-pregnancy pills be purchased? Where?—How can I get them? Please help me."[77]

For the growing army of women and men who came to view the Pill as their salvation, help was on its way. In the summer of 1957, the Food and Drug Administration approved Enovid and norethindrone, issued by Syntex's American partner, Parke-Davis, which had obtained exclusive rights from Syntex to market the drug. The FDA approved Enovid and norethindrone only as prescription treatments for gynecological disorders, such as infertility, habitual miscarriage, and excessive menstruation. But although the FDA limited legal licensure to gynecological disorders, nothing could prevent a woman from using the Pill for "off-label" uses. As Pincus told Sanger, "Any physician may prescribe it for any purpose for which he considers it valid."[78] A gleeful Katharine McCormick quickly grasped the revolutionary implications of the FDA's ruling. "Of course this use of the oral contraceptive for menstrual disorders," she wrote presciently, "is leading inevitably to its use against pregnancy."[79]

McCormick's instincts were right. Women patients across the country immediately began using the new drug for contraception. Not all doctors disapproved. Some, like Pincus, privately promoted Enovid's use for birth control. When women contacted Pincus to get information about oral contraceptives, he outlined the regimen they should follow. Take the Pill "on the fifth day after the start of a menstrual period," he instructed one woman in 1958. "Two or three days after cessation of the medication, a menstrual period will occur, and the pill-taking is resumed on the fifth day after the start of this period."[80] By late 1959, at least half a million women had gone on the Pill—far more than were thought to suffer from the disorders for which it was officially prescribed.[81] As they had throughout American history, women defined the meaning of this new technology on their own terms.

G. D. Searle was pleased with the trend. High sales, after all, supplied additional evidence that offering Enovid openly as birth control could be a profitable, albeit controversial, endeavor. Early consumer responses to Enovid shaped the company's production and marketing plans, providing yet another example of how women, as consumers, have shaped business practices and technological development.

In 1959, Searle decided to apply for FDA permission to market Enovid as an oral contraceptive. The decision reflected a careful accounting of the benefits and drawbacks to the company. In 1970, Searle's medical director, Irwin Winter, recalled what was at stake:

> The attitudes prevailing in 1959 . . . were vastly different from those which exist today. Contraception was not a word which was used freely, and that use in the lay press was circumspect indeed. No major pharmaceutical manufacturer had ever dared to put its name on a "contraceptive." The individual reaction of a very large religious minority in the United States could not be gauged. The possibility of losing overnight one fourth of all of our personnel, a considerable portion of our hospital business, and a crippling number of the physician prescribers of our products was not to be dismissed lightly. Indeed, there were those who considered this possibility to be not that but a probability. It was not an easy decision. Open association with "contraception" and its positive promotion was an activity which our government shunned like the plague and was regarded as unseemly by the vast majority of academicians and the practicing profession itself.[82]

The controversy over contraception helped keep potential Pill rivals at bay. Many American firms, including Upjohn, Pfizer, Parke-Davis, Ortho, and Merck, had turned down the opportunity to develop the first oral contraceptive. It was too controversial. Although most Americans had come to favor contraception by the late 1950s, most states—thirty in 1960—still had laws restricting contraceptive advertisement and sale.[83] In Massachusetts and Connecticut, two of the country's most Catholic states, their prescription was banned outright. Pharmaceutical firms feared the condemnation of the Catholic Church—and for good reason. Twenty-five percent of the American population was Catholic in 1960. It seemed prudent to businesses to avoid marketing products that might trigger a general Catholic boycott of company goods. Pfizer's president and Merck's chief executive were devout Roman Catholics. But even Ortho, the largest manufacturer of diaphragms and vaginal jellies at the time, expressed reservations. Ortho's research director, Carl Hartman, sat on the medical advisory committee of Planned Parenthood, but he doubted that women would embrace a once-a-day birth control method.[84] This question was of general concern. One financial analyst recalled that the main "issue among drug people was whether any woman would take a pill every day for twenty-one days to prevent the chance she might get pregnant. They believed nobody's going to do that, not when they're not sick—and they're not sick! This was a prevention drug—prevention as a social activity as opposed to prevention of cancer or something."[85]

Searle's only serious rival in the race for the Pill was the Mexican firm Syntex, which was disadvantaged because it did not have a retail marketing division in the United States. In 1956, the New York financier Charles Allen, who had previously made a fortune in the scrap-materials business, bought Syntex for about $2.5 million. The same year, the company began to manufacture its progestin, norethindrone, for commercial use. It licensed it to Schering A.G. in Germany, which sold it to European consumers for gynecological disorders, and to Parke-Davis, which in 1957 sold it in the United States under the trade name Norlutin. Then Syntex's plans to market Norlutin as birth control hit a snag. Parke-Davis, avowedly one of the most conservative pharmaceutical houses in America, informed Syntex it would not market Norlutin as a contraceptive. It had never planned to, of course, but official word left Syntex without a U.S. partner for a drug whose full market potential was unknown; in addition, Syntex's main rival, G. D. Searle, now possessed a variant of the drug. Syntex signed a contract with Ortho, but the Mexican company's problems were not over. Just when Syntex's American Pill seemed a done deal, Parke-Davis refused to release the results of its animal studies, required to secure FDA approval. Consequently, Ortho had to start several clinical investigations from scratch, creating a two-year time lag that cost Syntex and Ortho unquantifiable profits. In 1962, Ortho marketed Ortho-Novum, Syntex's American Pill. The delay had permitted G. D. Searle to reap the benefits of being the sole manufacturer of oral contraceptives in the U.S. market for two years.[86]

Syntex's interest in oral contraceptives kept pressure on G. D. Searle and helped nudge the Chicago firm from a position of caution to one of commitment. In December 1958, Irwin Winter contacted Pincus. "It is no news," he wrote, "that the powers that be are breathing down our neck in the hopes of speeding up our application to the Food and Drug Administration of the contraceptive utility of Enovid."[87] Searle was unsure how the FDA would react to its application. Enovid had already been sanctioned by the FDA for use for gynecological disorders, but Searle's new request—that the FDA approve its use for what was considered a "social" reason—was forcing the FDA into uncharted territory. Only a few months earlier, the science journalist Robert Sheehan had predicted a negative outcome. "There is a vast difference between dispensing the drug as a safe means of inducing temporary sterility for therapeutic purposes," he advised readers of an article on birth control pills for *Fortune*, "and dispensing it for 'habitual use' as a standard contraceptive. It will take perhaps five years of research to satisfy any drug firm that it is ready to apply to the Food and Drug Administration for permission to so label its product; and it would probably take five years after that before the FDA—which says it may well require clinical data on 'thousands of women,' not 500—would approve such applications."[88]

In the early 1960s, when reports of Pill-related medical problems surfaced, many wondered if FDA officials had failed women by approving Enovid as a contraceptive too hastily. But there is no evidence that the FDA rushed Searle's application through bureaucratic hoops or held Enovid to different, never mind inferior, standards. By law and custom, the FDA had only one mandate: to determine whether a manufacturer had proved the safety of a drug. At the time the FDA was evaluating Searle's application, the scope of its authority had remained unchanged since the passage of the 1938 Food, Drug, and Cosmetic Act, which had first imposed the "safety" requirement to regulate the patent medicine market. In October 1962, Congress strengthened FDA control over the approval of new drugs in the wake of Europe's thalidomide disaster. Thalidomide was a teratogenic drug introduced in 1956 as a sedative and widely prescribed to pregnant, predominantly western European, women to control morning sickness. Thousands of babies were born malformed as a result. Although the FDA did not approve the use of thalidomide in the United States, Europe's experience prodded Congress to broaden FDA authority. But in 1958, when Searle submitted its application, the events and concerns that gave rise to regulatory reform still lay ahead.

Was the clinical sample size for the Pill too small? Searle's application included data on 897 women. Tellingly, in the wake of the "Pill crisis," the FDA would impose tougher standards. In 1965, it stipulated that data on no fewer than a thousand women would be required before the FDA would consider an application for a new oral contraceptive. The new regulation reflected a concern, if not a consensus, that the medical experiences of 897 women were not enough.

But in the late 1950s, there were no fixed rules about what constituted an appropriate sample size for a new drug, a flexibility that permitted considerable variation from one drug application to the next. The size of the Pill sample was typical of that of other drug trials at the time.[89] In addition, the FDA had already pronounced Enovid safe for the treatment of gynecological disorders. Although Searle's contraceptive application was separate, FDA officials must have derived some reassurance from the absence of reports on serious Enovid-related troubles.

Telling, too, were the frequent frustrations expressed by those who brought Enovid to market. No one involved in the Pill project considered FDA officials pushovers or the application process easy. At one point, an exasperated Katharine McCormick declared the FDA approval mechanisms as "slow as molasses." Searle executives were furious when the FDA refused to review simultaneously three proposed Enovid doses—10, 5, and 2.5 milligrams. Because the FDA believed there was insufficient evidence to document the safety of the two smaller doses, Searle had to submit separate applications for these. The FDA's deliberations were comprehensive; Searle would later complain that it had taken nearly ten months for the agency to do its job. In truth, the FDA faced a herculean task, for Searle had submitted an astounding twenty volumes of data, the largest new drug application to date in American history. In addition to reviewing Searle's submission, the FDA contacted physicians who had prescribed the drug in private practice. In February 1960, it also sent out a questionnaire to seventy-five leading obstetrician-gynecologists at major medical schools, soliciting input on Enovid's prospective safety as a contraceptive. In May 1960, the FDA approved a 10-milligram daily dose of Enovid for contraceptive use. Concerned about potential long-term side effects, it limited consumer use to two sequential years.

Pasquale DeFelice, a staff physician at Georgetown University Medical Center, was in charge of assessing the initial application in 1959. His task was to decide whether the FDA should even consider Searle's application. A Catholic, he worked for the FDA as a part-time reviewer and was starstruck at meeting John Rock, who went to Washington in December 1959 with Irwin Winter to help present Searle's case before the FDA. DeFelice remembered that "the Searle people were very anxious to get the pill on the market." But DeFelice had his own anxieties. Although the important things "to us at the FDA were quality control, purity of product, and side effects," no one involved in the drug's approval was oblivious to the larger social issues at stake. "I knew what was going to happen once we licensed it," he recalled. "I knew that birth control pills would be flying out the windows. Everybody and her sister would be taking it. You know something; I was stupid. I should be a millionaire. I should have Searle stock, but I didn't. Somehow I thought I shouldn't since I was the person who approved it. But I often wondered why I never got an award for okaying the Pill. It changed the whole economy of the United States."[90] That, and it affected how millions of Americans experienced the 1960s.

TEN

The Pill in Practice

American women were quick to accept oral contraceptives into their lives. Within two years of FDA approval, 1.2 million women were taking the Pill, within five years, over six million.[1] Never just a medical event, Pill mania was a cultural and political phenomenon that joined journalists, scientists, politicians, and African-American and feminist activists in open and often heated debate about the social implications and larger meanings of oral contraception. As the nation's leaders wondered and worried, women registered their opinions at the pharmacist's counter, where they made the Pill one of the best-selling drugs in American history.

Elizabeth Linden remembers the unpleasant side effects she experienced when she first went on the Pill in 1960. She had headaches and bloating, and she gained almost fifteen pounds. But what she remembers most is the peace of mind an almost foolproof method of birth control gave her. The former schoolteacher had had three children in her first five years of marriage and had left the workforce to raise them. Her husband was finishing his residency in obstetrics and gynecology, and the family was struggling to pay the bills on a resident's salary. "He had jobs everywhere so we could make enough money to live," she recalled. And "I was just panicked that I might get pregnant."[2]

The couple had used condoms and spermicidal jelly for birth control when Jack first started medical school, but on June 23, 1960, a new product, one that Jack had heard a lot about, was released on the market. It was Searle's Enovid. Elizabeth had delivered her third baby in 1959, and when Jack told her about the new drug, she decided to give it a try. She stayed on it for ten years, stopping only when Jack had a vasectomy as a present for her on her fortieth birthday. During her decade on the Pill, Elizabeth commiserated about side effects with her female friends, most of whom took it, too. "I remember that I was very uncomfortable on it at first, that it was terrible," she said. But she refused to quit. She knew that next to abstinence, the Pill was the most effective birth control available. Despite the side effects, "I never stopped," she recalled. "I was afraid that if I went back to another method of birth control, then we'd get pregnant."[3]

Like Linden, women across the country exulted in the availability of a "magic pill" that, unlike any other contraceptive then available, prevented pregnancy almost 100 percent of the time. In Worcester, letters to Gregory Pincus arrived in droves. These were not the earlier missives of desperate women offering themselves as human subjects. These were fan letters sent by grateful women who had already discovered the wonders of Pincus's invention for themselves. "I would personally like to thank you for the marvelous contribution you have made to the world of medicine," wrote one from Van Nuys, California. Another concurred. The Pill had irrevocably improved the lot of womankind. "Not since they proved Pasteur's theory on childbirth death," she raved, "has anyone done more." The executive secretary of the St. Paul, Minnesota, branch of Planned Parenthood shared with Pincus a particularly memorable moment. "At a recent clinic session," she wrote, an Enovid user "told us that she has 'kissed' your picture (in our local newspaper)—she is so grateful to you, for this is the first year in her eight years of marriage that she has not been pregnant."[4]

Could a pill empower women? Some women certainly thought so. Clare Boothe Luce, the second American female ambassador, told a reporter in 1969 that with the Pill, "Modern woman is at last free, as a man is free, to dispose of her own body."[5] In her hit song "The Pill," Loretta Lynn sang of the advent of a new era of drug-induced sexual liberation. "All these years I've stayed at home while you had all your fun; / And ev'ry year that's gone by another baby's come," she belted. "There's gonna be some changes made right here on Nurs'ry Hill; / You've set this chicken your last time, 'cause now I've got the Pill."[6]

Here, finally, was a reliable method women could control without the fuss and mess of diaphragms. "It's the safest method of contraception," said one woman. "The only one I trust almost 100 per cent." Stated another: "As far as sex goes, well, we want to be able to do it in unexpected times and places. That's half the fun. We're finished with that greasy kid stuff forever." Joan, a thirty-six-year-old, was equally enthusiastic. She believed the Pill had saved her sex life and possibly her marriage. She had found use of her previous method, the diaphragm, laborious and had reserved insertion for occasions when sex with her husband seemed a "sure thing." Her husband yearned for spontaneity and asked her to "do it automatically. When you brush your teeth, put in the diaphragm. If we don't make love that night, so what? And if we do, we don't have to be bothered." Joan tried to be accommodating. But she felt rejected when "after I'd gone through the whole messy business of putting it in . . . he'd just turn over and go to sleep." The couple's sex life ground to a halt. Then Joan went on the Pill. Her husband thought the drug was "the greatest." Joan had reservations about its side effects, but five years after starting, she was still taking it.[7]

Some women complained about weight gain. Fad diets abounded in the 1960s as oral contraceptive users tried valiantly to fend off unwanted Pill poundage. But not every Pill user was bothered by her newfound plumpness. "Oh, I know, I've put on a little weight since I started on the pill," gushed one Chicago housewife in her late twenties, "but I think it's just from contentment."[8] As increased estrogen swelled women's breasts, brassiere designers scrambled to create undergarments that would comfortably accommodate them. The sale of C-cup bras increased 50 percent in the United States between 1960 and 1969.[9] "For the first time in my life, I have a real bosom," said one grateful woman. "I always felt so inferior. I used to wear falsies or at least a padded bra. . . . Once, in the swimming pool, one of my falsies came out and just floated away. I was a laughing stock."[10]

Women's testimonials and rising prescription rates demonstrated the new technology's appeal. By 1964, the Pill had become the most popular form of contraception in the country, used by one-fourth of all couples practicing contraception.[11] By 1968, American women were spending $150 million a year on oral contraceptives, almost as much as Americans in 1958 spent on all other contraceptive methods combined.[12]

Journalists added oral contraceptives to the long list of pharmaceutical triumphs Americans had come to expect from their Cold War scientists and engineers. Here was a technological breakthrough of global significance that confirmed Yankee ingenuity and the possibilities of a better world through chemistry. The Pill symbolized the redemption of science, showing it capable of developing a technology to stabilize a world order that it simultaneously threatened to destroy. As one journalist observed, "The promise of a simple way to control population has its ironic aspect . . . at a time when mankind is crouched in fear of wholesale destruction. . . . Science . . . seems to have discovered a method to limit the reproduction of people at the very time when the world is threatened by the self-annihilation of the species."[13]

But not everyone was so upbeat. As birthrates fell, businessmen who had prospered from the baby-boom economy worried about future earnings. Who would buy new homes, dolls, canned baby food?[14] Social conservatives blamed the Pill for relaxing moral standards, especially among the nation's youth. By removing the risk of unwanted pregnancy, oral contraception made promiscuity an easier choice. Nonsense, countered family planning advocates and the drug's inventors, who rushed to defend their creation. "Increased promiscuity has been voiced ever since the first contraceptive device was discovered," Gregory Pincus told one correspondent. "Countless studies . . . have shown that this fear is groundless."[15] John Rock agreed. The expense of the Pill and the fact that it was obtainable only by prescription prohibited its casual or "impulse" use. Besides, "low cost preventatives are already universally available for naughty little girls who want to use them."[16] After all, "any high school kid can get other contraceptives and probably knows about Saranwrap [for makeshift condoms] from the kitchen."[17] That fertility rates began to drop in 1957—three years before oral contraceptives were mass marketed—countered the assertion that the Pill was single-handedly responsible for ushering in new patterns of sexual behavior. "Women make decisions about the way they want to behave and then fit the pill in or not," insisted Ernst Prelinger, a Yale psychologist. A sociologist studying premarital sexuality agreed. Unmarried individuals were not blank slates over which the Pill exerted an almighty force. "Basic values, emotional involvement, and the courtship system," he argued, were the crucial variables determining how young women and men encountered this new technology.[18]

Meanwhile, the Catholic Church had its own worries. In 1958, a month before his death, Pope Pius XII outlined the Church's position on oral hormones. They could be used to treat reproductive disorders; but used for birth control, they were morally unacceptable. The Church was unpersuaded by John Rock's appeals, best articulated in his 1963 book, *The Time Has Come: A Catholic Doctor's Proposal to End the Battle over Birth Control*. Rock argued that because the Pill imitated the body's own chemistry to prevent an egg from maturing, its use was compatible with Church teachings.[19] In 1968, Pope Paul VI issued the encyclical *Humanae vitae*, affirming Pius's position. In this golden age of chemical contraception, the Catholic laity was admonished to stick with the rhythm method.

The Church met with a groundswell of resistance as women determined what was right and wrong for themselves. A majority of American Catholics favored a relaxation of Church rules; one 1964 survey found that those who did outnumbered those who did not by more than three to two. Catholic women openly defied Church teachings, taking oral contraceptives and defending their actions as morally just. "I don't confess that I take the pill," remarked a New Jersey mother of four, "because I don't believe it is a sin."[20] By 1970, an estimated 28 percent of all Catholic women of childbearing age had taken the Pill.[21]

Female enthusiasm was good news for pharmaceutical companies, especially G. D. Searle. The Illinois firm was rewarded handsomely for the risk it had incurred bringing the first oral contraceptive to market. In the two years that it took rival Johnson & Johnson's subsidiary, Ortho Pharmaceuticals, to launch its Ortho-Novum brand, Searle's was the only Pill that American women could buy. Searle's soaring sales—which rose from thirty-seven million dollars in 1960 to eighty-nine million in 1965—reflected the advantage of its initial monopoly status. Even after other brands were made available, many women remained loyal to Enovid.[22] In 1967, Searle claimed a 40 percent share of the ninety-million-dollar oral contraceptive market. The company made other best-selling proprietary drugs, including Dramamine for motion sickness, Lomotil for diarrhea, and Pro-Banthine for ulcers. But in 1965, half of its business came from oral contraceptives. Some industry analysts speculated that the company enjoyed the highest profit margin in the U.S. drug business.[23]

Not to be left out of the buying bonanza, other firms attempted to duplicate Searle's success. Disappointed by its failure to manufacture oral contraceptives first, Syntex rebounded. It supplied synthetic hormones to other manufacturers, principally Johnson & Johnson and Parke-Davis, which in 1964, as Carl Djerassi joked, "finally woke up to the facts of life and decided to enter the contraceptive market after all." Now equipped with a U.S. retail division, Syntex also introduced its own low-dose pill, Norinyl, in 1964.[24] In 1965, Eli Lilly and Company and Mead Johnson entered the fray with the first sequential, or phasic, oral contraceptives, which reduced the side effects associated with progestin intake.[25] In 1967, seven manufacturers were vying for a share of the lucrative Pill market, whose annual sales rose from $16 million in 1962 to $150 million in 1968, a nearly tenfold increase in just six years.[26]

Ironically, women's embrace of the Pill occurred within a business environment that impeded free and open contraceptive commerce. One barrier was advertising. Like other prescription drugs, the Pill could not be advertised directly to consumers. In addition, until 1965 in Connecticut and Massachusetts, obscenity laws prohibited even married women from acquiring birth control from doctors. Frustrated by Connecticut's contraceptive ban (part of a "mini" Comstock Law enacted in 1879), Estelle Griswold, executive director of the Planned Parenthood League of Connecticut, and C. Lee Buxton, chair of the Department of Obstetrics at the Yale University School of Medicine, decided to challenge the law's constitutionality. They opened a birth control clinic on November 1, 1961. Their prosecution resulted in the landmark 1965 ruling, *Griswold v. Connecticut*, in which the Supreme Court struck down the Connecticut law. The Court declared that a constitutional right to privacy for married couples fell within the "penumbra" of the Bill of Rights—understood in this context to be the right to matrimonial privacy in the bedroom, including the freedom to use contraceptives. It would take seven more years before the Supreme Court guaranteed the same rights to *unmarried* individuals in its 1972 ruling in *Eisenstadt v. Baird*. With this decision, the Supreme Court erased the last vestiges of Comstock's legal legacy.[27]

These Court victories were important, but it would be a mistake to assume that the laws they overturned had prevented women from learning about or acquiring the Pill. Women heard about the wonder drug from newspapers, magazines, television broadcasts, friends, relatives, and doctors. Even in Catholic Connecticut and Massachusetts, women got the Pill with the help of sympathetic doctors who avoided legal censure by "officially" prescribing it only for gynecological disorders. Not every doctor prescribed contraceptives, but those who would not frequently helped women locate doctors who did. Birgit Haus was a junior at Boston University in 1964 when she gave birth to her first child, the by-product of an unplanned pregnancy. ("Good girls didn't think about birth control," she recalled.) At her first postpartum checkup, Birgit and her OB-GYN discussed birth control. "I had the distinct sense that he wanted me to have this information," she remembers. Reluctant to give it to her, he referred her to another doctor who would.[28] Mary Calderone, the medical director of Planned Parenthood, speculated in 1961 that it was probably easier to get the Pill in Massachusetts and Connecticut than in other states where pharmacists who were uncomfortable with the drug's legal uses might refuse to fill prescriptions.[29]

By the mid-1960s, the Pill's popularity had proven that the over-the-counter condom had finally met its match, at least in the United States. In 1958, when sales of "ethical" female contraceptives (diaphragms, spermicidal jellies, creams, and tablets) accounted for $20 million, condoms were a $150 million business and the most frequently used contraceptive in the country. But the Pill displaced the condom, whose U.S. sales had plummeted to $85 million by 1963. In 1968, Americans were twice as likely to use the Pill as they were condoms.[30]

The country's love affair with the Pill was in many respects a quintessentially American phenomenon. Millions more women used the Pill in the United States than in any other country. In 1967, the Population Council estimated that of the 12.84 million women worldwide taking oral contraceptives, over half—6.5 million—were in the United States. Next highest on the list were Canada and Brazil, with 750,000 users each; Britain, with 700,000; and the rest of Europe, with 1.2 million. Developing nations accounted for only 2.9 million users, 23 percent of the total.[31]

In contrast, the condom remained the most popular global method in the late 1960s. Because the United States, with veteran manufacturers Julius Schmid and Youngs Rubber at the helm, led the way in worldwide condom production, American condom makers did not sustain heavy financial losses after the Pill took off at home. In 1968, the United States dominated international condom production, with 38 percent of the global market. Its biggest customers were West Germany, Canada, India, Ceylon, and Pakistan.[32]

In the United States, the Pill achieved what the prescription-only diaphragm had not: it medicalized birth control, transforming medical practice as much as it did women's lives. Suddenly physicians who had no training in hormonal birth control (and often only minimal professional experience with contraception more generally) found their days occupied with patient demand for and advice on the Pill. A Florida physician who graduated from medical school in 1954 recalled that early on "most methods of contraception were simple and commonly available without prescription at any drugstore." Contraceptive advice claimed no more than "1 percent of my practice time." Then came the Pill. "The time spent with advice and care related to contraception suddenly skyrocketed to 20 to 25 percent," he stated.[33]

Much has been made of the ways in which physicians ostensibly "pushed" oral contraceptives on women. Certainly, the decision by women to adopt the Pill entailed a trade-off. In exchange for more trustworthy contraception and spontaneous sex, women gave up some of the social control they had previously exercised over their own pregnancy prevention. Before 1960, because of the popularity of over-the-counter methods, the proportion of women who sought physicians' advice about birth control totaled no more than 20 percent. By the mid-1960s, the prescription-only Pill had made visits to the doctor routine for millions of American women and had made physicians the chief custodians of new contraceptive technologies, confirming and heightening their authority as experts. Women's vulnerability to pregnancy decreased even as their dependence on doctors and the biomedical industry grew.[34]

But doctors' recollections from this era suggest that many physicians felt pressured by women to prescribe oral contraceptives, not the other way around. As consumers, women were never just pawns of the reorientation of medical practice; they were its driving force.

Women's demands forced doctors who had been hesitant about prescribing birth control to accept family planning as a routine component of medical practice. A 1957 study of specialists and family practitioners in six communities showed that half were unwilling to initiate contraception counseling and that most viewed birth control as outside their professional scope. A 1971 study of 226 physicians in private practice revealed a dramatic change. When asked the question "Do you provide contraceptive service to your private female patients?" 98 percent of OB-GYNS, 95 percent of family physicians, and 87 percent of internists said they did. Even among Catholic physicians, the group least likely to support birth control, 78 percent replied affirmatively. Two-thirds of surveyed physicians stated that family planning was a "routine procedure" in their medical practices.[35]

The Pill changed the economics of medical practice, forcing doctors to comply with women's requests or lose business. This was an important consideration in a pre-HMO world, where a fee-for-service system gave patients more economic clout than they have today. In a 1967 poll of 2,515 obstetrician-gynecologists conducted by Ladies' Home Journal, 89 percent of respondents said that women expected them to prescribe the Pill. Although many physicians harbored misgivings about dispensing a drug whose long-term side effects were unknown, only a handful refused to prescribe oral contraceptives. To do so would result in the loss of patients.[36]

Jack Linden, the husband of Elizabeth Linden, experienced firsthand the myriad changes in medical practice spawned by the Pill. He graduated from medical school in 1954 and completed his residency in obstetrics and gynecology in 1959. He received little training in contraceptive medicine. When he began practice, his involvement with birth control was limited to fitting diaphragms and counseling women about condoms and the rhythm method, "which we euphemistically called 'Vatican Roulette.' " When Enovid arrived in 1960, "it was revolutionary. You couldn't avoid it." He remembers being pressured by women patients, who began calling his office and "just dropping by" en masse.[37]

A doctor's decision to prescribe oral contraceptives necessitated a long-term relationship with a patient. Medical protocol encouraged doctors to conduct an initial gynecological exam followed by periodic checkups once patients started taking the drug. This was necessary because of how oral contraceptives worked. Unlike barrier methods, the

Pill was systemic. Linden recalls: "The condom or the diaphragm had nothing to do with endocrinology, balancing your system. It was a simple mechanical device, and it was a no-brainer. When you put a woman on oral contraceptive pills, you are dabbling with a patient's physiologic mechanism, or endocrine system, not just the estrogen and progestin, you are finagling with her thyroid function, her reaction to other medications she may be taking, and things such as that. . . . If you compare the fitting of the diaphragm, overall, versus the need to write prescriptions and [have] consultations [with women] on their reaction to the Pill, the Pill is a bigger headache than the barrier method."[38]

Reports of Pill-related problems underscored the necessity of medical management. In late 1961, two young women in Los Angeles died of pulmonary embolisms, blood clots in arteries supplying the lungs, usually caused when a fragment of a larger blood clot in the veins (thrombophlebitis) breaks off and migrates. Both women had been taking Enovid, one for a month, the other for two. Both had been otherwise healthy. Alarmed by the possibility that the fatalities had been drug-induced, many physicians urged patients to discontinue oral contraceptives, and others began to monitor Pill patients more closely. Gregory Pincus defended the drug's safety. In a letter to Warren Nelson, the medical director of the Population Council, he described the two deaths as "either coincidences with nothing at all to do with the use of Enovid, or . . . if an Enovid effect is involved, it represents an incidence of approximately 1 in 500,000 which is so rare as to be scarcely investigatable."[39]

G. D. Searle reached similar conclusions. In 1962, it sponsored two conferences to discuss Enovid's safety. The first, attended by the company's medical staff, blood-coagulation experts, and representatives of the AMA's Council on Drugs, concluded that "no causal relationship between Enovid and thrombophlebitis had been demonstrated."[40] The second was attended by medical experts and well-known figures in the field of contraceptive research: Pincus, John Rock, Mary Calderone, and Christopher Tietze, research director of the Committee on Maternal Health. Conferees urged that more studies on the physiological and biochemical effects of Enovid be undertaken but concurred that the drug posed "no real immediate danger" to patients.[41]

The Food and Drug Administration was also forced to get involved. As of August 1, 1962, twenty-eight cases of blood clots among more than one million Enovid users had been reported in the United States. Following an article in the *British Medical Journal* indicating that four women had developed blood clots after taking the drug, Norway banned oral contraceptives. Family planning organizations and physicians in the United States turned to the FDA for guidance. On August 8, the FDA, finding no statistical correlation between the use of Enovid and the development of thrombotic disease, stated that Enovid could continue to be sold in the United States.

Soon circumstances would force the FDA to deliberate on Enovid's safety again. A precipitating factor was mounting political interest for legislation to expand FDA power in the wake of the thalidomide crisis. News about birth defects caused by the sedative first hit American newspapers in early 1962. The FDA's role in keeping the drug off the U.S. market earned the agency widespread praise and helped propel passage in October 1962 of new federal drug regulations, the Kefauver-Harris amendments. The amendments to the 1938 Food, Drug, and Cosmetic Act required pharmaceutical firms to demonstrate a new drug's effectiveness as a precondition of its approval. They also obligated manufacturers to inform doctors about the risks, as well as the benefits, of drugs in medical advertising. (Drug advertising to consumers was still forbidden.)[42] A milestone in the evolution of U.S. consumer regulation, the Kefauver-Harris amendments signaled the end of the postwar faith in pharmaceutical medicine and a growing suspicion of, even outright hostility toward, the drug industry.

The timing could not have been worse for G. D. Searle. Searle blamed mounting media scrutiny of the company and of Enovid on the thalidomide scare, a medical tragedy not of its making. Thalidomide, proclaimed John Searle, president of the company, had generated "mass hysteria on matters of medicine and health," creating an environment ripe "for sharp press, radio, TV, and public reactions to any news of an adverse nature involving *any* drug."[43] Certainly, it encouraged patients and physicians to report cases of blood clots among Enovid users to the FDA. By the end of 1962, the number of such reports had reached 272, up from only 28 in August.[44]

In August 1963, an ad hoc FDA committee pronounced Enovid safe for short-term use (two to four years) by women under age thirty-five. Finding no cause-and-effect relationship between Enovid and thrombotic disease in young women, it nevertheless urged Searle to send a "caution letter" to physicians, alerting them to the *possibility* of thrombophlebitis among Enovid users. Searle readily complied.[45] In 1966, a second FDA committee, the Advisory Committee on Obstetrics and Gynecology, released its *Report on the Oral Contraceptives*, addressing a possible link between the Pill and thromboembolic disease, cancer, and endocrine and metabolic disorders. The report was cautiously optimistic, concluding that there were "no adequate scientific data, at this time, proving these compounds unsafe for human use."[46]

When a British study contradicted these findings, the FDA was forced to reassess. The authors, two medical statisticians, examined the records of nineteen hospitals in southeastern England, earmarking those in which female patients had been admitted with thromboembolism. What they found was disturbing: women taking the Pill were nine times more likely to develop thrombophlebitis than those who were not. The study's findings triggered a maelstrom of debate in North America and Europe. By 1968, when the study's final report was published, it had become clear that there were more questions than answers about the safety of oral contraceptives.

The FDA took the British study seriously. It sent one of its infrequent "Dear Doctor" letters to every practicing physician in the country, announcing new oral contraceptive labeling requirements that included a summary of the findings on thromboembolism. It also launched its own study based on hospital admission records for women of childbearing age in five American cities. The FDA report, released in August 1969, corroborated the British study. It found that users of oral contraceptives were 4.4 times more likely than nonusers to develop thromboembolism. (Different risk rates between the two studies were attributed to sociocultural factors such as diet.) All told, it had taken the FDA more than eight years since the first reports of deaths among American Pill users to confirm a correlation between blood clots and oral contraceptives.[47]

Throughout this period of medical uncertainty, the number of American women taking the Pill continued to rise. We do not have an accurate count of how many women knew about the controversy, but we can reasonably assume that many, perhaps most, were aware that taking oral contraceptives posed certain health risks, even if they were uninformed about their scope or severity. Although most media accounts of oral contraceptives were favorable until the late 1960s, there were important exceptions, and even the most positive reports were punctuated by cautionary remarks. Women could learn about the pros and cons of the Pill in *Redbook, The Saturday Evening Post, Good Housekeeping, Ebony,* and *Ladies' Home Journal,* acquire information from concerned doctors, or discuss side effects with friends, as Elizabeth Linden did. By the end of the decade, they could also consult Barbara Seaman's pathbreaking 1969 book, *The Doctors' Case against the Pill,* which detailed the Pill's health risks so effectively that it established Seaman, in the words of one activist, as the "Ralph Nader of the birth control pill."[48] Seaman was a feminist journalist who worked as a columnist and contributing editor at *Ladies' Home Journal* from 1965 to 1969. Even before her book was published, she had alerted women to the Pill's potential dangers on radio and television and in magazine articles.

Seaman was dismayed to discover how many women knew about—or worse, suffered from—Pill-related problems but refused to give the contraceptive up. One mother of two, delighting in her more amply endowed bosom, was adamant. "I know the pill is dangerous," she told Seaman, "but I plan to stay on it come hell or high water. And if they withdraw it, I'm going to get those silicone shots. They're dangerous too. I know it. I don't care."[49] Another Pill user confided that when her doctor warned her of the drug's dangers, she retorted: "I don't care if you promise me cancer in five years, I'm staying on the pill. At least I'll enjoy the five years I have left. For the first time in eighteen years of married life I can put my feet up for an hour and read a magazine." Reminding the doctor that his services were replaceable, she added: "If you refuse to give me the pill, I'll go get it from someone else."[50]

Throughout the 1960s, dropout rates fluctuated, but a majority of women who tried the Pill stayed on it, for they believed the drug's benefits outweighed its risks. A Planned Parenthood study found an attrition rate of only 25 percent among Pill patients after several years of use, compared with 60 percent among women who used traditional methods.[51]

The availability of lower-dosed tablets minimized side effects and reassured women about the Pill's safety. The estrogen and progestin content of most oral contraceptives dropped during the 1960s. When Enovid was first released in May 1960, it contained 10 milligrams of progestin and .15 milligram of synthetic estrogen. By 1963, a tablet with 2 milligrams of progestin and .1 milligram of estrogen had become available. By 1970, the amount of estrogen (the cause of most women's side effects) in most oral contraceptives ranged from .05 to .1 milligram. (Today, oral contraceptives contain only 20 to 50 *micro*grams of estrogen.) Many women who switched to a lower-dosed oral contraceptive found that problems with weight gain, nausea, and headaches quickly subsided. Elizabeth Linden remembers that "as the dosage came down," life "got more comfortable."[52] By 1974, most women were taking low-dose formulations. In 1988, after pressure from the FDA, manufacturers removed high-dose estrogen contraceptives from the market.[53]

Not all women gave the Pill high marks. Although oral contraceptives had become the most popular form of birth control in the country by the mid-1960s, a majority of women of childbearing age did not take them. Most nonusers were not openly hostile to the Pill. They simply believed that it was not right for them. Some found oral contraceptives too expensive; others were satisfied with their traditional method. Women who had intercourse infrequently often viewed a daily drug regimen to prevent pregnancy as "pharmaceutical overkill." Still others were planning a family or were opposed, for personal or religious reasons, to birth control.

From the beginning, however, some women were vexed enough with the larger political issues posed by the Pill to voice their criticisms and concerns. Several sent angry letters to John Rock and Gregory Pincus. "Why don't you men take the contraceptive pills?" one irate mother asked Rock. "Stop making us—the women—guinea pigs in this experiment. . . . Why don't men mature and understand that there are desires in life besides excessive use of your love-stick?"[54] Addressing Pincus, a New York woman expressed concern over the feminization of birth control. "Why is it," she asked, "that the billions of words being written, printed, [and] spoken now on the subject of the Population Explosion, [are] directed to WOMEN? All about what Women can and should DO, but NOT ONE WORD have I read or heard directed towards MEN."[55] A grandmother of nine and mother of three from Ohio told Rock in 1963 that a pill for men was overdue: "The women more than do their share. The men are the most passionate, so why not control them for a change? . . . Please let us women have a rest from pills and put the cure where it belongs—on men!"[56]

Rock and Pincus defended the benefit to society of a "female" Pill with answers that by decade's end had become well-worn. Rock reassured the grandmother from Ohio that researchers were developing new and better male contraceptives. "It will not be long now when you can feel that you are getting even," he wrote. He also thanked her for her restraint. "You are somewhat gentler in approach than a correspondent from Kansas who suggested that clamps might be applied to appropriate places [on men] such as cattlemen use on bulls."[57] Pincus reminded one woman demanding more male methods that an excellent one, the condom, already existed. Worldwide, "men exercise control in far larger numbers than do women." The media excitement surrounding the Pill, he insisted, stemmed from the possibilities of female control over what had historically been a masculine domain. Like Sanger, Pincus had difficulties understanding why women would want to depend on men for contraception when "the woman bears the burden of pregnancy."[58]

By the late 1960s, the site of debate had shifted from private correspondence to public, national discussion. As questions about the Pill's safety escalated, so, too, did media attention to the problems and possibilities of contraceptive technology. Even more important to fomenting critical debate was the burgeoning feminist movement, which encouraged women to understand their individual experiences as part of broader social patterns. Women's frustrations with the Pill were parlayed into general indictments of sexism in American society. Why was birth control a female responsibility? Why did men control the medical profession and the pharmaceutical industry, and did women's health interests suffer as a result? Undergirding these questions was an unshakable conviction that when it came to the Pill, the personal was political.

In the late 1960s, the mainstream media were taking notice of the feminist movement even if, as the scholar Susan Douglas has shown, they also went to great lengths to contain it by legitimizing liberal, reform-minded views and denouncing those that called for a revolutionary overhaul of American society.[59] Television cameras rolled when busloads of women boycotted the Miss America Pageant in 1968. They were there again in 1970 to cover the speeches, rally, and march sponsored by the Women's Strike for Equality in New York City to commemorate the Nineteenth Amendment's fiftieth anniversary and to press for equal rights for working women. Newscasters debated the probable longevity of the new feminist magazine Ms., which hit newsstands on January 25,

1972. (Many who had predicted a short shelf life were embarrassed when it sold a whopping 250,000 copies in the first eight days.) Even before the first issue of *Ms.* appeared, its editor, Gloria Steinem, had graced the cover of *Newsweek* under the caption "The New Woman."

So it was no surprise that when the Senate held hearings on the safety of the Pill from January to March 1970, the media were there for that too. The hearings were conducted by the Wisconsin senator and Democrat Gaylord Nelson, chair of the Subcommittee on Monopoly of the Select Committee on Small Business. Since 1967, Nelson had been investigating competition in the pharmaceutical industry. He had already held hearings on antibiotics and psychotropic drugs such as barbiturates and tranquilizers. After reading Seaman's book, he decided to hold a similar inquiry into the use of oral contraceptives. Its two primary aims, he told the press, were: "First, whether they are dangerous for the human body, and, second, whether patients taking them have sufficient information about possible dangers in order to make an intelligent judgment whether they wish to assume the risk."[60]

Like Seaman, Nelson had misgivings about oral contraceptives. Influenced by the renascent consumer movement, he worried that the Pill had been inadequately tested, that its long-term effects were unknown, and that women were inadequately informed about the drug's risks. Still, Nelson won few feminist fans when he refused to ask a single woman to testify before the all-male committee in the first round of hearings, notwithstanding the fact that feminist organizations had asked to be heard. Altogether, only four women appeared before the Senate caucus. All were medical experts.[61]

The Pill hearings made the evening news on ABC, NBC, and CBS, and the camera captured for posterity women's anger at being so callously ignored. On the first day of testimony, women members of D.C. Women's Liberation, a group formed in 1969 to promote safe, legal abortions and feminist health care, disrupted the meeting with angry shouts. Yelled one member: "Women are not going to sit quietly any longer—you are murdering us for your profit and convenience." Nelson tried to restore order but made matters worse when he referred to the demonstrators as "girls," reproached them for their "unruly" behavior, and counseled them to sit down and be quiet. "No, we aren't going to sit down—why don't you give us some solid answers to our questions?" one demonstrator shouted back.[62]

Millions of women—an estimated 87 percent of women between the ages of twenty-one and forty-five followed the hearings—watched, listened, and learned. No new scientific evidence emerged, but for some women, the event itself was enough to persuade them to forgo oral contraceptives for another birth control method. Eighteen percent of women taking oral contraceptives quit during the Nelson hearings, and sales of diaphragms, contraceptive foam, intrauterine devices, and condoms increased. In April, however, only a month after the hearings concluded, a Gallup Poll found that the Pill was "coming back." Thirteen percent of dropouts had decided to return to the Pill, and another 26 percent were considering it. The poll foreshadowed future trends. In the long run, the Nelson hearings had little impact on retail sales. After a brief drop, prescription rates rebounded, and the number of users peaked in 1973 at approximately ten million.[63]

A more long-lasting effect of the Nelson hearings was their political mobilization of women. D.C. Women's Liberation held its own Pill hearings, inviting women to share their experiences with the drug—something Nelson's hearings had ignored. The statement issued by the group made clear that it was not opposed *a priori* to the Pill, only to "unsafe contraceptives foisted on uninformed women for the profit of the drug and medical industries and for the convenience of men." The statement invited women "to rise up, as women, and demand our human rights. . . . We will insist that the medical profession must meet our needs. We will no longer tolerate intimidation by white-coated gods, antiseptically directing our lives."[64]

In the intervening weeks and months, women took this invitation to activism to heart. In 1970, the feminist health care movement was in full swing. A year earlier, twelve young feminists had established the Boston Women's Health Book Collective to educate women about health and sexuality and to challenge conventional models of medicine that forced women into passive roles. In 1971, the collective published its pathbreaking *Our Bodies, Ourselves*, which went on to sell almost four million copies in twelve languages. The National Abortion and Reproductive Rights Action League was also formed in 1969 as an organization of grassroots activists committed to the provision of legal and safe abortions. In this period of feminist organization and health awareness, hundreds of women angered by the Pill hearings (in much the way that another generation of feminists would be angered by the Clarence

Thomas–Anita Hill hearings) decided to act. They wrote to the FDA demanding that the agency adopt a patient package insert that would inform women of the side effects, risks, and contraindications of oral contraceptive use. Wrote one: "I DEMAND,—that as a woman, having the option to take the pill or not, I have *all* facts in front of me!"[65]

The issue had been heatedly contested in the Nelson hearings, when an FDA witness first notified the committee of the agency's intent to require patient inserts. Committee member Bob Dole, then the junior senator from Kansas, wondered if informing women about the drug's potential hazards would make them unduly anxious: "We must not frighten millions of women into disregarding the considered judgments of their physicians about the use of oral contraceptives."[66] On another occasion, he joked that the hearings had "terrified a number of women. . . . I would guess they may be taking two pills now—first a tranquilizer and then the regular pill."[67] One equally paternalistic witness, a physician from Boston, warned that patient inserts would spawn unhealthy "placebo" side effects. "If you tell them they might get headaches," he warned, "they will."[68]

Despite such boorish proclamations, the FDA proceeded as planned. The end result was a compromise that largely conceded to the wishes of the pharmaceutical industry and the American Medical Association, both of which had opposed the insert. Doctors feared that consumer information undermined their professional credibility. Pill manufacturers worried that the patient insert would alarm consumers and reduce sales. Indeed, if manufacturers had had their way, not only would women have been kept in the dark, but also doctors would have received only select information about the drug's side effects. A 1961 volume of the *Searleman*, Searle's monthly organ for sales representatives, had instructed detail men to avoid mention of nausea and cancer when they promoted Enovid to doctors. Such conversations were classified as time-consuming, "unnecessary discussion[s]."[69]

The patient insert, required by the FDA after June 1970, was all of seven sentences long. It directed patients wanting more information to request an AMA-authored booklet from their physicians. At eight hundred words, the booklet was more comprehensive, but only a minority of Pill users saw it. Between 1970 and 1975, the AMA distributed only four million copies.[70] Not until 1978 did the FDA change its policy on patient inserts for oral contraceptives, requiring them to be included in every Pill package sold.

The Nelson hearings and the FDA's halfway acknowledgment of the importance of informed consent did not close debate about women and the Pill. They simply made it a more legitimate part of public discussion. The question of whether women were empowered or disserviced by oral contraceptives lingered throughout the 1970s. In *The Village Voice*, the journalist Jennifer Macleod urged readers blind to sex discrimination to envision a world in which men shouldered comparable contraceptive burdens. In such a world, the young bridegroom might receive the following advice:

> Most likely, you will choose one of the fine methods available to the modern husband. Consult a qualified urologist. She will explain to you several methods. . . . One widely used method is the insertion of sperm-killing liquid into the urethra before intercourse. She (your doctor) will show you how. . . . The other widely used method is of course the Capsule. . . . There are minor undesirable side-effects in some men: you may gain weight around the abdomen or buttocks, get white pigmentless patches on your face (which you may be able to conceal with a beard or face-bronzer), or suffer some morning nausea. But be patient— these effects often decrease or even disappear after a few months. The one serious drawback of the Capsule is that you are several times more likely than otherwise to suffer eventually from prostate cancer or fatal blood clots. But these ailments are relatively uncommon anyway, so that many couples consider it worth the risk, especially since this is the one method that is 100 percent effective.[71]

Macleod's depiction of a contraceptive world inverted by sex roles touched on a key issue in the 1960s and 1970s: the responsibilities of men in pregnancy prevention. Even as scientists, doctors, and patients discussed the adverse side effects of oral contraceptives on women, some critics bemoaned their negative impact on *men*. One psychoanalyst warned that a man's ability to impregnate unimpeded by technology was critical to his identity. "For a lot of men," he told *Redbook*, "masculinity is a purely physical matter. . . . They see their virility in terms of what they can do *to* women. A man like that used to be able to give his wife babies . . . lots of them . . . whether she wanted them or not. But the pills take this last bit of masculinity away from him."[72] An article in *Ladies' Home Journal* depicted men as the Pill's real victims. The author, Robert Kistner, was a professor of obstetrics and gynecology at the Harvard Medical School. He asserted that it "is generally accepted that the male is much more susceptible to psychological factors in his sexual activity than the female." By rendering sperm ineffectual, the Pill empowered women at men's expense. Men accustomed to a familial arrangement in which an active sex life made stay-at-home mothers out of wives had to adjust to a new set of rules. "Because the Pill eliminates even accidental pregnancies," Kistner stated, "career wives are able to postpone families indefinitely . . . and there isn't much [their] husband[s] can do about it."[73] This explained why there were so few contraceptives for men. Because man's "virility, sense of maleness, even his self-esteem are more closely allied to the sexual act than that of a woman . . . any method of contraception that diminished sperm count would create psychological problems for many men, leading to ego loss and impotence."[74] Apparently, these were more serious than an unwanted pregnancy.

Even scientists active in contraceptive research viewed men's psychological fragility as a significant impediment to the development of male contraceptives. At the 1968 meeting of the National Medicinal Chemistry Symposium of the American Chemical Society, a Merck researcher remarked that "the most difficult obstacle, perhaps, to a 'male' approach is the 'emotional-psychological' factor. The delicate male psyche equates virility with fertility, and it is believed that extensive education would be required to get men used to the idea of a 'male' contraceptive."[75] John Rock told one correspondent that developing new contraceptives for men was only half the battle. The real obstacle, he quipped, "is in prevailing upon the men to use them!"[76]

Others invoked biological rather than psychological explanations. But here, too, the preponderance of female methods was attributed to the "natural." It was not scientists or manufacturers who were at fault. If anyone—or anything—was to blame, it was the male genitals. It was easier to suppress the release of a solitary egg than to neutralize an army of sperm. Sheldon Segal, the vice president of the Population Council, referred to this and other biological differences to defend researchers' motives. There was no male conspiracy, he averred. It was simply that the number of "vulnerable links" in the female chain of reproductive events was greater, rendering the woman a more suitable subject of contraceptive research. A woman's cycle comprised myriad interwoven steps; only one had to be disrupted to prevent pregnancy.[77] With fewer points of vulnerability, the male reproductive system was less complicated but also harder to suspend. "Even the forces of women's liberation cannot change the fact that . . . the number of targets . . . is far more limited in males than females. It is not surprising then, that the number of approaches under study is fewer for male than for female methods."[78]

Segal accused feminist critics like Seaman of wanting to have it both ways. First they had complained of a paucity of good methods for women. Next they complained of a "male conspiracy" when scientists rectified this situation with the Pill. "Feminists, switched off from their decades-long battle to take the contraceptive decision away from men, . . . now demand more sharing by males of the responsibility and the risks of contraception," Segal charged. Segal ignored the nuances of the critique made by many feminist groups such as D.C. Women's Liberation, which condemned not the Pill but the way it had been tested, marketed, and distributed. And he discounted the extent to which the Pill, a systemic drug, represented a radical departure from contraceptive technology as generations of women had known it. Above all, he glossed over the fact that feminists were not a monolithic group and were entitled to divergent opinions. Margaret Sanger and Katharine McCormick had believed that female control of childbearing was nothing less than a precondition of the emancipation of women. It had never occurred to them to develop a contraceptive drug for men. McCormick remarked in 1958 that she "didn't give a hoot for a male contraceptive."[79] Both women's views were conditioned by the contraceptive choices of an earlier age, when women's options were fewer and condoms were king.

All the same, Segal and other luminaries in the family planning movement told women that new male methods—pills and injections—would soon be available. In 1963, promising clinical trials of a male contraceptive pill made national news. The drug, a diamine compound used to treat amoebic dysentery, was discovered to prevent sperm from maturing in laboratory animals. The compound was tested on thirty-nine convicts at the Oregon State Penitentiary, whose sperm production was halted by daily doses of the drug but whose libido was unaffected. (In previous tests on male prisoners, steroids, including the estrogen-progestin compound constituting Enovid, had suppressed the male sex drive to unacceptably low levels.) The diamine compound was economical too: a month's supply cost less than a dollar, compared with roughly $3.50 for the Pill. Then came disaster. When a doctor gave the drug to one of his patients, the man had a few drinks, became violently nauseated, experienced heightened blood pressure, and had to be hospitalized a few days later. His eyeballs also turned bright red. Outside the alcohol-free prison setting, it turned out, the diamine contraceptive could be safely used only by teetotalers.[80]

There were other leads. Scientists at Rockefeller University were experimenting with a reversible plug that blocked sperm production after liquid silicone was injected into men's testes. There were still several hitches. The plug deteriorated after six to eight months, and no one knew whether it harmed the testes. Researchers were also exploring immuno-contraception, hoping to discover a way of immunizing a man against his sperm in much the way that the body could be immunized against polio. In the meantime, the perpetually innovative John Rock found that sperm production decreased in men who wore an insulated scrotal supporter continuously. The supporter, which relied on heat and constriction to inhibit sperm production, became affectionately known as the "Rock strap." Because results varied by user, the strap was deemed unreliable for contraceptive use (although, even today, fertility experts warn men wanting families to avoid constricting underwear and hot baths before intercourse).[81] By the mid-1970s, most of these initiatives had been placed on the back burner as funding for contraceptive research dried up and as manufacturers, nervous about liability issues, expressed growing reservations about bringing new products to market.

The sex of contraceptive users was not the only issue that framed political debate. Just as the feminist movement seized on the Pill as a symbol of gender inequality, the burgeoning black nationalist movement portrayed the Pill as a technology of genocide. Throughout the 1960s and 1970s, black nationalists reiterated the long-standing fear that birth control would lead to race suicide by subduing the size and strength of the black population. African-Americans could not afford attrition at a time when blacks had finally gained, through the Voting Rights Act of 1964, the promise of universal suffrage.[82] Large black families were the community's best insurance against racial extermination, its best promise for political and social gain. A May 1969 issue of *The Liberator* told readers, "For us to speak in favor of birth control for Afro-Americans would be comparable to speaking in favor of genocide."[83] In 1967, a Black Power conference held in Newark, New Jersey, passed a resolution denouncing birth control, setting the movement in opposition to the National Association for the Advancement of Colored People, which had endorsed a resolution at its fifty-seventh annual meeting to "support the dissemination of information and materials concerning family health and family planning to all those who desire it."[84]

Black militants pointed to history as evidence of the true intentions of whites who promoted contraception in the black community. In a cover story in *Ebony* in 1971, one journalist justified his suspicions:

> For years [whites] told us where to sit, where to eat, and where to live. Now they want to dictate our bedroom habits. First the white man tells me to sit in the back of the bus. Now it looks like he wants me to sleep under the bed. Back in the days of slavery, black folks couldn't grow kids fast enough for white folks to harvest. Now that we've got a little taste of power, white folks want us to call a moratorium on having children.[85]

In articles and cartoons in the black press, the Pill was depicted as a wolf in sheep's clothing: a technologically upgraded but no less malevolent weapon in whites' war to exterminate blacks. A poster circulated by the Berkeley, California–based group EROS—Endeavor to Raise Our Size—likened the Pill to lynching. Lynching represented "Birth Control Then . . . The Crude Way." Under the image of a woman reaching for her oral contraceptives was the caption: "Now, the Smooth Way."[86] A cartoon in the Nation of Islam's *Muhammad Speaks* proffered a similar warning, depicting a bottle of oral contraceptives marked with a skull and crossbones.[87]

Despite the harsh rhetoric and images, there were signs of dissent, even at high levels of leadership. When a Planned Parenthood representative interviewed Black Muslim leader Malcolm X, she found him unexpectedly supportive of the idea of contraception. But he had a suggestion. He urged that Planned Parenthood use the term "family planning" rather than "birth control" when dealing with blacks, because "Negroes [are] more willing to plan than to be controlled." Female leaders were especially sympathetic to the importance of contraception to black women. Frances Beal, head of the Black Women's Liberation Committee of the Student Nonviolent Coordinating Committee, insisted, "Black women have the right and the responsibility to determine when it is in the interests of the struggle to have children or not."[88] The activist and author Toni Cade agreed. "I've been made aware of the national call to Sisters to abandon birth control . . . and to raise revolutionaries," she wrote. "What plans do you have for the care of me and the child?"[89]

Black women found themselves pulled by competing loyalties. A social worker in 1966 noted that many of her clients, "impoverished and poorly educated Negroes," took the Pill but resented it. They felt "that a main purpose of the pill is to reduce the number of Negroes in the world."[90] Planned Parenthood admitted its attempts to introduce contraceptive services to some neighborhoods had been hampered by the fact that "some Negroes . . . [are] influenced by 'black power' arguments that birth-control drives among the poor are attempts to keep Negro numbers down."[91]

Although feelings of disloyalty to the movement may have preyed on them, most African-American women seem to have supported contraception both in theory and in practice. In a Pittsburgh neighborhood, black women banded together and rallied for the return of a mobile Planned Parenthood clinic that had shut down after receiving bomb threats from the male leader of a local militant group.[92] A 1970 study found that 80 percent of African-American women surveyed in Chicago supported contraception, and 75 percent practiced it.[93]

Still, a disproportionate number of Pill users were white. One 1965 investigation found that white couples were 20 percent more likely than blacks to use oral contraceptives. Birth control practices had long been shaped by race and ethnicity. In a study undertaken right before the release of the Pill, Planned Parenthood found striking differences in favored methods among racial groups, with white patients preferring the condom, African-Americans the douche, and Mexican-Americans the diaphragm.[94] But the Pill was supposed to overcome these differences, fulfilling Sanger's dream of a simple and cheap contraceptive that would be embraced by women of color and the working poor around the globe.

Instead, the Pill became the darling of middle-class white women who could afford it. The wide profit margins enjoyed by Pill manufacturers shut many poor persons and persons of color out of the market. Although the average annual retail price of oral contraceptives plummeted within a few short years—from one hundred dollars in 1960 to twenty-five dollars in 1965—until the late 1960s, the Pill was often too expensive for working-class women.[95] Women could get discounted pills from Planned Parenthood, whose medical advisory committee formally approved their prescription at each of its hundred affiliates on August 4, 1960.[96] But not every woman had access to the clinics, only twenty-four of which had begun dispensing Enovid by early December that year. Those women who did, moreover, frequently found even the discounted price—less than half that of retail—prohibitively high. Maurice Sagoff, the executive director of the Planned Parenthood League of Massachusetts, complained in 1961 to the medical director of Searle that "even at the present consumer price . . . [Enovid] is beyond the reach of many of our low-income inquirers."[97] Adding to the cost of filling prescriptions were the costs of doctors visits. As the price of oral contraceptives dropped, the number of Planned Parenthood patients using them increased. Between 1961 and 1966, the proportion of new patients choosing oral contraceptives rose fivefold, from 14 to 70 percent. Still, women who got their prescriptions from clinics represented a minority of total Pill users, only 4 percent in 1969.[98]

But it was not price alone that cemented the Pill's middle-class identification. Also critical was birth control promoters' fear that oral contraceptives, although almost 100 percent effective when used as directed, would be misused by uneducated and poor women. Mary Calderone, the medical director of Planned Parenthood, recalled an encounter with a female student at a public junior high school in New York City. Observing the girl drop her handbag during a break between classes, Calderone stopped to help her assemble its contents and "was astonished to see a package of birth control pills." "I asked the child," Calderone told a reporter at *The Saturday Evening Post*, "Do you really know about these things? 'Oh, yes,' she replied, 'I take them every Saturday night when I go on a date.' " Calderone lamented, "If it weren't so funny, it would be tragic."[99]

Presumably the "problem" of patient compliance was remedied by the Dialpak, an oral contraceptive package introduced in 1963 to remind women to take their Ortho-Novum. Instead of getting a vial of undifferentiated pills, women could get the Dialpak, permitting them to check at a glance if they had taken their daily tablet. Designed by David P. Wagner to help his wife remember to take the Pill, the Dialpak established a model that was soon emulated by other manufacturers. But it did little to quell doubts about patient compliance. To underscore the importance of and need for memory aids, Pill manufacturers emphasized the gravity of female forgetfulness, heightening alarm about the very problem they claimed to have solved.[100]

Not everyone believed that women, especially the "forgetful poor," were incompetent Pill users. Edris Rice-Wray, involved in the original clinical trials of oral contraceptives, stated, "It's extremely rare to find a woman willing to accept another method once she knows that 'the Pills' exist. . . . Even the poorest, with little or no schooling, are found to be faithful and conscientious users."[101]

Such views were discounted by votaries of population control and the growing army of critics who blamed the "problem" of unwed motherhood on poor, black women. As the historian Rickie Solinger has shown, racist characterizations of female sexual behavior anchored political discussions of illegitimacy and fertility control in the 1950s and 1960s. Resurrecting the arguments of early eugenicists, policy makers urged that irresponsible women, presumed to be black, be sterilized to prevent burdening society with unwanted and costly offspring. In 1958, the Mississippi state legislator David H. Glass proposed a bill, "An Act to Discourage Immorality of Unmarried Females by Providing for Sterilization of the Unwed Mother under Conditions of the Act; and for Related Purposes." Justifying its need, Glass wrote, "The Negro woman because of child welfare assistance [is] making it a business, in some cases, of giving birth to illegitimate children."[102] Glass's failure to enact the bill did not deter lawmakers in eighteen other states from proposing similarly punitive measures in the late 1950s and early 1960s.

Within a political environment replete with racist and elitist stereotypes regarding women's procreative identity, policy makers, legislators, and population control proponents evaluated the Pill. Fears of the consequences to *taxpayers* of noncompliance among women of color and poor women exaggerated suspicions that only middle-class women, presumed to be white, educated, and responsible, could be "trusted" to swallow a pill a day for twenty consecutive days. As Alan Guttmacher put it in 1960, "Although many modern contraceptive devices are highly effective, they are not the answer for the poor or the uneducated. They are too expensive for budgets that deal in pennies a day [and] they require intelligence and instruction."[103] Hugh Davis, the director of the Family Planning Clinic at the Johns Hopkins University and IUD inventor, brought this argument into even sharper relief when he testified at the Nelson hearings:

> It is especially tragic that for the individual who needs birth control the most—the poor, the disadvantaged, and the ghetto-dwelling black—the oral contraceptives carry a particularly high hazard of pregnancy as compared with methods requiring less motivation. . . . [I]t is the suburban middle-class woman who has become the chronic user of the oral contraceptives in the United States in the past decade, getting her prescription renewed month after month and year after year without missing a single tablet. Therein, in my opinion, lies the real hazard of the presently available oral contraceptives.[104]

But what was to be done? Amid the confluence of several events—support for population control at home and abroad, the perceived inability of oral contraceptives to become a birth control for the masses, and the medicalization of contraceptive technology spawned by oral contraceptives—researchers and scientists went back to the drawing board. With financial support from the government and the Population Council, they breathed new life into an old contraceptive, the IUD.

ELEVEN

Searching for Something Better

The early 1970s were heady times for family planning advocates, pharmaceutical firms, and women and men who waited expectantly for news of the next contraceptive breakthrough—perhaps a reversible sterilant, a contraceptive vaccine, or the much-anticipated male pill.[1] Thirteen companies—eight of them American—were on the job.[2] Already journalists were hailing a new plastic IUD as a cheap solution to overseas population growth and the presumed financial drain of "welfare" babies at home. In 1971, some twelve million women around the world, over three million in the United States alone, were wearing IUDS. Most of these were American-made.[3]

The bubble of enthusiasm popped suddenly and tragically in 1974, when reports of deaths and injury resulting from the Dalkon Shield, the most popular IUD of the day, prompted its manufacturer, A. H. Robins, to remove it from the market. By the time the dust had settled, more than eleven thousand lawsuits had been filed, and the company had declared bankruptcy.

By the late 1960s, the federal government had begun to aid in the dissemination of contraceptives to the nation's poor, a practice that was already in place in several, mainly Southern, states. In 1945, Alabama was the first to establish a tax-supported family planning program to reduce state poverty and "illegitimacy" rates.[4] As politicians in the 1960s recognized poverty and illegitimacy to be national rather than regional problems, they introduced federally funded programs. Under the 1967 child health provision of the Social Security Act, the federal government assumed up to 75 percent of the costs of birth control services for the poor in state, city, and nonprofit programs.[5] In 1969, Congress appropriated fifty million dollars for family planning programs operating under services such as Medicaid and Aid to Families with Dependent Children (AFDC), which provided low-income Americans with birth control supplies and advice. Even the Department of Defense got involved, purchasing oral contraceptives for 200,000 military wives.[6]

The new government policy was sold to taxpayers not as sexual emancipation but as a cost-saving measure to tamp the procreative power of the poor. Proponents of government-backed family planning argued that cash spent on birth control would cost considerably less than AFDC outlays, which in 1965 were estimated to be $1.6 billion. In Mecklenburg County, North Carolina, a sharp drop in welfare costs—from 27 to 10 percent of the county's budget—was attributed to the establishment of free birth control services. According to Wallace Kuralt, the director of public welfare, "It is currently costing less than one twenty-fifth as much to prevent unwanted births" among relief claimants as "it costs the public to support the children."[7] Dr. Joseph D. Beasley, the director of the Louisiana Family Planning Program, reported similar results in his state, where, in 1969, one in thirteen residents was on relief and the illegitimacy rate among the impoverished was estimated at 30 percent. Sixteen months after family planning clinics began dispensing free contraceptives to the needy in thirty-five "test-case" parishes, births among low-income families had declined by 32 percent, illegitimate births by 40. Beasley told the story of a blind and mentally retarded woman, aged twenty-one, who had three children, "all illegitimate." He calculated that "the cost of that girl and her children to the State, not to mention the cost in human suffering, eventually will be $800,000. You could educate 500 normal persons at Louisiana State University for that amount."[8]

Underlying these cost accountings was a widely shared view that the procreative agency of poor and black women cost taxpayers too much. This belief meshed easily with foreign policy objectives, which supported contraceptive distribution to developing nations partly because of the long-term costs—poverty, political upheaval, and the threat of communism—associated with nonintervention. Domestic and foreign birth control objectives were merely different sides of the same coin, for "skyrocketing relief costs in the U.S. [and] mushrooming population overseas [are] twin problems now costing taxpayers billions."[9] Presidents John F. Kennedy, Lyndon Johnson, and Richard Nixon—who in 1969 unveiled his five-year plan to make contraceptives available to all low-income families—were less sexual revolutionaries than cold warriors who endorsed family planning for political reasons that played well economically at home.

Widespread support for birth control as a palliative for poverty was clouded by doubts that oral contraceptives were up to the task. If women could be trusted to swallow a pill a day, some argued, they would not be so "irresponsible" as to need public assistance. In this political climate, the development of intrauterine devices seemed a godsend. Cheaper than the Pill, virtually impossible for a woman to remove, and requiring only a single "motivated" act—the decision to have one inserted—the IUD seemed almost too good to be true.

Long-standing medical opposition to IUD contraception had thawed only gradually in the United States. In the 1930s, when thousands of European and Japanese women were using IUDs, American physicians continued to denounce the device's safety and efficacy. The most popular model at the time, and the first IUD to be commercially manufactured as birth control, was the Gräfenberg ring, invented in the 1920s by Dr. Ernst Gräfenberg, a Berlin gynecologist in private practice. Gräfenberg fashioned a contraceptive IUD made of silkworm gut shaped with silver wire into ring form, and tested it on more than two thousand patients without incident. The ring was an excellent contraceptive, but it was not without complications. Its rigidity and size, measuring one inch in diameter, required the cervix to be dilated to about one hundred millimeters before insertion. With anesthesia, dilation and insertion were pain-free but medically complicated; without anesthesia, they were agonizingly painful. The ring also caused and worsened endometriosis in some women and increased all users' susceptibility to pelvic inflammatory disease.[10] Still, the Gräfenberg ring eliminated many of the safety problems associated with the older and larger stem pessaries, especially the risk of uterine perforation and infection. Subsequent versions made the ring even safer by the use of "German silver," an alloy of copper, nickel, and tin less likely to corrode than pure silver IUDs.[11]

As medical evidence of the ring's efficacy mounted, and as a host of knockoffs appeared on the U.S. birth control market, American physicians clung to their condemnations. Linking IUDs to a tradition of female-controlled, illicit birth control, they blamed the ring's surging popularity in the United States on the crass commercialism of "illegitimate faddists." The renowned obstetrician J. Whitridge Williams was one such critic. A professor of obstetrics at the Johns Hopkins Medical School during the 1920s, Williams carried a watch adorned with a gold intrauterine ring. When questioned about the ring's significance, Williams would explain that he had personally extracted it from a "placenta at term." Its visibility on his chain, he believed, supplied enduring proof that IUDs did not work.[12]

But as early as the 1950s, several technological advances encouraged a handful of scientists in the United States to engage in IUD research. The availability of antibiotics in the 1940s made pelvic inflammatory disease and other IUD-related infections curable for the first time. In addition, the invention of malleable plastic in the 1950s enabled scientists to make IUDs with "memory," devices that could stretch into linear form before insertion but regain their original shape in the uterus. Because compressible IUDs could be inserted into an undilated cervix, they were easier and cheaper to use than models requiring anesthesia. In 1959, the Margulies spiral, invented by the gynecologist Lazar Margulies of the Mount Sinai Hospital in New York City, became the first of a new generation of plastic IUDs to be tested. Margulies's invention was not only the first non-ring plastic IUD; it was also the first to use a straight inserter tube. Made of polyethylene and a small amount of barium sulfate that permitted radiological detection in the event of suspected expulsion, the spiral's tail, designed to protrude into the vagina, also enabled women to confirm the IUD's presence. Unfortunately, the length and rigidity of the tail caused "discomfort and trauma to male partners," destining Margulies's first model to a short life (although its companion inserter tube became a staple of IUD paraphernalia). Nonetheless, the possibilities of plastic encouraged further American IUD experimentation, as did a favorable 1959 report on the Gräfenberg ring by an Israeli gynecologist;

published in the *American Journal of Obstetrics and Gynecology*, it was the first clinical evaluation of intrauterine birth control to appear in an American scientific journal.[13]

The stage was set for a modification of American medical views when the Pill was unleashed on the American public in 1960. The changes to contraceptive practice wrought by the popularity of oral contraceptives had important consequences for how American society came to view IUDs. After 1965, when IUDs first became widely available, physicians' authority to manage female contraception, the superiority of scientifically engineered birth control (a superiority celebrated by both women and scientists), and the image of female birth control users as patients went largely uncontested. The medicalization of contraception spawned by the Pill made it that much easier for IUDS, yet another scientifically engineered, doctor-controlled contraceptive used by women, to gain acceptance.[14]

Americans' experiences with oral contraceptives were the seedbed for support of IUDs in yet another way, for they underscored the impossibility of the Pill's becoming the contraceptive for the masses so critical to the agenda of population control. In 1961, the Population Council, the most active organization in IUD promotion in the 1960s, began funding the IUD research of Margulies and the obstetrician Jack Lippes, medical director of the Planned Parenthood Federation of Buffalo. With the council's financial help and institutional support, Margulies's new-and-improved spiral, the Gynekoil, and Lippes's loop would become two of the most commercially successful IUDs of all time.[15] Before the Dalkon Shield was marketed in January 1971, the Lippes loop was the most popular IUD in the country.[16] The Population Council was enamored with the idea of a "simple, inexpensive, and reliable permanent contraceptive" better suited to the "unmotivated," prolific underclass than the Pill.[17] In 1962, the council sponsored the first international conference on intrauterine contraception in New York and launched a research program that included both laboratory studies and clinical trials with promising IUDs. By July 1963, it was underwriting the costs of the insertion and medical monitoring of IUDs in 3,750 female patients at twelve medical centers across the country.[18]

In 1965, the Population Council launched a campaign to distribute American-made IUDs to developing nations. By 1967, six million devices had been either supplied directly by the council or manufactured locally with its assistance. In 1964, the council entered into an agreement with Jack Lippes that divided the global IUD market into high- and low-profit sectors and assigned the council patent rights in over a dozen developing countries, including India, Pakistan, Egypt, and Turkey.[19] Lippes retained rights for the wealthier sector, which included the United States, Canada, and Great Britain. By the end of the year, the council had helped five countries to make their own IUDs by issuing nonexclusive licenses to manufacture the Lippes loop and providing technical support. Unlike the Pill, IUDs were simple to manufacture in any country with a plastics industry. In the United States, they were made on assembly lines, but in poorer nations, the Population Council advocated the use of hand-operated, one-cavity injection molding machines as a low-cost alternative. In India, the council supplied 1.2 million American-made devices before helping local family planning organizations open their own factory, equipped to churn out 14,000 loops a day. To drum up local support, the council distributed small gold-plated loops as souvenirs on opening day.[20]

Following the council's lead, the U.S. government, having only recently endorsed international birth control aid as vital to national security, began to bankroll efforts at global IUD distribution. In 1965, under the Johnson administration, the Agency for International Development (AID) began to funnel money to family planning projects overseas. Funds were initially reserved for the provision of "research, training and communications," but by the end of the decade, AID had also become involved in the direct distribution of birth control devices. By 1969, AID had helped supply 14 million women with contraceptives, many of them IUDs. Indeed, by 1974, an estimated 697,000 Dalkon Shields had been purchased with AID money for global use. The collaboration of the federal government, the Population Council, and other organizations such as International Planned Parenthood and the Pathfinder Fund had enabled some 7.5 million women to be fitted with IUDs in developing countries by 1974.[21]

In the United States, IUDs first became widely available to women at Planned Parenthood clinics and other low-cost or free health centers in the mid-1960s. By 1965, half of Planned Parenthood's 128 affiliates were providing women with one or more models. Initially, most IUD wearers

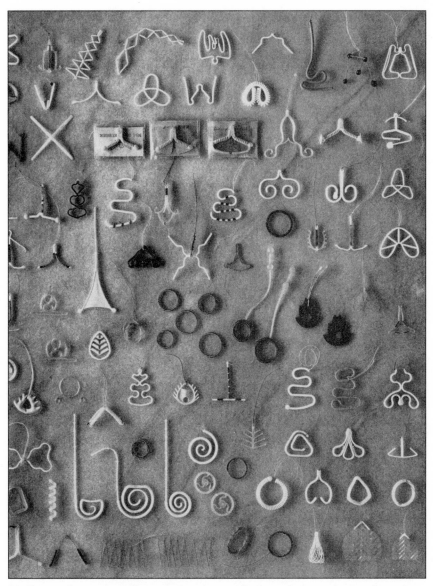

30. Twentieth-century IUDs, including the metal rings and plastic devices shown here, came in a range of shapes and sizes (Courtesy of the History of Contraception Museum, Janssen-Ortho Inc., Toronto, Canada)

were patients at public clinics. As supporters of population control had hoped, the rate of adoption was highest among African-American women, who were more likely than whites to rely on public health facilities for birth control. Over time, as a growing number of private doctors came to prescribe IUDs and as word of their benefits spread, IUD technology became more widely diffused. Between 1965 and 1970, adoption rates by both black and white women increased significantly—almost threefold among blacks and, confounding expectations, more than sixfold among whites. By the end of 1970, over three million women had been fitted with IUDs in the United States.[22]

As they had with the Pill, women sought doctors who would insert the new IUDs, which were the subject of numerous laudatory articles in women's magazines and in newspapers in the late 1960s. In Boston, one physician had to install a second telephone line to handle the volume of calls he received from women eager to be fitted with the plastic devices.[23] Some scholars have viewed such women as victims of corporate and medical manipulation, but it is important to evaluate the decision to use an IUD in the context of the time. In the late 1960s, evidence abounded that the Pill was not the birth control panacea for which many women had hoped. The method's expense, the necessity of ongoing medical monitoring, and health problems ranging from migraines to nausea to the threat of stroke occupied women's discussions of oral contraceptives and framed their search for something better. For some women, the IUD seemed an alternative well worth trying. Locally acting, it did not tamper with a woman's chemical system. It was cheaper too. In 1966, most women could expect to pay a combined onetime insertion and device fee of thirty dollars. The IUD promised one-stop birth control; in theory, once the device was inserted, a woman need not worry about contraception again. Many wearers must have shared the sentiments of one young mother of three who commented: "I've heard much about the emancipation of American women . . . but I had my doubts until this new kind of birth control came along."[24]

The dramatic escalation in the number of IUD wearers in the late 1960s and early 1970s thus must be understood as the intersection of a technological revolution and a growing demand from women for improved contraceptives. What women could not control, however, was the disparity between their objectives and those of population control advocates, whose dollars drove IUD invention and distribution. Whereas women selected birth control on the basis of individual preferences and needs, proponents of IUDs typically identified prospective wearers as a monolithic group: impoverished, irresponsible, and too prolific. Although women of all socioeconomic backgrounds appreciated the low cost of IUDs, proponents of population control equated cheapness with birth control for the poor. What women construed to be the simplicity of IUDs as contraception meant to its professional advocates a form of contraception whose efficacy, unlike that of the Pill, could not be altered by female behavior.

IUD inventors routinely invoked metaphors of violence to trumpet the power and control that masculine technologies wielded over women's uteri. In so doing, they borrowed from and perpetuated a long history of medical representation of the female body that cast women's reproductive organs as a passive, natural sphere (the very anchor of all that defined "woman") readily controlled by masculine technological might. Applied to IUDs, such an account encouraged the telling of war stories in which aggressive, battle-hungry IUDs invade, irritate, infect, and finally subdue the ultimately powerless uteri. Responding to concerns in the late 1960s that small, compressible IUDs, of particular appeal to women because they caused less pain and cramping, were too easily expelled, IUD inventors championed the "staying power" of new meaner, larger models. One was configured with "two pairs of arms . . . stiffened with wiring springs to provide anchoring mechanisms." The Dalkon Shield, its very name suggesting a weapon of war, would likewise stay intact because of the IUD's "plurality of spurs . . . [which are] slanted in a given direction so as to impede expulsion." The technological superiority of another, particularly large device was attributed to its sporting "substantial surface areas for uterus *wall-engaging* purposes *strategically disposed* for maximum effectiveness."[25] The meanest of the bunch was an IUD patented on August 10, 1971, containing a stainless barb, shaped like a fishhook, and a balloon-like vane. The physician inserting the device was instructed to push the tube and its contents into the uterus, applying enough force to inflate the vane and to ensure that the "barb pierces into, but not through the muscular wall and retains the device securely in place." And so it was that, pierced by a stainless steel barb and lined with plastic, a woman's uterus was made safe from unwanted pregnancy. The inventor made no mention of the need for painkillers or anesthesia in his patent application.[26]

Mercifully, the uterus-piercing IUD was never mass manufactured. But the spirit behind its design, which relegated women to a passive role as receptors of technological violence, endured. Describing IUD insertions in Hong Kong, Alan Guttmacher of Planned Parenthood saw ballet in what is better described as gynecological Taylorism:

> The best IUD manipulator I have ever observed was in Hong Kong. . . . Her record was seventy-five insertions in three hours[,] . . . that is one every two minutes and twenty-four seconds. Dr. Wong kept three nurses busy helping her. One was supervising the removal of the panties of the next patient, the second nurse soothed the brow of the patient on the table and the third passed instruments to Dr. Wong. I have never seen such graceful hands, such exquisite economy of finger movement; there wasn't a false motion. I regret that I am not a choreographer, for a ballet of IUD patients with the ballerina making Dr. Wong's finger and hand movements would be a sensation.[27]

In a radio broadcast in New York City, Christopher Tietze, the research director of the Committee on Maternal Health, explained how class and education factored into calculations of contraceptive efficacy:

> I stress the fact that purely from the point of view of effectiveness . . . an intelligent highly motivated couple would not necessarily fare better with intrauterine contraception than with traditional contraception. But the situation is quite different when you come to populations that are not accustomed to "the contraceptive way of life," whether you find populations in an Indian village or in an American slum. Then you would expect at least 20 to 40 pregnancies per 100 women per year and if you in fact get only 2 by using IUD's, you are way ahead.[28]

In a letter to John Searle, the president of G. D. Searle, Guttmacher made a similar point. He confided that the device did not meet middle-class expectations of reliability:

IUD's have special application to underdeveloped areas where two things are lacking: one, money, and the other sustained motivation. No contraceptive could be cheaper, and also, once the damn thing is in, the patient cannot change her mind. In fact, we can hope she will forget that it is there and perhaps in several months wonder why she has not conceived. I do not believe the IUD's will cut into the competitive pill market materially in industrialized, more sophisticated regions. The big difference is that the IUD's are not as effective as the pill in preventing conception. If Mrs. Astorbilt, or Mrs. Searle or Mrs. Guttmacher gets pregnant while using an IUD, there is quite a stink— the thing is no good and a lot of people will hear about it. However if you reduce the birth rate of . . . the Korean, Pakistanian or Indian population from 50 to 45 per 1,000 per year to 2, 3, or 5, this becomes an accomplishment to celebrate.[29]

Viewing IUDs as birth control for the masses made it easier for physicians designing and inserting them to deem irrelevant the unique attributes and varied responses of individual wearers. As Guttmacher's letter suggests, what defined IUD efficacy in the 1960s depended entirely on who was doing the defining.

Guttmacher's words were prescient. By the time A. H. Robins began marketing the Dalkon Shield in 1971, a majority of IUD users in the United States were middle-class women. When the device made hundreds of them sick and allowed numerous pregnancies, when eighteen died, there was indeed "quite a stink," one that sent shock waves through the birth control community and forever changed the face of American contraceptive research and development.

The story of the Dalkon Shield begins with Hugh Davis, who in the mid-1960s was one of many gynecologists working to design a better IUD. A native of Puerto Rico, Davis had received his medical degree from the Johns Hopkins University in 1953. He very quickly demonstrated a flair for invention. Early in his career, he became a pioneer in laparoscopic

United States Patent

[11] 3,633,574

[72]	Inventor	Irwin S. Lerner Greenwich, Conn.
[21]	Appl. No.	775,729
[22]	Filed	Nov. 14, 1968
[45]	Patented	Jan. 11, 1972
[73]	Assignee	A. H. Robbins Company, Incorporated Richmond, Va.

[54] INTRAUTERINE CONTRACEPTIVE DEVICE
30 Claims, 12 Drawing Figs.

[52]	U.S. Cl.	128/130
[51]	Int. Cl.	A61f 5/46
[50]	Field of Search	128/127, 128, 129, 130, 132, 136, 138, 139, 130; 46/30, 31; 74/490; 151/35

[56] References Cited
UNITED STATES PATENTS

1,874,596	8/1932	Olson	151/35
3,422,564	1/1969	Izumi	46/31 X
3,454,004	7/1939	Leininger	128/130
3,537,445	11/1970	Burnhill	128/130
3,256,878	6/1966	Schwartz et al	128/130
2,122,579	7/1938	Meckstroth	128/130
2,432,770	12/1947	Kurkjian	128/128
2,875,755	3/1959	Heubonki et al.	128/127
3,253,590	5/1966	Birnberg et al.	128/130
3,371,664	3/1968	Pleshette	128/127

OTHER REFERENCES

Time magazine of 7/31/64

Primary Examiner—Richard A. Gaudet
Assistant Examiner—G F. Dunne
Attorney—Strauch, Nolan, Neale, Nies & Kurz

ABSTRACT: An intrauterine contraceptive device comprises an outer ring formed with a central membrane to prevent tissue obtrusion and control the deflection characteristics of the device, and lateral spurs slanted in a retrograde direction to impede expulsion through the cervical os. The device is molded of a plastic material and may be coated with a metal film as a barrier against calcium deposits and provide radio-opacity.

31. The patent for the Dalkon Shield made no mention of Hugh Davis's involvement

surgery, a less invasive alternative to prevalent forms of abdominal and uterine surgery, and patented more than thirty laparoscopy-related devices. After a research stint in Denmark, Davis joined the Johns Hopkins medical faculty in 1962 and in 1964 became director of the university's new Family Planning Clinic.[30]

Davis soon developed a reputation as an international expert on contraception. Fluent in Spanish, he served as a medical consultant to several Latin American countries and to the health departments of Maryland and the District of Columbia. Invited to testify at the Nelson hearings in 1970, Davis warned of the dangers of oral contraceptives and their misuse by "the poor, the disadvantaged, and the ghetto-dwelling black." He proposed instead the wholesale adoption of intrauterine devices, which he had been inserting into patients at the Johns Hopkins clinic. He claimed that the best IUDs provided 99 percent protection against pregnancy with minimal risk. "I think you can safely state that the major hazards of the use of an intrauterine device are related to the technical act of insertion, that if you carry out technical precautions, it carries less risk than a smallpox vaccination," he asserted.[31]

At the time of the hearings, Davis had a commercial interest in the Dalkon Shield, but he denied it. Committee member James P. Duffy III pointedly asked Davis whether it was true that he had recently patented such a device. Davis responded: "I hold no recent patent on any intrauterine device." Duffy followed up: "Then you have no particular commercial interest in any of the intrauterine devices?" Davis replied: "That is correct."[32]

As history would show, Davis liked to play loose with the truth. Years earlier, he and a colleague had applied for a patent for the Incon Ring, a plastic IUD to which Johns Hopkins was granted licensing rights. In 1967, Davis patented a second IUD, a dime-sized plastic device that he called the "shield" because it resembled a policeman's badge. Davis showed the IUD to Irwin Lerner, an electrical engineer and family friend. Lerner modified the shield, adding five fins on each side to reduce the likelihood of accidental expulsion. In November 1968, a patent application was filed listing Lerner as sole inventor, a move that hid Davis's involvement and freed him from his obligation to share profits from the device with his employer, Johns Hopkins.[33]

In the fall of 1968, Davis, Lerner, and an attorney, Robert E. Cohn, formed the Dalkon Corporation and assigned to it all future profits from the sale of the Dalkon Shield. Lerner and Davis arranged for several hundred devices to be manufactured at a plastics factory in Brooklyn, New York. When enough inventory was on hand, Davis began a twelve-month experiment in Baltimore on clinic patients, mainly poor African-American women. Between September 1968 and September 1969, he fitted 640 women with the Dalkon Shield. They would be the first of over two million American women to use it.[34]

This yearlong study provided the empirical data for Davis's first report on the device's safety and efficacy. Davis's article "The Shield Intrauterine Device: A Superior Modern Contraceptive" was published in the *American Journal of Obstetrics and Gynecology* on February 1, 1970. As in the Nelson hearings, Davis did not disclose his commercial interest in the Dalkon Shield. Adopting the guise of the impartial scientist, he trumpeted the superiority of his device. Of all the benefits he cited—a low expulsion rate, patient satisfaction—the one that most enthused readers was the annual pregnancy rate: only 1.1 percent, significantly lower than that of any other IUD on the market. The article so masterfully promoted the Shield that a year later, when A. H. Robins mass marketed the device, the company sent over 190,000 reprints to prospective customers.

Davis had again withheld vital information. Not only had he concealed his financial stake in the device, but he had failed to report several methodological problems that invalidated his findings. He made no mention, for instance, of his having advised patients to use contraceptive foam for the first two to three months after insertion. Instead, he gave full credit to the Shield for low pregnancy rates. In addition, although he boasted of a 1.1 percent *annual* pregnancy rate, Davis had stopped tracking pregnancies three days after the end of the twelve-month study period. As a result, pregnancies in women who had been fitted with an IUD at the end of the study did not factor into his computation. In fact, the average length of Shield use in Davis's study was only six months. Follow-up research would show a much higher pregnancy rate within the study group. Davis's omissions undermined both his credibility and the veracity of his claims.[35]

Davis's manipulation of the evidence came to light only later. In February 1970, news of an IUD almost as effective as oral contraceptives was golden. Davis's article was published during the height of American enthusiasm for IUDs. Because of the Nelson hearings, Pill attrition rates were at an all-time high. Thousands of former oral contraceptive users were searching for a different method. The IUD was already a known (and media-approved) contraceptive, used by more than a million American women. The technology had the backing of family planning organizations, government programs, and population control advocates. Amid the fanfare, along came Davis, a renowned contraceptive expert who had denied before a Senate committee that he maintained a commercial interest in the very device he now praised in the country's most respected gynecology journal.

It was small wonder that A. H. Robins immediately bid for the right to manufacture and distribute the heralded Shield. Founded in 1866 by Albert Hartley Robins, an ex-Confederate soldier, A. H. Robins began as a small pharmacy in Richmond, Virginia. By the late 1890s, it had become a separate business, operating on the second floor above the family apothecary shop and manufacturing and distributing drugs exclusively to physicians. In the 1930s, Albert's son Claiborne, who had received his pharmacy degree in 1933 from the Medical College of Virginia, took over the business. During the next fifty years, under Claiborne's leadership, Robins evolved from a small family outfit to one of the four hundred largest corporations in the United States. In the early 1970s, the pharmaceutical powerhouse had distribution systems and subsidiaries around the world. Its products included Robitussin cough syrup, Dimetapp cold remedies, and Chap Stick lip balm.[36]

On June 12, 1970, the company outbid Upjohn Pharmaceuticals to purchase rights to the Dalkon Shield. The deal was a lucrative one for the Dalkon Corporation, which received $750,000 plus 10 percent of future royalties. Davis was hired as a salaried consultant, an association that was kept from the public. The purchase proceeded despite warnings from executives at A. H. Robins that Davis's follow-up studies had revealed a pregnancy rate of 5.3 percent, not 1.1. Dismissing executives' concerns, A. H. Robins forged ahead. Company engineers modified Davis and Lerner's design, adding barium sulfate to enhance the device's visibility in X rays and rounding out the prongs. Robins also created a smaller "nullip" version for women who had never carried a pregnancy to term. Most doctors believed that it was dangerous for women who had not given birth to wear an IUD, but Robins hoped to overturn this consensus and open up a new segment in the IUD market. Neither the new-and-improved Dalkon Shield nor the specially sized "nullip" model was tested before A. H. Robins began marketing them in January 1971. The company advertised Davis's original pregnancy rate of 1.1 percent, which it knew to be false, to promote the newly engineered devices.[37]

There were two structural problems with the Dalkon Shield. One was the series of prongs on each side, which gave the device a fishlike appearance. Many IUD users in the 1960s had discovered, often when it was too late, that uterine contractions—the natural reaction of the uterus to the presence of a foreign object—had expelled their IUDs, leaving them vulnerable to pregnancy. The prongs corrected this flaw, but their downward angle made insertion and removal of the device difficult and painful. They were also responsible for the tendency of the device to embed itself in or perforate the uterine wall.[38]

The second, more serious problem was the design of the tail string, which passed through the cervix into the vagina. Tail strings permitted patients to determine if the device was in place and enabled doctors to remove IUDs efficiently. But whereas other inventors had used a monofilament tail string to prevent the absorption of moisture and bacteria into the uterus, Davis and Lerner had used a multifilament made of hundreds of tiny nylon strands encased in a nylon sheath. Davis and Lerner had worried that a monofilament string would break when the Shield was removed because of the resistance action of the prongs. They ruled out a thicker monofilament because of the discomfort it might cause male partners, a problem that had surfaced during clinical trials of the original Margulies spiral. Their compromise was the multifilament. But because they did not seal its ends, they unwittingly created a biological expressway for the transmission of bacteria from the vagina directly into the uterus, a process called "wicking." Wicking was a major cause of potentially life-threatening uterine infections. In addition, the sheath encasing the multifilament began to deteriorate after insertion, creating holes that also enabled bacteria to spread into the uterus. Wayne Crowder, a quality-control manager at A. H. Robins, had advised company management of the potential hazards of the Shield multifilament in the spring of 1971, after independent tests had revealed a rapid transfer of moisture from one end of the string to the other. Not wanting to slow down Dalkon Shield production, A. H. Robins management ignored

Crowder's warnings and reminded him that safeguarding tail string safety was not part of his job.[39]

Thus in the spring of 1971, the Dalkon Shield was a medical disaster waiting to happen. The crisis might have been averted by premarket FDA scrutiny, but in the early 1970s the FDA had limited authority over the medical device industry. Whereas drug manufacturers were required to demonstrate a new drug's safety and efficacy *before* it was marketed, medical devices were not subjected to premarket approval. The FDA could remove unsafe devices only after they were marketed, and then only if the agency could document that the device was sold "under false and misleading claims, that it is adulterated, or that it is unsafe for the intended use." In contrast with drug regulation, the burden of proof resided with the FDA, not manufacturers.[40]

A. H. Robins aggressively publicized its first contraceptive. The IUD market was highly competitive in the United States, with at least seventy other models. A. H. Robins worked overtime to win converts and customers. Although the company's medical advisory board had recommended marketing the device only to gynecologists, warning that under no circumstances should the Dalkon Shield be "pushed on a physician who is just casually familiar with pelvic anatomy," the company promoted the Shield to general practitioners.[41] More doctors meant more sales. The Dalkon Shield was advertised in medical and trade journals, as was customary. But it was also advertised directly to women in magazines and on radio and television. Advertisements proclaimed the Shield to be "safe and effective," "trouble free," and "truly superior." Potential side effects were downplayed or ignored. Although the Dalkon Corporation had recommended that physicians be instructed to administer a painkiller prior to insertion (Davis injected patients with the narcotic Demerol before insertion), A. H. Robins ignored the suggestion to boost sales. It did not want to frighten women or physicians. The patient brochure promised that "the insertion procedure is generally well tolerated by even the most sensitive women. . . . Some women have cramps for a short time after insertion, but these are generally mild and usually pass in a few minutes."[42]

Between January 1971 and May 1974, 2.2 million Dalkon Shields were sold in the United States, more than all other IUDs combined. Another 1.5 million were sold abroad.[43] Major Russel J. Thomsen, a physician in Fort Polk, Louisiana, recalled how easy it was to be seduced by Robins's promotional campaign. "Like many physicians trained in the 1960s, I was introduced to the new generation of plastic IUD's without the inherent bias against intrauterine contraceptives which older practitioners held," he said. "Within the context of the raging furor over the oral contraceptive tablet, the IUD and its promotional claims made good sense. . . . I inserted hundreds."[44]

Thomsen soon realized he had been misled. Many women were physically and emotionally traumatized by the pain of insertion. "I have seen a number of women faint following IUD insertion and particularly from Dalkon Shield insertion," he stated in 1973. "Many patients—especially those having undergone severe pain during insertion—look forward to its removal with such apprehension as to request to be 'put to sleep' during that fateful event. This, of course, is rarely done, but many patients benefit by being given pain medication prior to the removal of the IUD. In fact, pain medication, a lead bullet to bite on, and a short memory are the requisites of some IUD removals, particularly with the Dalkon Shield." Attempting to understand the disjunction between insertion reality and the upbeat patient brochure promising women at worst minor cramps, he concluded that the "person who wrote [the brochure] was probably a man and most certainly had never undergone the experience of receiving a Dalkon Shield." As for the physician literature characterizing the Dalkon Shield as "Designed for Greater Comfort," Thomsen had only this to say: "I have seen a number of women pass out from Dalkon Shield insertion. If that is designed for comfort, then I would hate to see one that was not designed for comfort."[45]

Other physicians and patients reported similar experiences. Indeed, A. H. Robins began receiving complaints within a month after it had first marketed the Shield. One doctor wrote that although he had inserted thousands of other IUDs without incident, he had found the insertion of a Dalkon Shield to be "the most traumatic manipulation ever perpetrated upon womanhood."[46] One woman, a patient of Dr. Davis's, discovered the hard way that even a Demerol injection was not enough to dull insertion pain. When her husband complained of his wife's suffering, Davis advised him to "take her out for a 'stiff drink.' "[47] Another woman's bad experience with the Dalkon Shield compelled her to contact her congressman:

When I was attending the University of Virginia, I used the clinic facilities for a regular gynecology checkup. During one of these checkups a nurse encouraged me to have an IUD inserted and told me there was only "slight discomfort" involved in insertion. She gave me some literature prepared by the A. H. Robins Company and I took it home and discussed it with my husband. We carefully read the literature and having no other source of information, we decided that I would try it. Upon returning to the clinic for the IUD I was astonished when the same nurse gave me a shot of codeine and told me, when I asked why, that it was "for the pain." Having been told nothing of what was to come I was indeed stunned but I was still unprepared for what came afterward. It's hard for me to describe the pain, but I can honestly say it was like no other I have ever experienced. I did not faint but I have known women who did.[48]

Pain alone did not kill, but other problems resulting from the Dalkon Shield did. The device's tendency to become embedded in the endometrium and to wick caused eighteen known deaths. The greatest risk stemmed from septic abortions. In women who got pregnant while wearing the device, miscarriages frequently occurred. In some cases, these miscarriages caused an infection of the uterine lining, which can cause septicemia, a serious infection of the blood system. Unless an afflicted patient is treated with immediate and aggressive antibiotic therapy, she dies. In addition to being responsible for at least eighteen deaths, the Dalkon Shield caused over 200,000 infections, miscarriages, hysterectomies, and other gynecological complications and led to an untold number of birth defects, caused by contact between the device and the developing fetus.[49] Early on, A. H. Robins defended the safety of the Dalkon Shield by insisting that its popularity, accounting for two-thirds of IUDs distributed between 1971 and 1973, explained the high number of septic abortions. This was untrue. A report issued by the Centers for Disease Control in 1983 concluded that the Dalkon Shield was four times more likely to cause complications than any other IUD.[50]

By the spring of 1974, A. H. Robins had received over four hundred complaints about the Shield. These included reports of thirty-six septic abortions, four of them fatal, among women who became pregnant wearing the IUD. Word of a forthcoming and highly critical journal article linking the Dalkon Shield to maternal deaths prodded A. H. Robins to send letters to physicians on May 8, 1974, warning them of possible complications with the device. After pressure from the FDA, A. H. Robins stopped marketing the Shield on June 28, 1974, but continued foreign sales. Finally, in April 1975, two months after the esteemed contraceptive expert Dr. Howard Tatum published a devastating report on his experiments with the Dalkon Shield tail string in the *Journal of the American Medical Association*, the company suspended foreign sales. But it refused to recall the device, for to have done so would have been to admit that the product was flawed. By this time, fifteen wearers of the Dalkon Shield had died.[51]

In 1975, A. H. Robins lost its first lawsuit and faced hundreds more.[52] Women's claims revealed the scope of human suffering inflicted by the device. In one case, a woman conceived while wearing the Dalkon Shield. Despite the promotional literature's claim that the IUD would inflict no harm on a developing fetus and could safely remain *in utero*, the baby was born severely brain damaged.[53] In another instance, a woman who had the Shield inserted when she was eighteen immediately began to suffer from recurring pelvic infections. Eight months later, she had the Shield removed. Even then, her problems did not go away. Years later, she started getting "sick cramps, vomiting, high fever, the same spells that had come up periodically." Her doctor told her that she was infected with "tubo-ovarian abscesses, one the size of a grapefruit, one the size of an orange. I was apparently about ready to explode." At the age of twenty-five, she was given a total hysterectomy and placed on hormone-replacement therapy.[54]

A. H. Robins defended the integrity of its actions and the safety of the Shield. Early on, its defense was an aggressive offensive. Company lawyers accused women with medical problems of sexual promiscuity. Frequent sex with multiple partners, not the Dalkon Shield, had led to sexually transmitted diseases that caused pelvic infections. Robins's lawyers also blamed doctors for inserting Shields into "unsuitable" female candidates. This blame-the-victim strategy humiliated the women who were forced to recount their sexual histories on the stand. Fortunately, it backfired. By the end of 1985, A. H. Robins and the Shield insurer, Aetna Life and Casualty Company, had paid out $378.3 million to settle women's claims plus $107.3 million in legal costs. In those cases that had gone to trial, Robins had lost more than it had won.[55]

In June 1970, Aetna began providing product-liability insurance to Robins, which it renewed annually. But in 1977, the insurance company saw the writing on the wall. The volume of awards to Shield victims and the number of lawsuits being filed were on the rise, with no end in sight. Aetna notified Robins that it would cancel its insurance policy, effective February 28, 1978. It also contended that it would not be held legally responsible for claims filed after the cutoff date. Robins sued Aetna, insisting that Aetna's liability in Shield cases covered litigation initiated after the insurance cutoff date if a plaintiff had been wearing the Shield when Aetna's policy was in force. On March 9, 1977, the two companies reached a cost-sharing pact, whereby Aetna agreed to pay compensatory awards for bodily injuries and Robins agreed to pay for punitive damages, which juries award to punish defendants for wanton or reckless behavior.[56] After 1978, Robins was unable to secure an insurer.

By the early 1980s, Robins had gone on the defensive. In September 1980, following two devastating court verdicts, the company sent another "Dear Doctor" letter advising two hundred physicians to remove the Dalkon shield from their patients. The letter did not acknowledge product defects but rather mentioned the higher risk of infection posed by long-term use of *any* IUD.[57] In 1984, the company's legal team was rattled by the actions of Judge Miles Lord, a federal judge in Minnesota who had been assigned to hear twenty-three Dalkon Shield cases. Lord had consolidated the cases for trial, to be followed by separate hearings on damages. The judge's consolidation order denied the company the opportunity to defend itself by examining and attacking each plaintiff's sexual history. Suspicious of a corporate cover-up, Lord also issued a discovery order that forced top company officials to be subject to deposition and obligated Robins to produce documents that had hitherto been concealed, including damning in-house studies of the Shield's tail string troubles. The discovery results were incriminating, and the company doled out millions—more even than claimants had requested—to settle the cases out of court. Before he approved the final settlement agreement, Lord condemned the company, represented by president E. Claiborne Robins, Jr., general counsel William Forrest, and research director Carl Lunsford, for its actions. His statement stands out as one of the most impassioned speeches delivered by a judge in American history:

> Gentlemen . . . as you sit here attempting once more to extricate yourself from the legal consequences of your acts, none of you has faced up to the fact that more than nine thousand women have made claims that they gave up part of their womanhood so that your company might prosper. . . . I dread to think what would have been the consequences if your victims had been men rather than women, women who seem through some strange quirk of our society's mores to be expected to suffer pain, shame, and humiliation. . . . Your company, without warning to women, invaded their bodies by the millions and caused them injuries by the thousands. And when the time came for these women to make their claims against your company, you attacked their characters. You inquired into their sexual practices and into the identity of their sex partners. You exposed these women—and ruined families and reputations and careers—in order to intimidate those who would raise their voices against you. . . . The only conceivable reason you have not recalled this product is that it would hurt your balance sheet and alert women who already have been harmed that you may be liable for their injuries. You have taken the bottom line as your guiding beacon, and the low road as your route. This is corporate irresponsibility at its meanest.[58]

Lord's statement, the spiraling cost of settlements, and the thousands of cases still pending had shaken the company's resolve to absorb the financial and public relations damage of litigation one case at a time. Then, in the summer of 1984, a devastating attack on the company's refusal to recall the Dalkon Shield aired on CBS's 60 *Minutes*. In October 1984, following reports of more Shield-related deaths, A. H. Robins recalled the Shield and offered to pay for the costs of removal. Within a few months, five thousand women had had the Shield removed at the company's expense.[59]

Less than a year later, on August 21, 1985, A. H. Robins filed for reorganization under Chapter 11 of the Bankruptcy Code, a move calculated to limit the number of future claims against it. Two months later a deadline of April 30, 1986, was set for claimants to file personal-injury claims. After that time, "any person that has a claim against Robins . . . shall be forever barred from participating in the Chapter 11 estate." The company had estimated that no more than 35,000 claims would be filed by the deadline. Instead, over 325,000 were filed, roughly 8 percent of those thought to be wearing Dalkon Shields worldwide. In 1989, as A. H. Robins was trying to determine how it could honor these claims under its proposed reorganization, the American Home Products Corporation came up with a winning offer. The wealthy company, best known as a manufacturer of health care and household products that included Advil, Anacin, and Chef Boyardee, would establish a $2.5 billion trust fund to compensate women as part of its purchase of A. H. Robins. The trust fund barely dented the annual profits of the American Home Products Corporation.[60]

Epilogue:
The Contraceptive Conundrum

Readers may remember a *Seinfeld* episode that aired shortly after the V. L. I. Corporation of California announced that it would stop manufacturing the Today Sponge. In the episode, Elaine buys as many boxes of the disposable sponge as she can find, depleting her precious reserve only when she meets a man she deems "spongeworthy." The episode resonated with loyal users and woman's rights activists distressed by the sudden withdrawal of one of the few new contraceptives since plastic IUDs and the Pill. The sponge was approved by the FDA in 1983, and its disappearance in 1995 had nothing to do with the device's safety or reliability. Rather, the manufacturer decided not to upgrade its factory's air and water supply, which the FDA had cited as substandard. That left women with only one nonprescription female method, the Reality condom.[1]

Available in the United States since 1993, Reality has had its own share of problems. Described by its manufacturer, a small Chicago firm, as a "soft, loose-fitting plastic pouch that lines the vagina," it is more popular in overseas markets, especially in Africa, than in the United States. Despite its obvious benefits to women—Reality is female-controlled and can protect women from STDs such as AIDS—it is "not popular," one Planned Parenthood spokeswoman recently admitted. It is big and bulky, and it makes some women squeamish. Some women have reported that it squeaks during sex. The condoms are expensive too. Through the assistance of the United Nations AIDS program, women in

Zimbabwe, South Africa, and Zambia can get them free or at cost. In the United States, the one-use condoms cost about three dollars each.[2]

At the dawn of a new millennium, we are faced with a contraceptive conundrum of far-reaching import. On the one hand, the United States has one of the highest unwanted-pregnancy rates in the Western world. Fully 60 percent of all pregnancies in the United States are unplanned or unwanted. On the other hand, recent developments have yielded a dizzying array of new, effective female technologies. These include Norplant, six soft plastic capsules containing the synthetic progesterone levonorgestrel that are surgically inserted in a patient's upper arm, releasing hormones over five years, and Depo-Provera, a high-progestin contraceptive injected into a woman's arm or buttocks every three months. Both methods are reversible and have a success rate exceeding 99 percent in the first year of use. And, after a five-year hiatus, the disposable sponge is back. There are also a number of new birth control devices on the horizon: hormone-releasing patches, gels, and vaginal rings; a new IUD; a one-size-fits-all diaphragm that works; a silicone-rubber cervical cap; and male injections and implants.[3] One wonders what George Bernard Shaw, who considered the rubber condom the greatest invention of the nineteenth century, would say of the state of contraceptive technology now.

How do we explain the disjunction between the availability of a cornucopia of effective technologies and patterns of everyday use? One answer is that Americans want more and better options. Although there is no such thing as a perfect contraceptive, we yearn for methods that have fewer side effects and aesthetic drawbacks. Americans desire contraceptives that will do more than prevent pregnancy—like protect us from STDs, clear up acne, and prevent cancer. We are discontented with methods that fall short of our high—some would say unrealistically high—expectations. A 1985 poll found that 60 percent of American women were dissatisfied with contraceptive options.[4] Since then, four new female methods have been marketed (the female condom, the sponge, Norplant, and Depo-Provera), but only a minority of women—less than 6 percent—use them.[5] No new male methods have been marketed. In the early 1980s, a government report predicted that there would be twenty new contraceptives available by the year 2000.[6] Despite important product breakthroughs, we have fallen short of that goal. It is ironic that in a post–*Roe* v. *Wade* world that celebrates reproductive choice, the most frequently used contraceptive in the country—by a wide margin—is irreversible female sterilization. In a very real sense, Americans are still waiting for the heralded "second contraceptive revolution" to arrive.

One problem is that the pace of contraceptive research slowed in the late 1970s and early 1980s. The biggest deterrent to new product development was the increased cost of liability insurance. Litigation was the only recourse for women injured by the Dalkon Shield. But women's legal successes caused insurance premiums to skyrocket. Contraceptive research in the United States ground almost to a halt as the nation's leading pharmaceutical firms swapped birth control initiatives for less risky ventures. Promising projects were tabled or scrapped. Leading scientists left the field. The number of American companies active in contraceptive research fell from a dozen in the early 1970s to two in the late 1990s.[7]

The cost of product liability insurance affected various contraceptives differently. Some methods, such as the Pill, enjoyed a wide enough profit margin to be self-insured. Manufacturers of oral contraceptives, for instance, spent only a few cents to manufacture a month's supply of oral contraceptives in the 1980s but charged several dollars. Because the Pill requires repeat purchases, pharmaceutical companies can set aside some of their profits to cover the cost of potential lawsuits. The same cannot be said for long-acting methods such as the IUD that necessitate only a onetime purchase.[8] In the late 1980s, more research money was being spent on modifications of existing steroidal contraceptives—especially differently formulated oral contraceptives—than on new methods that might cost less to consumers.[9] And, of course, the staggering cost of product research and development and the risk of lawsuits effectively preclude the possibility of an entrepreneurial renaissance—a contraceptive research program powered by small-business people. In the near future, we can expect to see no Rosemarie Lewis or Julius Schmid taking up the cause.

Government grants to academic centers and the work of nonprofit groups like the Population Council can go only so far to fill the product development void. Government funding tends to be short-term. New medical technologies are rarely developed in a few years, and contraceptives are no exception. In addition, funding for contraceptive research is highly politicized and inherently unstable. The strength of the pro-life movement, for instance, has stymied government-backed research on methods that work after fertilization has occurred. The Agency for International Development is barred by law, and the National Institutes of Health by policy, from funding research into any method that interrupts pregnancy.[10] Nonprofit organizations such as the Population Council have stayed active in the field of contraceptive research. But like universities and development agencies, they have been hit hard by the liability issue. Without profits with which they can compensate potential injured users, they must rely on private-sector partners to bring products to market.

For example, the Population Council developed Norplant, but it needed a pharmaceutical firm to handle distribution and marketing. It found one in Wyeth-Ayerst Laboratories, a division of the American Home Products Corporation and one of the few pharmaceutical firms actively engaged in contraceptive research in the late 1980s. The company marketed the subcutaneous implant in 1990. But when silicone-gel breast implants began to be taken off the market in 1992, Norplant fell under suspicion because its rods were made of silicone (although not silicone gel). Insertions of Norplant fell from eight hundred a day in 1990 to fewer than sixty in 1995. In addition, women scarred by the insertion and especially the removal of Norplant filed hundreds of lawsuits against Wyeth.[11] Inadequate physician training was one reason for the problem. As has been the case throughout American history, medical education lagged behind technological development. But another reason for the problem was that women's health groups had lobbied manufacturers not to develop biodegradable implants. They feared that capsules that dissolved would rob women of the option of having Norplant removed before the drug's five-year term was up.[12]

Manufacturers called the mass filing of product-liability lawsuits against Wyeth the "Norplant syndrome." Women's health groups called it justice. Separating these opposing views is a question that remains unresolved: What defines the threshold between acceptable risk and product liability? In 1970, Carl Djerassi astutely predicted that unless consumer attitudes changed, lawsuits would thwart reproductive research. Women expect too much, he complained. If they want more and better contraceptives, they must be content with a higher degree of medical risk. "The consumer . . . suffers from the delusion that drug safety and drug efficacy are all-or-none propositions," he argued. "The fact that people experience side effects from 'safe' drugs should be no more surprising than the fact that occasionally some people die when 'safe' airplanes crash."[13]

Many scientists, doctors, and family planning advocates agree. In 1996, the Committee of the Institute of Medicine, a branch of the National Academy of Sciences, renewed its 1990 recommendation that Congress enact tort reform to shield manufacturers of contraceptives from costly product-liability lawsuits. Women's groups vigorously object to this proposal. The right to sue and collect damages is the only recourse available to consumers who have been injured or hurt, and it must be preserved, they say. The fear of lawsuits might limit women's birth control options, but it also keeps them safe. The history of contraceptives tells a story of technological triumph, but also of too much grief.[14]

On August 15, 1996, Wyeth-Ayerst received good news from the FDA. Its second-generation version of Norplant had been declared safe and effective. It could be released on the market. Instead of celebrating FDA clearance, Wyeth hesitated. "We're evaluating whether to introduce it," admitted Audrey Ashby, a company spokesperson. "Frankly, we have to assess the environment of the U.S. market—including litigation. We're looking at what has happened."[15]

But if product development troubles and a corresponding dissatisfaction with existing methods explain some of the contraceptive conundrum, they do not explain it all. The technologies available in the United States also exist in countries that have much lower rates of unwanted pregnancy. In fact, pregnancy rates among women under age twenty are higher in the United States than in any other developed country except Hungary. This is not because young adults in the United States have more sex than they do elsewhere. In Sweden, for instance, sex among young adults is more prevalent, yet rates of pregnancy, birth, and abortion are significantly lower. The reason is simple. Young adults in Sweden use contraceptives more frequently than their American counterparts.[16]

It is not the availability of technology that determines patterns of contraceptive use but the specific contexts in which women and men encounter it. In Sweden, contraceptive supplies and services are available at cost, and sex education, including contraceptive instruction, is compulsory. In the United States, more than seventy years after the military quietly acknowledged that asking young male recruits "to just say no" does little except increase the incidence of VD, we still cling to the belief that abstinence is an effective medical and social policy. Birth control education in U.S. public schools is minimal, the distribution of free contraceptives unheard of. Many politicians expressed moral outrage when the former surgeon general Joycelyn Elders, emphasizing the importance of adolescent pregnancy prevention, declared she would happily coronate herself the "condom queen" and "wear a crown on my head with a condom on it" if only she could "get every young person in the United States who is engaging in sex to use a condom." At the same time, politicians opposed to the diffusion of contraceptive programs profess great shock when teenage girls become "welfare moms."

Of course, few women yearn for the indignities that are part and parcel of accepting welfare payments, just as no woman is born *wanting* to have an abortion. If we want to reduce the frequency of these events, we must multiply our efforts to make contraceptives accessible to all.

Empowering women and men to exercise freedom of contraceptive choice is not the same as choosing methods for them. The history of contraceptives is replete with examples of birth control coercion, perpetuated in the name of the public good and usually carried out at the expense of poor women and women of color. Since the 1970s, when the worst sterilization abuses were checked by new, rigid federal guidelines, other concerns have surfaced. Health care activists, feminists, and minority rights advocates have warned about the abuse of Norplant and Depo-Provera, contraceptives that, though reversible, are still long-term. One legislator in Kansas proposed that welfare mothers be offered a lump cash payment for using Norplant—a suggestion that pressures financially vulnerable women to undergo a surgical procedure to save taxpayers money. It may not be eugenics, but it is certainly not freedom of choice.[17]

In this country, when it comes to contraceptives, accessibility means affordability. It is not enough to promote sex instruction. We must make sure that contraceptive technologies are available to women and men regardless of their financial situation. I recently interviewed Lorraine, a mother of three. She is one of the millions of working Americans caught in the health care crisis. She works full-time in the service industry. Her employer offers her no health care; he himself is a struggling small-business man. For years, Lorraine made too much money to qualify for Medicaid but not enough to afford over-the-counter contraceptives—never mind a visit to the doctor. She has had four abortions. One was caused by the ingestion of the abortifacient pennyroyal, which grows wild in the area where she lives. It almost killed her. Recently, her circumstances changed. She applied for Medicaid and had her tubes tied.[18]

Lorraine's lot improved significantly once she got health care, but even Americans with health insurance often discover that coverage for contraceptives is limited. HMOs and traditional fee-for-service plans generally cover prescription drugs. But a 1998 study by the Women's Research and Education Institute in Washington found that two-thirds of the nation's largest group health plans exclude reversible contraceptives, classifying them as an unnecessary drug. This exclusion forces women to pay, on average, 68 percent more on out-of-pocket prescription expenses than men. And it encourages women who cannot afford to dole out hundreds of dollars for the Pill to undergo sterilizations, which more insurance plans cover. With access to reversible methods tied to income, it is not surprising that sterilizations are more popular among low-income women, especially Hispanics and blacks, than they are among affluent women and non-Hispanic whites. When HMOs do cover reversible contraceptives such as the Pill, they usually cover only part of the cost, and then only the (typically) few brands included in the HMO's formulary. Should a woman need a differently formulated Pill, for instance, she often must shoulder the full expense of her prescription. "We allow our insurance companies to be biased against women," noted Dr. Mitchell Creinin, the director of family planning at the University of Pittsburgh. "If men were the ones who got pregnant, you know it would be different."[19]

Nothing illustrates the veracity of Creinin's claim more than the willingness of insurance companies to cover the expensive new anti-impotence drug Viagara (which currently costs about ten dollars *per pill*) but not reversible contraceptives such as the Pill. Apparently, enabling a man to achieve orgasm rates higher on our list of priorities than protecting a woman from the long-term consequences of his short-term delight.

In the absence of universal health care or prescription drug coverage, one way out of the contraceptive conundrum may be the development of more affordable over-the-counter methods, which would increase men's and women's options without tethering contraceptive use to the medical marketplace from which millions are excluded. In the 1920s, Margaret Sanger demonized the over-the-counter birth control trade, believing that the surest way of making contraceptives respectable was to place control of their distribution in doctors' hands. Today, to meet the needs of women and men who lack sufficient resources, we must supplement reliable medical methods with inexpensive over-the-counter options. Imagine Anthony Comstock's world with a twist: not just cheap contraceptives on every street corner, but cheap contraceptives *that work* on every street corner, finally freed from the risk of injury and the stigma of illegitimacy that, even today, thwart the best efforts of many Americans to take charge of their procreative destinies and their lives.

$\mathcal{N}otes$

INTRODUCTION

1. Diane Lore, "Insurers Slow to See Benefits of the Pill," *Atlanta Journal-Constitution*, May 9, 2000.

1. 1873

1. *Chicago Tribune*, March 5, 1873, p. 1; *Chicago Tribune*, March 4, 1873.
2. D. M. Bennett, *Anthony Comstock: His Career of Cruelty and Crime* (1878; reprint, New York: Da Capo Press, 1971), p. 1017.
3. The congressmen were not to be that lucky. When the salary raise made headline news, the public outcry ensured the law's repeal.
4. Comstock Act, chap. 258, 17 Stat. 598 (1873). The ban on contraceptives remained on the books until 1970, when Congress struck birth control from the obscenities list. James Reed, *From Private Vice to Public Virtue: The Birth Control Movement and American Society since 1830* (New York: Basic Books, 1978), p. 377.
5. Mary Ware Dennett, *Who's Obscene?* (New York: Vanguard Press, 1930), p. 210. The bill, introduced in Congress, was defeated by the opposition of Henry Clay and Daniel Webster.
6. James C. N. Paul and Murray L. Schwartz, *Federal Censorship: Obscenity in the Mail* (New York: Free Press, 1961), p. 12.
7. On print culture, regulation, and the evolution of the U.S. postal system, see Richard R. John, *Spreading the News: The American Postal System from Franklin to Morse* (Cambridge, Mass.: Harvard University Press, 1995); Dorothy Fowler, *Unmailable: Congress and the Post Office* (Athens: University of Georgia Press, 1977). The 1792 Post Office Act institutionalized a two-tiered rate system, but only news-

paper readers and printers benefited. The measure admitted every newspaper into the mail, charging one to one and a half cents postage, depending on the distance traveled. Until the Post Office Acts of 1845 and 1851, sending a letter was prohibitively costly for many social groups. Prior to these measures, postal rates were calculated on the basis of distance and the number of sheets of correspondence contained, but not on weight. The 1845 and 1851 acts adopted a weight-based formula that assigned a flat rate irrespective of distance, with only a few exceptions. John, *Spreading the News*, pp. 36, 160. In 1863, mailable matter had been broken down into the following categories: first class (all correspondence); second class (regularly printed matter); and third class (pamphlets, books, maps, photographs, seeds, and such). See Fowler, *Unmailable*, p. 55.

8. John D'Emilio and Estelle B. Freedman, *Intimate Matters: A History of Sexuality in America* (New York: Harper and Row, 1988), p. 158; on venereal disease during the Civil War, see James Boyd Jones, Jr., "A Tale of Two Cities: The Hidden Battle against Venereal Disease in Civil War Nashville and Memphis," *Civil War History* 31 (1985): 270–76.

9. *Congressional Globe*, February 8, 1865, p. 661.

10. Ibid.; Paul and Schwartz, *Federal Censorship*, p. 17. As initially proposed, the bill would have empowered the Post Office to open mail and seize and destroy confiscated material. Reservations expressed by Senators Reverdy Johnson of Maryland and John Sherman of Ohio ensured that these provisions were struck. Johnson worried that postal workers would get "censorship happy." "It is true that most of the printed matter that is sent is sent without being covered or sealed up," he cautioned, "but if there is any danger of this kind those who send this species of publications will no doubt soon begin to seal them, and then the postmaster, whenever he suspects that an envelope contains anything which is obnoxious to objection, will break the seal." The amendment, proposed by Sherman, dropped all references to seizure and confiscation and left the detection of obscene publications to individual postal workers' wits. See *Congressional Globe*, February 8, 1865, p. 661.

11. The new law criminalized the mailing of any "book, pamphlet, picture, print, or other publication of a vulgar or indecent character, or any letter upon the envelope of which, or postal card upon which scurrilous epithets may have been written or printed." It would be this clause, contained in section 148 of the Post Office Act of 1872, that the Comstock Law would significantly expand. *Appendix to the Congressional Globe*, June 8, 1872, p. 790.

12. Janet Farrell Brodie, *Contraception and Abortion in Nineteenth-Century America* (Ithaca, N.Y.: Cornell University Press, 1994), p. 259; Nicola Beisel, *Imperiled Innocents: Anthony Comstock and Family Reproduction in Victorian America* (Princeton, N.J.: Princeton University Press, 1997), pp. 22–24, 37–38; Heywood Broun and Margaret Leech, *Anthony Comstock: Roundsman of the Lord* (New York: Albert and Charles Boni, 1927), p. 38.

13. Homer B. Sprague, "Societies for the Suppression of Vice," *Education* (September 1882): 76; Register of Post Office Inspectors, box 16, Postal Inspection Service

Records, Post Office Department Records, RG 28, National Archives; Broun and Leech, *Anthony Comstock*, chap. 4.

14. Brodie, *Contraception and Abortion*, p. 259; Beisel, *Imperiled Innocents*, p. 37; Bennett, *Anthony Comstock*, p. 1012; C. G. Trumbull, *Anthony Comstock: Fighter* (New York: Fleming Revell Company, 1913), passim.

15. Timothy Gilfoyle, *City of Eros: New York City, Prostitution, and the Commercialization of Sex, 1790–1920* (New York: W. W. Norton, 1992), p. 58, table 1, p. 177.

16. Ibid., p. 234.

17. Brodie, *Contraception and Abortion*, p. 259.

18. Broun and Leech, *Anthony Comstock*, p. 81.

19. One biography has suggested that Maggie Comstock's age rendered her infertile. This seems unlikely: when her daughter died in 1872, she was thirty-eight, young enough to conceive even by the standards of the 1870s. Ibid., p. 67.

20. Brodie, *Contraception and Abortion*, p. 260.

21. Trumbull, *Anthony Comstock*, passim; Broun and Leech, *Anthony Comstock*, p. 91.

22. Brodie, *Contraception and Abortion*, pp. 261–62.

23. Ibid., p. 261; Paul Boyer, *Purity in Print: The Vice Society Movement and Book Censorship in America* (New York: Scribner, 1968), p. 5; Anthony Comstock, "The Suppression of Vice," *North American Review* 135 (November 1882): 484–85; Sprague, "Societies for the Suppression of Vice," pp. 78–79.

24. Lawrence M. Friedman, *Crime and Punishment in American History* (New York: Basic Books, 1993), pp. 127–42.

25. Comstock quoted in Broun and Leech, *Anthony Comstock*, p. 224; Friedman, *Crime and Punishment*, p. 130.

26. D'Emilio and Freedman, *Intimate Matters*, p. 160.

27. "Milestone 65: A Brief Survey of the New York Society for the Suppression of Vice," box 17, Medical Interests, Rockefeller Family Collection, Rockefeller Archives, Tarrytown, N.Y.; Boyer, *Purity in Print*, pp. 5–6.

28. *Sixth Annual Report of the New York Society for the Suppression of Vice* (New York, 1880), pp. 27–28; Mary Ware Dennett, *Birth Control Laws: Shall We Keep Them, Change Them, or Abolish Them?* (New York: Grafton Press, 1926), p. 31.

29. Dennett, *Birth Control Laws*, p. 32. The Criminal Code specified that "any agent of the New York Society for the Suppression of Vice upon being designated thereto by the sheriff of any county in the State may within such county make arrests and bring before any court or magistrate thereof having jurisdiction, offenders found violating the provisions of any law for the suppression of the trade in and circulation of obscene literature and illustrations, advertisements and articles of indecent or immoral use, as it is or may be forbidden by the laws of the State or of the United States."

30. Register of Post Office Inspectors, RG 28.

31. Anthony Comstock, *Frauds Exposed* (Montclair, N.J.: Patterson Smith, 1880), p. 389.

32. *Appendix to the Congressional Globe*, March 1, 1873, p. 168.

33. Fowler, *Unmailable*, p. 60; Broun and Leech, *Anthony Comstock*, p. 122.

34. Norman Himes, *Medical History of Contraception* (Baltimore, Md.: Williams and Wilkins Company, 1936), pp. 59–63; Linda Gordon, *Woman's Body, Woman's Right: A Social History of Birth Control in America* (New York: Penguin, 1974), pp. 42–43; Percy Skuy, *Tales of Contraception* (Ortho, 1995), p. 11.

35. Peter James and Nick Thorpe, *Ancient Inventions* (New York: Ballantine, 1994), pp. 187–88; Gerald I. Zatuchni, "Contraceptive Technologies for the Future," in John M. Leventhal, ed., *Current Problems in Obstetrics and Gynecology* (Chicago: Year Book Medical Publishers, 1984), pp. 7–9; Himes, *Medical History of Contraception*, p. 80; Gordon, *Woman's Body, Woman's Right*, pp. 43–44.

36. Stopes's findings are reported in Marie C. Stopes, "Positive and Negative Control of Conception in Its Various Technical Aspects," *Journal of State Medicine* (London) 39 (1931): 354–60, and discussed in Gordon, *Woman's Body, Woman's Right*, p. 44.

37. As with herbal decoctions and douching techniques, abortifacient recipes were readily obtained from midwives, female friends, and kin; popular medical guides, by identifying substances to be avoided during pregnancy, unwittingly served as an additional source of information. Although the outcome, the termination of a pregnancy, made their pharmacological impact unique, abortifacients were considered (at least at the time of their ingestion) indistinguishable from other emmenagogues, medicines widely used in the colonial era and early Republic to bring on a late or irregular menstrual period. Susan Klepp, "Lost, Hidden, Obstructed, and Repressed: Contraceptive and Abortive Technology in the Early Delaware Valley," in Judith A. McGaw, ed., *Early American Technology: Making and Doing Things from the Colonial Era to 1850* (Chapel Hill: University of North Carolina Press, 1994).

38. Brodie, *Contraception and Abortion*, pp. 190–91.

39. Andrea Tone, ed., *Controlling Reproduction: An American History* (Wilmington, Del.: Scholarly Resources, 1997), p. 101; Brodie, *Contraception and Abortion*, pp. 191–92.

40. Ezra Heywood, *Uncivil Liberty: An Essay to Show the Injustice and Impolicy of Ruling Woman without Her Consent* (Princeton, Mass.: Cooperative Publishing Co., 1872), p. 21.

41. Todd quoted in Shirley Green, *The Curious History of Contraception* (London: Ebury Press, 1971), p. 14.

42. Ely Van de Warker, "The Criminal Use of Proprietary or Advertised Nostrums," *New York Medical Journal* 17 (1873): 23.

43. But this middle ground was contested indeed: the politics of supporting a woman's *right* to time her pregnancies were considered, given the standards of the day, quite radical. In short, if we subject past actors to a present-day litmus test, we ignore the ways in which the politics of reproductive control in the 1870s were differently gauged and we overlook the diversity of opinion that occupied this middle ground.

44. Tone, ed., *Controlling Reproduction*, p. 138. Generally, these early statutes sought to protect women from poisonous abortifacients and dangerous procedures, and punished individuals responsible for providing them, not the women who had abor-

tions. On antebellum abortion criminalization, see James Mohr, *Abortion in America: The Origins and Evolution of National Policy, 1800–1900* (New York: Oxford University Press, 1978).

45. Mary Alden Hopkins, "Birth Control and Public Morals: An Interview with Anthony Comstock," *Harper's Weekly*, May 22, 1915, p. 490.

46. Sexual radicals, such as Ezra Heywood and Victoria Woodhull, shared Comstock's views on abortion. Heywood described abortion as a "murderous practice . . . unworthy of free lovers [who] accept and rear the child, but take precautions that the next one be born of choice, not by accident." Ezra Heywood, *Cupid's Yokes; or, The Binding Forces of Conjugal Life* (Princeton, Mass.: Cooperative Publishing Co., 1877), p. 20. Woodhull regarded the moment of conception as "the greatest of all constructive processes—the formation of an immortal soul"—but also believed that women should be given the power to determine under what circumstances this "fearful responsibility" occurred. Victoria Woodhull, "And the Truth Shall Make You Free" (New York: Woodhull and Claflin, 1874), p. 36.

47. Claflin quoted in Gordon, *Woman's Body, Woman's Right*, p. 97.

48. Nicholas Francis Cooke, *Satan in Society: By a Physician* (Cincinnati and San Francisco: Edward F. Hoovey, 1882), pp. 24, 150. Although the book was published in 1882, it was written in 1870.

49. Quoted in D'Emilio and Freedman, *Intimate Matters*, p. 146. Physicians' acceptance of a reproductive explanation for physiological, intellectual, and emotional maladies promoted medical interventions to cut, burn, remove, or otherwise manipulate the offending organ. In an article praising gynecologists' ability to "correct" female deviance, Storer boasted of his success curing an unmarried schoolteacher's nymphomania (manifested in "excessive masturbation" and a purported inability to "restrain herself from soliciting the approach of the other sex") by chemically burning her cervix with *potassa fusa*. Horatio Storer, "The Relations of Female Patients to Hospitals for the Insane: The Necessity on Their Account of a Board of Consulting Physicians to Every Hospital," *Transactions of the American Medical Association* 15 (1865): 125.

The frequency of "curative" gynecological interventions prompted one doctor to caution satirically in 1868 that the unharmed American uterus was fast becoming an endangered species. The uterus, he wrote, "is a harmless, unoffensive little organ, stowed away in a quick place. Simply a muscular organ, having no function to perform, save at certain periods of life, . . . [it is] nowadays subject to all sorts of barbarity from surgeons anxious for notoriety. Had Dame Nature foreseen this, she would have made it iron clad. What with burning and cauterizing, cutting and slashing and gouging, and spitting and skewering, and pessarying, the old-fashioned womb will cease to exist, except in history." Quoted in Green, *Curious History of Contraception*, p. 114.

50. Edward H. Clarke, M.D., *Sex in Education; or, A Fair Chance for the Girls* (Boston: James R. Osgood and Company, 1873), pp. 23, 33. Emphasis added.

51. Cooke, *Satan in Society*, p. 152. In *Is It I? A Book for Every Man*, his companion vol-

ume to his 1867 guide for women, Storer added to this list of afflictions "the un-steady step, gray hairs, and premature decrepitude of many of our men." Horatio Storer, *Is It I? A Book for Every Man* (Boston: Lee and Shepard, 1868), p. 94. Also see Thomas E. McArdle, "The Physical Evils Arising from the Prevention of Conception," *American Journal of Obstetrics* 21 (1881): 934–39.

52. Karen Lystra, *Searching the Heart: Women, Men, and Romantic Love in Nineteenth-Century America* (New York: Oxford University Press, 1989).

53. Anthony Comstock, *Traps for the Young*, ed. Robert Bremner (1883; reprint, Cambridge, Mass.: Harvard University Press, 1967), p. 133.

54. Beisel, *Imperiled Innocents*, p. 40; *Second Annual Report of the New York Society for the Suppression of Vice* (New York, 1876), p. 5.

55. *Index to the Congressional Globe*, 42nd Cong., 2nd sess., 1872, p. xiii.

56. Broun and Leech, *Anthony Comstock*, pp. 130–31; Trumbull, *Anthony Comstock*, p. 85; C. Thomas Dienes, *Law, Politics, and Birth Control* (Urbana: University of Illinois Press, 1972), p. 37.

57. *Congressional Globe*, February 18, 1873, p. 1436; Broun and Leech, *Anthony Comstock*, p. 135.

58. *Congressional Globe*, February 20, 1873, p. 1525.

59. *Congressional Globe*, March 1, 1873, p. 2004.

60. Ibid., p. 2005.

61. Comstock Act, chap. 258, 17 Stat. 598 (1873).

62. Broun and Leech, *Anthony Comstock*, p. 142.

63. Shaw quoted in ibid., pp. 229–30.

64. Constance B. Backhouse, "Involuntary Motherhood: Abortion, Birth Control, and Law in Nineteenth Century Canada," *Windsor Yearbook of Access to Justice* 3 (1983): 117; Angus McLaren, "Birth Control and Abortion in Canada, 1870–1920," *Canadian Historical Review* 59 (1978): 323.

65. Mary Alden Hopkins, "The Control of Births," *Harper's Weekly*, April 10, 1915, p. 342.

66. Dennett, *Birth Control Laws*, pp. 268–71; Carol Flora Brooks, "The Early History of the Anti-contraceptive Laws in Massachusetts and Connecticut," *American Quarterly* 18 (Spring 1966): 3–23. Twenty-two other states passed or strengthened existing obscenity statutes, enabling prosecution for the purchase or sale of contraceptives by applying the federal law's definition of "obscene."

2. THE LIMITS OF THE LAW

1. Credit reports for George Brinckerhoff, vol. 370, p. 700 a/64 (entries for May 27, 1875, August 30, 1875, October 10, 1881), p. 700 a/145 (entry for October 6, 1883), R. G. Dun and Company Collection, Baker Library, Harvard Business School, Boston, Mass.; "Report of Persons Arrested under the Auspices of the New York Society for the Suppression of Vice for the Year 1873," Records of the New York Society for the Suppression of Vice, container 1, Manuscript Division, Library

of Congress, Washington, D.C. (hereafter cited as Records of the NYSSV); "Indictment of George Brinckerhoff," October 7, 1873, box 12, Criminal Case Files of the
U.S. Circuit Court for the Southern District of New York, National Archives, Regional Office, New York.

2. Margaret Sanger, *Margaret Sanger: An Autobiography* (New York: W. W. Norton,
   1938), pp. 93–95. A recent book-length history of fertility control, for instance,
   while offering important new insights on the practice of birth control and abortion
   in the nineteenth-century United States, concludes that the new laws of the
   1870s "overrode a generation of commercialization and growing public discourse
   and drove reproductive control, if not totally back underground, at least into a
   netherworld of back-fence gossip and back-alley abortion." Janet Farrell Brodie,
   Contraception and Abortion in Nineteenth-Century America (Ithaca, N.Y.: Cornell
   University Press, 1994), p. 288. Brodie acknowledges that Sanger's remarks were
   exaggerated but accepts their basic premise. See also Carl N. Degler, *At Odds:
   Women and the Family in America from the Revolution to the Present* (New York: Oxford University Press, 1980), p. 222; Shirley Green, *The Curious History of Contra-
   ception* (London: Ebury Press, 1971), p. 15; Carol Flora Brooks, "The Early History
   of the Anti-contraceptive Laws in Massachusetts and Connecticut," *American
   Quarterly* 18 (Spring 1966): 22; Kathleen Endres, " 'Strictly Confidential': Birth-
   Control Advertising in a Nineteenth-Century City," *Journalism Quarterly* 63 (Win-
   ter 1986): 748–51; and C. Thomas Dienes, *Law, Politics, and Birth Control* (Urbana:
   University of Illinois Press, 1972), pp. 50–73. Two notable exceptions, neither of
   which explores the social or economic context of criminalization in depth, are
   Michael Grossberg, *Governing the Hearth: Law and the Family in Nineteenth-Century
   America* (Chapel Hill: University of North Carolina Press, 1985), pp. 175–95; and
   John D'Emilio and Estelle B. Freedman, *Intimate Matters: A History of Sexuality in
   America* (New York: Harper and Row, 1988).

3. Embezzling letters and mail and post office robberies accounted for 259 arrests; embezzling government funds, 11; using the mail for fraudulent purposes, 18; other of-
   fenses, 95. U.S. Post Office Department, *Annual Report of the Postmaster-General
   of the United States for the Fiscal Year Ended June 30, 1873* (Washington, D.C.:
   Government Printing Office, 1873), p. xxii. Also see C. G. Trumbull, *Anthony
   Comstock: Fighter* (New York: Fleming Revell Company, 1913), p. 188; Mary Ware
   Dennett, *Birth Control Laws: Shall We Keep Them, Change Them, or Abolish Them?*
   (New York: Grafton Press, 1926), p. 30; P. H. Woodward, *The Secret Service of the
   Post-Office Department* (Columbus, Ohio: Estill and Company, 1886), p. 20.

4. Grossberg, *Governing the Hearth*, pp. 187–93; Dennett, *Birth Control Laws*, pp.
   268–71; Brooks, "Early History of the Anti-contraceptive Laws in Massachusetts
   and Connecticut"; Leslie J. Reagan, *When Abortion Was a Crime: Women, Medicine,
   and Law in the United States, 1867–1973* (Berkeley: University of California Press,
   1997); H. S. Pomeroy, *The Ethics of Marriage* (New York: Funk and Wagnalls,
   1888), pp. 185–97; Dienes, *Law, Politics, and Birth Control*, pp. 42–47. My analysis
   of criminal litigation reveals that of 105 persons arrested for birth control crimes

between 1873 and 1898 by NYSSV agents, all but 12 were prosecuted in federal courts. "Report of Persons Arrested under the Auspices of the New York Society for the Suppression of Vice for the Years 1873–1898," containers 1–3, Records of the NYSSV.

5. The geographic breakdown of arrests recorded in the NYSSV arrest ledger between 1873 and 1898 is, by state: New York, 57; Illinois, 12; Massachusetts, 9; Pennsylvania, 7; New Jersey, 6; Connecticut, 3; Indiana, 3; Ohio, 2; New Hampshire, 2; Michigan, 1; Kentucky, 1; Tennessee, 1; Iowa, 1. "Report of Persons Arrested under the Auspices of the New York Society for the Suppression of Vice for the Years 1873–1898," containers 1–3, Records of the NYSSV. Comstock also depended on postal agents to enforce obscenity laws where NYSSV agents could not be present as easily, particularly in western and southern states.

6. These include those whose primary offense was making or selling birth control as well as those whose inventory included contraceptives, evidence that would lead to an additional criminal charge of violating birth control laws.

7. Comstock to S. Murphy, Esq., December 11, 1905, box 17, Medical Interests, Rockefeller Family Collection, Rockefeller Archives, Tarrytown, N.Y.; "Report of Persons Arrested under the Auspices of the New York Society for the Suppression of Vice for the Years 1873–1898," containers 1–3, Records of the NYSSV; Anthony Comstock, *Frauds Exposed* (Montclair, N.J.: Patterson Smith, 1880), pp. 5, 308, 434; *The Second Annual Report of the New York Society for the Suppression of Vice* (New York, 1876), pp. 11, 14.

8. The promotional pamphlet is quoted in D. M. Bennett, *An Open Letter to Samuel Colgate* (New York, 1879), pp. 8–9. Edward B. Foote, *The Radical Remedy in Social Science; or, Borning Better Babies through Regulating Reproduction by Controlling Conception* (New York: Murray Hill Publishing, 1886), p. 90; Edwin C. Walker, *Who Is the Enemy; Anthony Comstock or You?* (New York, 1903), p. 16.

9. Bennett, *Open Letter to Samuel Colgate*, p. 9; Heywood Broun and Margaret Leech, *Anthony Comstock: Roundsman of the Lord* (New York: Albert and Charles Boni, 1927), p. 189; Anthony Comstock, *Traps for the Young*, ed. Robert Bremner (1883; reprint, Cambridge, Mass.: Harvard University Press, 1967), p. 148.

10. Credit report for Morris Glattstine, vol. 257, p. 3342 (entries for January 29 and August 31, 1881), R. G. Dun and Company Collection; "Report of Persons Arrested under the Auspices of the New York Society for the Suppression of Vice for the Year 1878," container 1, Records of the NYSSV; Comstock to David B. Parker, March 21, 1878, box 27, Postal Inspection Service Records, Post Office Department Records, RG 28, National Archives; Brodie, *Contraception and Abortion*, p. 234. The company went unnamed in Comstock's letter to Parker, although Comstock's notes in the NYSSV 1878 arrest record indicate that he knew it at the time he wrote the letter.

11. See, for example, "Preliminary Hearing of William C. Halleck," 1919, pp. 118, 140, box 11, Transcripts of Hearings on Fraud Cases, 1913–1945, Post Office Department Records, RG 28, National Archives; Goodyear Rubber Company, *Physician's*

Friend and Nurse's Guide (Washington, D.C., 1898), pp. 1–7, 9, pamphlet, box 2, Rubber Trade Catalogues, Warshaw Collection of Business Americana, National Museum of American History, Smithsonian Institution, Washington, D.C.; B. F. Goodrich Company, *India Rubber Druggists' Sundries* (n.p., c. 1895), pp. 23–24, 33–47, 74–76, 81–83, 87, box 1, ibid.; Perry, Stearns & Company, *Rubber Goods of Every Description* (Chicago, 1890), pp. 28–34, box 8, ibid.; Tyer Rubber Company, *Illustrated Catalogue and Price List of Druggists' Sundries and Miscellaneous Rubber Goods* (Andover, Mass., 1908), pp. 10, 10a, 40, 40a, 88, 88a, box 8, ibid.; McKesson & Robbins, *Illustrated Catalogue of Druggists' Sundries, Fancy Goods, Surgical Instruments, Sponges, Chamois etc.* (New York: Daniel G. F. Class, 1883), pp. 112, 132, 151, 191; Sears, Roebuck & Co., *1897 Sears Roebuck Catalogue*, ed. Fred L. Israel (reprint, New York: Chelsea House Publishers, 1968), p. 32; Sears, Roebuck & Co., *1902 Sears Roebuck Catalogue*, ed. Cleveland Amory (reprint, New York: Gramercy Books, 1993), p. 455; Sears, Roebuck & Co., *1908 Sears Roebuck Catalogue*, ed. Joseph J. Schroeder, Jr. (reprint, Chicago: Follett Publishing Co., 1981), p. 795; James MaHood and Kristine Wenburg, *The Mosher Survey: Sexual Attitudes of 45 Victorian Women* (New York: Arno Press, 1980), case 47. On the social camouflaging of other medical devices in this era, see Rachel P. Maines, *The Technology of Orgasm: "Hysteria," the Vibrator, and Women's Sexual Satisfaction* (Baltimore, Md.: Johns Hopkins University Press, 1999).

12. *National Police Gazette*, January 3, 1885, pp. 14–15, November 16, 1889, p. 14, and March 24, 1900, pp. 14–15.
13. "Male pouch" by Uberto Ezell. U.S. Patent 824,634, June 26, 1906.
14. "Pessary" by G. J. Gladman, U.S. Patent 544,091, August 6, 1895. Also see "Pessary" by T. Brauns, U.S. Patent 168, 711, October 11, 1875.
15. "Report of Persons Arrested under the Auspices of the New York Society for the Suppression of Vice for the Years 1873–1898," containers 1–3, Records of the NYSSV.
16. "Report of Persons Arrested under the Auspices of the New York Society for the Suppression of Vice for the Years 1873, 1876," container 1, Records of the NYSSV; credit report for George Brinckerhoff, vol. 370, p. 700 a/145 (entry for October 6, 1883), R. G. Dun and Company Collection.
17. Comstock, *Traps for the Young*, p. xx; Anthony Comstock, "The Suppression of Vice," *North American Review* 135 (November 1882): 486.
18. Broun and Leech, *Anthony Comstock*, pp. 160, 164.
19. Comstock to Parker, June 1, 1878, box 27, Postal Inspection Service Records, Post Office Department Records, RG 28, National Archives; *New York Times*, May 10, 1878, p. 1; *National Police Gazette*, May 21, 1878, p. 14; D. M. Bennett, *Anthony Comstock: His Career of Cruelty and Crime* (1878; reprint, New York: Da Capo Press, 1971), p. 1074. Sarah Chase listed herself as a physician in the city directory. See *1882–83 New York City Directory* (New York, 1882), s.v. "Chase, Frank B."
20. "Report of Persons Arrested under the Auspices of the New York Society for the Suppression of Vice for the Year 1878," Records of the NYSSV; Comstock to

Parker, June 1, 1878, box 27, Postal Inspection Service Records; Bennett, *Anthony Comstock*, pp. 1074–75; *New York Times*, May 10, 1878, p. 1; *National Police Gazette*, May 21, 1878, p. 4.

21. Broun and Leech, *Anthony Comstock*, pp. 156–57; Grossberg, *Governing the Hearth*, p. 190; "Report of Persons Arrested under the Auspices of the New York Society for the Suppression of Vice for the Year 1878," Records of the NYSSV.

22. "Report of Persons Arrested under the Auspices of the New York Society for the Suppression of Vice for the Year 1878," container 1, Records of the NYSSV; Comstock to Parker, June 1, 1878; Bennett, *Anthony Comstock*, pp. 1074–75; *New York Times*, May 10, 1878, p. 1; *National Police Gazette*, May 21, 1878, p. 4.

23. "Report of Persons Arrested under the Auspices of the New York Society for the Suppression of Vice for the Year 1878," container 1, Records of the NYSSV; *National Police Gazette*, July 20, 1878; Bennett, *Anthony Comstock*, p. 1080; Comstock to Parker, June 1, 1878.

24. "Report of Persons Arrested under the Auspices of the New York Society for the Suppression of Vice for the Year 1900," container 3, Records of the NYSSV; Brodie, *Contraception and Abortion*, p. 132.

25. "Report of Persons Arrested under the Auspices of the New York Society for the Suppression of Vice for the Years 1873–1898," containers 1–3, Records of the NYSSV; Broun and Leech, *Anthony Comstock*, p. 167; Dennett, *Birth Control Laws*, p. 48.

26. *New York Times*, February 6, 1878, pp. 2–6.

27. *Ex parte Jackson*, 96 U.S. 727, 733 (1877).

28. *U.S.* v. *Adams*, 59 Fed. 674, 675 (1894).

29. *U.S.* v. *Bott*, 24 Fed. Cas. 1204, 1205 (1873).

30. *U.S.* v. *Whittier*, 28 Fed. Cas. 592 (1878).

31. Ezra Heywood, *Free Speech: Report of Ezra H. Heywood's Defense* (Princeton, Mass.: Cooperative Publishing Co., [1883?]), pp. 6, 14–18; Martin Henry Blatt, *Free Love and Anarchism: The Biography of Ezra Heywood* (Urbana: University of Illinois Press, 1989), pp. 144–45.

32. Heywood, *Free Speech*, pp. 17–18; Blatt, *Free Love and Anarchism*, pp. 144–45. On Americans' preoccupation with hygiene and cleanliness at this time, see Nancy Tomes, *The Gospel of Germs: Men, Women, and the Microbe in American Life* (Cambridge, Mass.: Harvard University Press, 1998), pp. 1–67.

33. Heywood, *Free Speech*, p. 43; Blatt, *Free Love and Anarchism*, p. 144.

34. Foote, *Radical Remedy in Social Science*, p. 98. Edward Bond Foote was the son of the contraceptive entrepreneur and prolific author Edward Bliss Foote.

35. "Report of Persons Arrested under the Auspices of the New York Society for the Suppression of Vice for the Year 1873," container 1, Records of the NYSSV; Broun and Leech, *Anthony Comstock*, p. 168; Ezra Heywood, *Cupid's Yokes; or, The Binding Forces of Conjugal Life* (Princeton, Mass.: Cooperative Publishing Co., 1877); Rutherford B. Hayes diary, January 10, 1879, in *Diary and Letters of Rutherford Birchard Hayes*, ed. Charles Richard Williams (Ohio State Archaeological and Histor-

ical Society, 1924), p. 518. *Index to the Congressional Record*, 43rd Cong., 1st sess., 1873, p. x.

36. Comstock's biographers Heywood Broun and Margaret Leech note that of all Comstock-initiated arrests, conviction rates were lowest for those who violated birth control and abortion restrictions. Broun and Leech, *Anthony Comstock*, pp. 160, 164–66.

37. Credit report for George Brinckerhoff, vol. 202, p. 577, vol. 370, pp. 700 a/64, a/145 (entries for September 25, 1867, May 27, August 30, 1878, December 19, 1879, October 10, 1881), R. G. Dun and Company Collection; "Indictment of George Brinckerhoff," October 7, 1873, box 12, Criminal Case Files of the U.S. Circuit Court for the Southern District of New York, National Archives, Regional Office, New York; "Report of Persons Arrested under the Auspices of the New York Society for the Suppression of Vice for the Year 1873," container 1, Records of the NYSSV.

38. "Report of Persons Arrested under the Auspices of the New York Society for the Suppression of Vice for the Year 1878," container 1, Records of the NYSSV; credit reports for Sarah B. Chase, vol. 389, p. 2293 (entries for October 20, 1879, March 8, 1889, February 12, 1890), R. G. Dun and Company Collection; Manuscript Population Schedules, Enumeration District 406, New York City, Tenth Census of the United States, 2880, Chase household. On the culture of female entrepreneurship, see Kathy Peiss, *Hope in a Jar: The Making of America's Beauty Culture* (New York: Metropolitan Books, 1998); Wendy Gamber, *The Female Economy: The Millinery and Dressmaking Trades, 1860–1930* (Urbana: University of Illinois Press, 1997); Lucy Eldersveld Murphy, "Business Ladies: Midwestern Women and Enterprise, 1850–1880," *Journal of Women's History* 3, no. 1 (1991): 65–89.

39. Credit report for Morris Glattstine, vol. 257, p. 3342 (entries for January 29, August 1, 1881), R. G. Dun and Company Collection; Brodie, *Contraception and Abortion*, p. 234; "Report of Persons Arrested under the Auspices of the New York Society for the Suppression of Vice for the Year 1878," container 1, Records of the NYSSV.

40. "Report of Persons Arrested under the Auspices of the New York Society for the Suppression of Vice for the Years 1873, 1874, 1878," container 1, Records of the NYSSV.

41. "The Fashionable Crime," *Michigan Medical News* 3 (1880): 341. On doctors who ignored birth control laws, see Frederick A. Blossom, "Some Medico-Legal Aspects of the Birth Control Question," *Medico-Legal Journal* 33 (January 1917): 7.

42. Although many doctors' views of birth control were dictated by conscience and not AMA policy, it is equally the case that, as a spate of family planning studies shows, it took until the mid-1960s for a majority of family practitioners and internists to endorse contraception openly as a legitimate field of medical practice. Physicians' opposition and ambivalence, far from deterring sexually active individuals from using birth control, amplified the importance of over-the-counter methods. See, for example, S. S. Spivack, "The Doctor's Role in Family Planning," *Journal of the American Medical Association* 188 (1964): 152; N. H. Wright, M.D., G. Johnson,

and D. Mees, "Physicians' Attitudes in Georgia toward Family Planning Services," in *Advances in Planned Parenthood*, ed. Aquiles J. Sobrero and Sarah Lewit Tietze, 3 vols. (New York: Excerpta Medica Foundation, 1968), vol. 3, p. 37. Morton A. Silver, "Birth Control and the Private Physician," *Family Planning Perspectives* 4 (April 1972): 43; Pomeroy, *Ethics of Marriage*, pp. 56, 59–60, 185–97.

43. Albert Janin to Violet Blair Janin, July 3, 1874, and Violet Blair Janin to Albert Janin, August 22, 1874, Janin Family Collection, Huntington Library and Archives, San Marino, Calif. Although some doctors doubted the existence of a safe time, most agreed that it occurred in the middle of a woman's menstrual cycle. On medical views of and women's firsthand experiences with the safe period, see Margaret Marsh and Wanda Ronner, *The Empty Cradle: Infertility in America from Colonial Times to the Present* (Baltimore, Md.: Johns Hopkins University Press, 1996), pp. 84–85; Eric Matsner and Frederick Holden, *The Technique of Contraception* (Baltimore, Md.: Williams and Wilkins Company, 1938), p. 33; John Rock and Marshall K. Bartlett, "Biopsy Studies of Human Endometrium," *Journal of the American Medical Association* 108 (June 12, 1937); Irving F. Stein and Melvin R. Cohen, "An Evaluation of the Safe Period," *Journal of the American Medical Association* 110 (January 22, 1938); David M. Kennedy, *Birth Control in America: The Career of Margaret Sanger* (New Haven, Conn.: Yale University Press, 1970), p. 210; Abe Laufe, ed., *An Army Doctor's Wife on the Frontier: Letters from Alaska and the Far West, 1874–1878* (Pittsburgh, Pa.: University of Pittsburgh Press, 1962), p. 165.

44. Violet Blair Janin to Albert Janin, November 23, 1874, November 26, 1874, and Albert Janin to Violet Blair Janin, November 24, 1874, Janin Family Collection.

45. Quoted in Elizabeth Hampsten, ed., *Read This Only to Yourself: The Private Writings of Midwestern Women, 1880–1910* (Bloomington: Indiana University Press, 1982), p. 104.

46. Degler, *At Odds*, pp. 224–25.

3. CONTRACEPTIVE ENTREPRENEURS

1. "Report of Persons Arrested under the Auspices of the New York Society for the Suppression of Vice for the Year 1885," container 2, Records of the New York Society for the Suppression of Vice, Manuscript Division, Library of Congress, Washington, D.C. (hereafter cited as Records of the NYSSV).

2. See, for example, "Preliminary Hearing of William C. Halleck," 1919, pp. 118, 140, box 11, Transcripts of Hearings on Fraud Cases, 1913–1945, Post Office Department Records, RG 28, National Archives; Goodyear Rubber Company, *Physician's Friend and Nurse's Guide* (Washington, D.C., 1898), pp. 1–7, 9, pamphlet, box 2, Rubber Trade Catalogues, Warshaw Collection of Business Americana, National Museum of American History, Smithsonian Institution, Washington, D.C.; Louis Galambos with Jane Eliot Sewell, *Networks of Innovation: Vaccine Development at Merck, Sharp & Dohme, and Mulford, 1895–1995* (New York: Cambridge University Press, 1995), p. 17; Janet Farrell Brodie, *Contraception and Abortion in Nineteenth-Century America* (Ithaca, N.Y.: Cornell University Press, 1994), p. 215.

3. In the words of one early birth control historian, the condom industry was "anarchical." Norman Himes, *Medical History of Contraception* (Baltimore, Md.: Williams and Wilkins Company, 1936), pp. 204–5.

4. Linda Gordon, *Woman's Body, Woman's Right: A Social History of Birth Control in America* (New York: Penguin, 1974), pp. 63–64.

5. "Report of Persons Arrested under the Auspices of the New York Society for the Suppression of Vice for the Year 1889," container 2, Records of the NYSSV; Manuscript Population Schedules, Enumeration District 622, Borough of Queens, New York City, Twelfth Census of the United States, 1900, Schmid household; "The Accident of Birth," *Fortune*, February 1938, p. 108.

6. "Report of Persons Arrested under the Auspices of the New York Society for the Suppression of Vice for the Year 1889," container 2, Records of the NYSSV; Manuscript Population Schedules, Enumeration District 622, Borough of Queens, New York City, Twelfth Census of the United States, 1900, Schmid household; William H. Robertson, *An Illustrated History of Contraception* (London: Parthenon, 1990), p. 113; Jeannette Parisot, *Johnny Come Lately: A Short History of the Condom* (1985; reprint, London: Journeyman, 1987), p. 11; Timothy Gilfoyle, *City of Eros: New York City, Prostitution, and the Commercialization of Sex, 1790–1920* (New York: W. W. Norton, 1992), pp. 203–9.

7. Robertson, *Illustrated History of Contraception*, p. 112; Parisot, *Johnny Come Lately*, p. 1; Himes, *Medical History of Contraception*, p. 186.

8. Parisot, *Johnny Come Lately*, p. 5; Himes, *Medical History of Contraception*, p. 188; Eric Chevallier, *The Condom: Three Thousand Years of Safer Sex* (London: Puffin, 1995).

9. John Peel, "The Manufacture and Retailing of Contraceptives in England," *Population Studies* 17 (1963–1964): 113.

10. Quoted in ibid., p. 113.

11. Himes, *Medical History of Contraception*, p. 195.

12. T. J. B. Buckingham, "The Trade in Questionable Rubber Goods," *India Rubber World*, March 15, 1892, p. 164.

13. *Druggists' Circular and Chemical Gazette* 15, no. 1 (January 1871): 1.

14. *The United States Practical Receipt Book: or, Complete Book of References* (Philadelphia: Lindsay and Blakiston, 1844), p. 29, quoted in Gordon, *Woman's Body, Woman's Right*, pp. 44–45.

15. Brodie, *Contraception and Abortion*, p. 208.

16. Ibid., p. 208.

17. Ibid., pp. 207–9.

18. Howard Wolf and Ralph Wolf, *Rubber: A Story of Glory and Greed* (New York: Covici, Friede, 1936), pp. 15–29; P. Schidrowitz and T. R. Dawson, eds., *History of the Rubber Industry* (Cambridge, U.K.: W. Heffer and Sons Ltd., 1952), p. 40; H. J. Stern, "History," in C. M. Blow and C. Hepburn, eds., *Rubber Technology and Manufacture* (London: Butterworth Scientific, 1982), pp. 1–7; Paul Gilmore, "The Strange History of the Vulcanization of Rubber," unpublished paper in author's possession.

19. James Reed, *From Private Vice to Public Virtue: The Birth Control Movement and American Society since 1830* (New York: Basic Books, 1978), p. 13.

20. "Charles Goodyear's Fame," *Druggists' Circular* 64 (September 1920): 345; Wolf and Wolf, *Rubber*, p. 310.

21. "Charles Goodyear's Fame," *Druggists' Circular*, p. 345. Many of the companies they established were short-lived. Others, like L. Gandee & Co. of New Haven, Connecticut, the first to license Goodyear's vulcanization patent, lasted long enough to amalgamate with nine other firms to form the U.S. Rubber Company in 1892. Census enumerators counted twenty-nine rubber firms in 1860 and fifty-six in 1870. Some were small-scale producers, with as few as two, four, or nine workers; others, especially garment manufacturers, had labor forces numbering in the hundreds. *The Statistics of the Wealth and Industry of the United States*, Ninth Census, vol. 2 (Washington, D.C.: Government Printing Office, 1872), pp. 600, 820.

22. Brodie, *Contraception and Abortion*, p. 210; Vern L. Bullough, "A Brief Note on Rubber Technology and Contraception: The Diaphragm and the Condom," *Technology and Culture* 22 (January 1981): 108.

23. Buckingham, "Trade in Questionable Rubber Goods."

24. Ibid., p. 164.

25. Ibid., pp. 104–5.

26. Ibid., p. 104.

27. Brodie, *Contraception and Abortion*, p. 211.

28. John H. Nelson, *The Druggist's Cost Book* (Cleveland, Ohio: J. B. Savage, Printer, 1879), pp. 25–26.

29. Reed, *From Private Vice to Public Virtue*, p. 115.

30. Bullough, "Brief Note on Rubber Technology and Contraception," p. 105; Robertson, *Illustrated History of Contraception*, p. 114.

31. Bullough, "Brief Note on Rubber Technology and Contraception," p. 105; Robertson, *Illustrated History of Contraception*, p. 114.

32. Bullough, "Brief Note on Rubber Technology and Contraception," p. 105; J. Rutgers, "Clinics in Holland," *Birth Control Review* 4 (April 1920): 9–10; Gerald I. Zatuchni, "Contraceptive Technologies for the Future," in John M. Leventhal, ed., *Current Problems in Obstetrics and Gynecology* (Chicago: Year Book Medical Publishers, 1984), p. 9; "Contraceptive Devices," *Human Fertility* 10 (September 1945): 69–70; Robert L. Dickinson, "Contraception: A Medical Review of the Situation," *American Journal of Obstetrics and Gynecology* 8 (November 1924); Le Mon Clark, "Two Types of Vaginal Diaphragms," *Journal of Contraception* (November 1938): 199–201; Holland-Rantos, *Report on Physicians' Replies to Questionnaire concerning Their Experience with the Vaginal Diaphragm and Jelly* (New York, 1929), p. 19.

33. Rutgers, "Clinics in Holland," pp. 9–10; Dorothy Bocker, *Birth Control Methods* (New York: Birth Control Clinical Research, 1924); Bullough, "Brief Note on Rubber Technology and Contraception," p. 105; Reed, *From Private Vice to Public Virtue*, pp. 97–99; Holland-Rantos, *Suggestions for Contraceptive Practice* (New York, 1930), p. 3.

34. U.S. Patent Office, patent no. 4,729, August 28, 1846.

35. Quoted in Brodie, *Contraception and Abortion*, pp. 217–18. Tarbox was found guilty, but his conviction was overturned by the state supreme court.

36. "Report of Persons Arrested under the Auspices of the New York Society for the Suppression of Vice for the Year 1876," container 1, Records of the NYSSV; Reed, *From Private Vice to Public Virtue*, p. 16.

37. "Report of Persons Arrested under the Auspices of the New York Society for the Suppression of Vice for the Year 1876," container 1, Records of the NYSSV.

38. Brodie, *Contraception and Abortion*, p. 240.

39. Credit report for E. B. Foote, vol. 380, p. 001 (entries for May 26, 1869, April 14, 1873, November 3, 1875, July 11, 1876), and vol. 381, p. 200a/156 (entries for November 28, 1877, June 11, 1880, October 26, 1881), R. G. Dun and Company Collection, Baker Library, Harvard Business School, Boston, Mass.

40. U.S. Patent Office, patent no. 202,037, April 2, 1878. Lockwood's device, patented after the Comstock Act, made no mention of contraception or the covering that would have made his instrument an effective occlusive device. But it would have been simple to add more to the rubber already needed to cover the spring cover before vulcanization to transform his device into an effective contraceptive.

41. Credit report for H. Gustavas Farr, vol. 69, p. 667 (entries for September 27, 1872, May 3, 1876), R. G. Dun and Company Collection; "Report of Persons Arrested under the Auspices of the New York Society for the Suppression of Vice for the Year 1876," container 1, Records of the NYSSV.

42. Michael A. La Sorte, "Nineteenth-Century Family Planning Practices," *Journal of Psychohistory* 4 (Fall 1976): 176.

43. "Report of Persons Arrested under the Auspices of the New York Society for the Suppression of Vice for the Year 1885," container 2, Records of the NYSSV.

44. U.S. Food and Drug Administration, Advisory Committee on Obstetrics and Gynecology, *Report on Intrauterine Contraceptive Devices* (Washington, D.C.: U.S. Department of Health, Education, and Welfare, 1968), p. 3.

45. U.S. Food and Drug Administration, Medical Device and Drug Advisory Committee on Obstetrics and Gynecology, *Second Report on Intrauterine Contraceptive Devices* (Washington, D.C.: U.S. Department of Health, Education, and Welfare, 1978); Howard Tatum, "Intrauterine Contraception," *American Journal of Obstetrics and Gynecology* 112 (1972): 1000; Brodie, *Contraception and Abortion*, p. 222.

46. Shirley Green, *The Curious History of Contraception* (London: Ebury Press, 1971), p. 114.

47. Quoted in Gordon, *Woman's Body, Woman's Right*, p. 67.

48. Orin Davis, M.D., *Welcome Words to Women* (Attica, N.Y., n.d.), p. 35, pamphlet, box 68, Patent Medicine Catalogues, Warshaw Collection of Business Americana.

49. Quoted in Brodie, *Contraception and Abortion*, p. 221.

50. B. F. Goodrich Co., *India Rubber Druggists' Sundries* (n.p., c. 1895), pp. 23–24, 81–83, box 1, Rubber Trade Catalogues, Warshaw Collection of Business Americana.

51. Tyer Rubber Company, *Illustrated Catalogue and Price List of Druggists' Sundries and Miscellaneous Rubber Goods* (Andover, Mass., 1908), and Davol Rubber Company, *Davol Rubber Goods* (1914), both in box 8, Rubber Trade Catalogues, Warshaw Collection of Business Americana; Perry, Stearns, and Company, *Rubber Goods of Every Description* (Chicago, 1890), p. 34.

52. Goodyear syringes were advertised in the Sears, Roebuck Catalogue, including the 1897 volume. Sears, Roebuck & Co., *1897 Sears Roebuck Catalogue*, ed. Fred L. Israel (reprint, New York: Chelsea House Publishers, 1968). Also see Tyer Rubber Company, *Illustrated Catalogue and Price List of Druggists' Sundries and Miscellaneous Rubber Goods*, p. 40.

53. B. F. Goodrich Co., *India Rubber Druggists' Sundries*, pp. 33–40.

54. McKesson & Robbins, *Illustrated Catalogue of Druggists' Sundries, Fancy Goods, Surgical Instruments, Sponges, Chamois etc.* (New York: Daniel G. F. Class, 1883).

55. Brodie, *Contraception and Abortion*, p. 73.

56. John Wyeth & Brothers Manufacturing Chemists, *Prices Current* (Philadelphia, 1891).

57. Detroit Pharmacal Company, *Catalogue of Physicians' Supplies* (Detroit, 1894), p. xii.

58. Galambos with Sewell, *Networks of Innovation*, p. 17.

59. Ibid., passim; Brodie, *Contraception and Abortion*, p. 215. Mulford's successor, Sharp & Dohme, continued the tradition. In a 1919 fraud case initiated by the U.S. Post Office, the Hygiene and Kalology Company, a smaller outfit, named Sharp & Dohme as the manufacturer of contraceptive goods it sold directly to consumers. "Preliminary Hearing of William C. Halleck," 1919, box 11, Transcripts of Hearings on Fraud Cases, 1913–1945, Post Office Department Records.

60. "Preliminary Hearing of William C. Halleck," 1919, box 11, Transcripts of Hearings on Fraud Cases, 1913–1945, Post Office Department Records.

61. Hearings of Mrs. A. S. Hon, September 21, 1917, box 35, Transcripts of Hearings on Fraud Cases, 1913–1945, Post Office Department Records.

62. On the history of gender and entrepreneurship, see Alice Kessler-Harris, "Ideologies and Innovation: Gender Dimensions of Business History," *Business and Economic History* 20 (1991): 46; Wendy Gamber, "A Gendered Enterprise: Placing Nineteenth-Century Businesswomen in History," and Kathy Peiss, " 'Vital Industry' and Women's Ventures: Conceptualizing Gender in Twentieth-Century Business History," both in *Business History Review* 72 (Summer 1998): 188–241; Wendy Gamber, *The Female Economy: The Millinery and Dressmaking Trades, 1860–1930* (Urbana: University of Illinois Press, 1997); and Kathy Peiss, *Hope in a Jar: The Making of America's Beauty Culture* (New York: Metropolitan Books, 1998).

Unfortunately, the number of women involved in the contraceptive business cannot be identified. Men's use of female aliases, entrepreneurs' intentional cloaking of their activities, and the absence of census enumeration for this illegal enterprise make an accurate measurement of the extent of female involvement impossible.

63. Quoted in Gordon, *Woman's Body, Woman's Right*, p. 68.

64. Gordon, *Woman's Body, Woman's Right*, p. 68; Brodie, *Contraception and Abortion*, pp. 72–73; U.S. Patent Office, patent no. 208,883, July 25, 1878.

65. Hearings of Mrs. A. S. Hon, September 21, 1917, box 35, Transcripts of Hearings on Fraud Cases, 1913–1945, Post Office Department Records.

66. Ibid.

67. Ibid.; Department of Commerce, *Fourteenth Census of the United States Taken in the Year 1920*, vol. 2 (Washington, D.C.: Government Printing Office, 1922), table 15.

68. Hearings of Mrs. A. S. Hon, September 21, 1917, box 35, Transcripts of Hearings on Fraud Cases, 1913–1945, Post Office Department Records.

69. Ibid. The federal mail-fraud statute under which Hon was prosecuted was enacted in 1872. It prohibited fraud executed through the use of the mail or through a private interstate carrier. Geraldine Szott Moohr, "Mail Fraud Meets Criminal Theory," *University of Cincinnati Law Review* 67 (Fall 1998): n. 2.

4. BLACK-MARKET BIRTH CONTROL

1. Jeannette Parisot, *Johnny Come Lately: A Short History of the Condom* (1985; reprint, Journeyman, 1987), p. 13; William H. Robertson, *An Illustrated History of Contraception* (London: Parthenon, 1990), p. 113; Norman Himes, *Medical History of Contraception* (Baltimore, Md.: Williams and Wilkins Company, 1936), p. 195.

2. Parisot, *Johnny Come Lately*, p. 13.

3. Air-burst tests and ratings are discussed in "How Reliable Are Condoms?" *Consumer Reports*, May 1995.

4. This practice is described by Helena Wright in *The Sex Factor in Marriage* (New York: Vanguard Press, 1938), p. 163. Also see John Peel, "The Manufacture and Retailing of Contraceptives in England," *Population Studies* 17 (1963–1964): 117; Parisot, *Johnny Come Lately*; Michael A. La Sorte, "Nineteenth-Century Family Planning Practices," *Journal of Psychohistory* 4 (Fall 1976): 17–18; Vern L. Bullough, "A Brief Note on Rubber Technology and Contraception: The Diaphragm and the Condom," *Technology and Culture* 22 (January 1981): 107.

5. La Sorte, "Nineteenth-Century Family Planning Practices," p. 173; Bullough, "Brief Note on Rubber Technology and Contraception," p. 107.

6. Parisot, *Johnny Come Lately*, p. 13.

7. Quoted in ibid., p. 17.

8. Quoted in ibid., p. 26.

9. Quoted in Janet Farrell Brodie, *Contraception and Abortion in Nineteenth-Century America* (Ithaca, N.Y.: Cornell University Press, 1994), p. 210.

10. Robert A. Hatcher, James Trussell, Felicia Stewart, Gary K. Stewart, Deborah Kowal, Felicia Guest, Willard Cates, Jr., and Michael S. Policar, *Contraceptive Technology*, 16th rev. ed. (New York: Irvington, 1994), p. 167.

11. T. J. B. Buckingham, "The Trade in Questionable Rubber Goods," *India Rubber World*, March 15, 1892, p. 164; Bullough, "Brief Note on Rubber Technology and Contraception," p. 108.

12. Because warmed natural rubber is adhesive, it could be worked around a penis-

shaped mold until its edges stuck together, creating a seamless condom upon vul-canization. Goodyear patented this technique in 1848 to make hollow items, such as rubber balls, that were airtight enough to prevent deflation. In addition, by the 1880s, a process pioneered in Germany in which glass molds were dipped into a so-lution of liquefied rubber mixed with petroleum solvent, dried, and then vulcanized by exposure to sulfur dioxide gas, had provided another technique for manufactur-ing seamless condoms. When this technique was adopted in the United States is unknown. Seamless rubber gloves were made this way starting in the 1880s, but Buckingham's 1892 description of condom production refers to glass dipping as a rumored but untried method. "Several years ago a foreign chemist in New York made no secret of the fact that he was about to put upon the market a line of goods made from dissolved [rubber] . . . and dipped on glass formers," he reported. But the goods never came. Contemporary reports indicate that by the 1920s most condoms manufactured in the United States were made this way. U.S. Patent Office, patent no. 5,536, 1848; Buckingham, "Trade in Questionable Rubber Goods," p. 165; Bul-lough, "Brief Note on Rubber Technology and Contraception," p. 109.

13. Norman Himes, *Practical Birth Control Methods*, discussed in James Reed, *From Pri-vate Vice to Public Virtue: The Birth Control Movement and American Society since 1830* (New York: Basic Books, 1978), p. 15.
14. *Druggists' Circular and Chemical Gazette* 15 (January 1871): 1.
15. Robert L. Dickinson, "Contraception: A Medical Review of the Situation," *Ameri-can Journal of Obstetrics and Gynecology* 8 (November 1924): 585–87.
16. Judith Walzer Leavitt, *Brought to Bed: Childbearing in America, 1750 to 1950* (New York: Oxford University Press, 1986), p. 268.
17. "Prophylactic Sheaths," *Journal of Contraception* (May 1938): 111; Rachel Lynn Palmer and Sarah Koslow Greenberg, *Facts and Frauds in Woman's Hygiene: A Med-ical Guide against Misleading Claims and Dangerous Products* (Garden City, N.Y.: Gar-den City Publishing Co., 1938), p. 272.
18. "How Reliable Are Condoms?" *Consumer Reports*, May 1995, p. 320.
19. Hatcher et al., *Contraceptive Technology*, pp. 113, 341–44; Dickinson, "Contracep-tion," p. 602.
20. On the medical hazards of withdrawal, see X. Y. Z., "The Prevention of Concep-tion," *Medical and Surgical Reporter*, November 10, 1888, p. 600; W. R. D. Black-wood, "The Prevention of Conception," *Medical and Surgical Reporter*, Novem-ber 10, 1888, p. 698; James MaHood and Kristine Wenburg, *The Mosher Survey: Sexual Attitudes of 45 Victorian Women* (New York: Arno Press, 1980), case 9.
21. O. E. Herrick, "Specialties," *Michigan Medical News* 4 (1881): 41.
22. Margaret Marsh and Wanda Ronner, *The Empty Cradle: Infertility in America from Colonial Times to the Present* (Baltimore, Md.: Johns Hopkins University Press, 1996), p. 85; Eric Matsner and Frederick Holden, *The Technique of Contraception* (Baltimore, Md.: Williams and Wilkins Company, 1938), p. 37; John Rock and Marshall K. Bartlett, "Biopsy Studies of Human Endometrium," *Journal of the Amer-ican Medical Association* 108 (June 12, 1937): 2022–28; Irving F. Stein and Melvin R. Cohen, "An Evaluation of the Safe Period," *Journal of the American Medical As-*

sociation 110 (January 22, 1938): 257–61; David M. Kennedy, *Birth Control in America: The Career of Margaret Sanger* (New Haven, Conn.: Yale University Press, 1970), p. 210.

23. Abe Laufe, ed., *An Army Doctor's Wife on the Frontier: Letters from Alaska and the Far West, 1874–1878* (Pittsburgh, Pa.: University of Pittsburgh Press, 1962), p. 165. A woman interviewed in 1913 regarded the safe period as equally unreliable. She and her husband resorted to it only when they "could afford chance." MaHood and Wenburg, *Mosher Survey*, case 45.

24. MaHood and Wenburg, *Mosher Survey*, pp. xii–xviii.

25. Ibid., pp. xii–xviii.

26. Ibid., cases 1, 8, 41.

27. Ibid., case 45.

28. Dickinson, "Contraception," p. 586; Bullough, "Brief Note on Rubber Technology and Contraception," pp. 104–6; Hatcher et al., *Contraceptive Technology*, pp. 195–212, 639.

29. Brodie, *Contraception and Abortion*, pp. 221–24; Andrea Tone, "Violence by Design: Contraceptive Technology and the Invasion of the Female Body," in Michael Bellesiles, ed., *Lethal Imagination: Violence and Brutality in American History* (New York: New York University Press, 1999).

30. Boston Women's Health Book Collective, *The New Our Bodies, Our Selves: A Book by and for Women* (New York: Simon and Schuster, 1992), pp. 294–95; Hatcher et al., *Contraceptive Technology*, pp. 347–48.

31. Warren E. Leary, "A Look at Douches' Safety," *New York Times*, April 30, 1997; Hatcher et al., *Contraceptive Technology*, p. 508; M. J. Rosenberg and R. S. Phillips, "Does Douching Promote Ascending Infection?" *Journal of Reproductive Medicine* (1992): 930–38.

32. Leary, "A Look at Douches' Safety"; Hatcher et al., *Contraceptive Technology*, p. 508; Boston Women's Health Book Collective, *New Our Bodies, Our Selves*, p. 300; Robert L. Dickinson and Louise Stevens Bryant, *Control of Conception: An Illustrated Medical Manual* (Baltimore, Md.: Williams and Wilkins Company, 1931), pp. 39–45, 69–74; Dorothy Dunbar Bromley, *Birth Control: Its Use and Misuse* (New York: Harper, 1934), pp. 92–98; Palmer and Greenberg, *Facts and Frauds in Woman's Hygiene*, p. 18; Dorothy Bocker, *Birth Control Methods* (New York: Birth Control Clinical Research, 1924), p. 5.

33. Dickinson, "Contraception," p. 586; Bocker, *Birth Control Methods*, p. 5.

34. Dickinson, "Contraception," pp. 585–87.

35. Ibid., p. 586; Bocker, *Birth Control Methods*, p. 5.

36. Dickinson and Bryant, *Control of Conception*, p. 42; Robert L. Dickinson, "Household Contraceptives," *Journal of Contraception* (February 1936): 43–44; MaHood and Wenburg, *Mosher Survey*, case 10.

37. Bocker, *Birth Control Methods*, p. 5.

38. Ibid., p. 5; Brodie, *Contraception and Abortion*, p. 77; Matsner and Holden, *Technique of Contraception*, p. 33.

39. Dickinson and Bryant, *Control of Conception*, pp. 78–80; Bromley, *Birth Control*,

pp. 99–100; Palmer and Greenberg, *Facts and Frauds in Woman's Hygiene*, pp. 242–50; Bocker, *Birth Control Methods*, pp. 6–7, 27; Dickinson, "Household Contraceptives," pp. 43–44; Irving F. Stein and Melvin R. Cohen, "Jelly Contraceptives," *American Journal of Obstetrics and Gynecology* 5 (May 1941): 852; Leo Shedlovsky, "Some Acidic Properties of Contraceptive Jellies," *Journal of Contraception* 2 (August–September 1937): 147–55.

40. Hatcher et al., *Contraceptive Technology*, p. 113. Some notable exceptions include the sponge and cap, if used by women who have borne children.

41. MaHood and Wenburg, *Mosher Survey*, cases 17, 29, 45.

42. Stein and Cohen, "Jelly Contraceptives," pp. 580–82.

43. MaHood and Wenburg, *Mosher Survey*, case 15.

44. Bocker, *Birth Control Methods*, p. 4.

45. H. S. Pomeroy, *The Ethics of Marriage* (New York: Funk and Wagnalls, 1888), p. 59.

46. MaHood and Wenburg, *Mosher Survey*. Of the forty-five women surveyed, thirty-seven used contraception. Of these thirty-seven, twenty-six used contraceptives. The other eleven used nonmarket methods such as withdrawal or the safe period.

47. Margaret Sanger, "The Prevention of Conception," *Woman Rebel* 1 (March 1914): 8. On Sanger's early career, see Ellen Chesler, *Woman of Valor: Margaret Sanger and the Birth Control Movement in America* (New York: Simon and Schuster, 1992), chaps. 2–5; Kennedy, *Birth Control in America*, pp. 1–35; Reed, *From Private Vice to Public Virtue*, pp. 67–88.

48. See, for instance, Kennedy's discussion of Sanger's difficulties tracking down contraceptive information in 1913 or her reaction to the death of Sadie Sachs in *Birth Control in America*, pp. 17–19, and Chesler's observations in *Woman of Valor*, p. 63.

49. The incident and its possible dramatization by Sanger are discussed in Kennedy, *Birth Control in America*, pp. 16–18; Chesler, *Woman of Valor*, pp. 62–63; Reed, *From Private Vice to Public Virtue*, pp. 82–83.

50. *Journal of the American Medical Association* 94 (1930): 2806.

51. *Michigan Medical News* 5 (1882): 37.

52. Letter of David E. Matteson, November 29, 1888, *Medical and Surgical Reporter* 59 (1888): 760; Thomas E. McArdle, "The Physical Evils Arising from the Prevention of Conception," *American Journal of Obstetrics* 21 (1888): 936.

53. American shoppers have never made price and income the only criteria for consumption. The phenomenal market success of some products (like Barbie or Beanie Babies) but not others, the overuse of credit cards to the point of bankruptcy: these are modern examples of the subjective considerations that inform consumer behavior.

54. *Birth Control Review* (March 1923): 69.

55. In the survey of birth control, of 1,208 patients, 800 stated that they had used contraceptives. Of these, the douche was used by 60 percent, the condom by 42 percent, the sponge by 4 percent, the IUD by 2 percent, the cervical cap by 10 percent, the tablet by 2 percent, the powder by 5 percent, the suppository by 12 percent, and the "douche plus chemical" by 50 percent. Among nonmarket methods used by the

800, "nursing baby" was used by 30 percent, male withdrawal by 40 percent, "holding back" by 30 percent, and complete abstinence by 4 percent. See Bocker, *Birth Control Methods*, pp. 4–7.

56. *National Police Gazette*, November 16, 1889, p. 14; *1897 Sears Roebuck Catalogue*, ed. Fred L. Israel (reprint, New York: Chelsea House Publishers, 1968).

57. Scott Derks, ed., *The Value of a Dollar: Prices and Incomes in the United States, 1860–1989* (Detroit: Gale Research, Inc., 1994), p. 15.

58. Linda Gordon, *Woman's Body, Woman's Right: A Social History of Birth Control in America* (New York: Penguin, 1974), p. 70.

59. Brodie, *Contraception and Abortion*, p. 191.

60. Elliott Gorn, *The Manly Art: Bare-Knuckle Prize Fighting in America* (Ithaca, N.Y.: Cornell University Press, 1986), p. 181; Brodie, *Contraception and Abortion*, pp. 190–91.

61. E. C. Allen Company, scrapbook of unpublishable advertisements, Baker Library, Harvard Business School, Boston, Mass.

62. Hearings of Mrs. A. S. Hon, September 21, 1917, box 35, Transcripts of Hearings on Fraud Cases, 1913–1945, Post Office Department Records, RG 28, National Archives.

63. Birth Control Collection, box 85, American Medical Association Health Fraud Archives, American Medical Association, Chicago. My thanks to Johanna Giebelhaus for identifying the language used in the Septigyn ad.

64. Before the U.S. Birth Registration Area was established in 1915, there was no record of live births, and only in 1890 did the federal census provide information on the number of children ever born per woman. As a result, demographic historians cannot tally "true" birthrates. Instead, they estimate fertility rates by calculating the ratio of children under five to women ages fifteen to forty-nine (or, in some cases, twenty to forty-nine). This computation, a reasonable approximation of true fertility, does not take into account changing infant mortality rates over time or possible differences among socioeconomic groups. Nor does it factor in the chronic undercounting of blacks, workers, and mobile groups by census takers, a problem that persists today.

65. See Wilson H. Grabill, Clyde V. Kiser, and Pascal K. Whelpton, *The Fertility of American Women* (New York: John Wiley and Sons, 1958); Yasukichi Yasuba, *Birth Rates of the White Population in the United States, 1800–1860: An Economic Study* (Baltimore, Md.: Johns Hopkins Press, 1962); Susan E. Bloomberg, Mary Frank Fox, Robert M. Warner, and Sam Bass Warner, Jr., "A Census Probe into Nineteenth-Century Family History: Southern Michigan, 1850–1880," *Journal of Social History* 5 (1971): 26–45; Maris A. Vinovskis, "Socioeconomic Determinants of Interstate Fertility Differentials in the United States in 1850 and 1860," *Journal of Interdisciplinary History* 4 (Winter 1976): 375–96; Charles Tilly, ed., *Historical Studies of Changing Fertility* (Princeton, N.J.: Princeton University Press, 1978); Stanley P. Engerman, "Changes in Black Fertility, 1880–1940," and Tamara Hareven and Maris A. Vinovskis, "Patterns of Childbearing in Late Nineteenth-Century Amer-

ica: The Determinants of Marital Fertility in Five Massachusetts Towns in 1880," both in Tamara K. Hareven and Maris A. Vinovskis, eds., *Family and Population in Nineteenth-Century America* (Princeton, N.J.: Princeton University Press, 1978); Xarifa Sallume and Frank W. Notestein, "Trends in the Size of Families Completed prior to 1910 in Various Social Classes," *American Journal of Sociology* 38 (November 1932): 398–408.

An additional disadvantage of household census data is that they include information about occupation but not income, making determinations of class difficult.

66. Carl N. Degler, *At Odds: Women and the Family in America from the Revolution to the Present* (New York: Oxford University Press, 1980), p. 222.

67. Hareven and Vinovskis, "Patterns of Childbearing," p. 123.

68. Gordon, *Woman's Body, Woman's Right*, p. 48; Engerman, "Changes in Black Fertility," p. 132; Stewart Tolnay, "The Decline of Black Marital Fertility in the Rural South: 1910–1940," *American Sociological Review* 52 (April 1987): 211; Jesse Rodrigue, "The Black Community and the Birth Control Movement," in Kathy Peiss and Christina Simmons, eds., *Passion and Power: Sexuality in History* (Philadelphia: Temple University Press, 1989), pp. 138–39.

69. Raymond Pearl, "Contraception and Fertility in 2,000 Women," *Human Biology* 4 (1932): 395, quoted in Rodrigue, "Black Community and the Birth Control Movement," pp. 138–39. Also see Dorothy Roberts, *Killing the Black Body: Race, Reproduction, and the Meaning of Liberty* (New York: Vintage, 1997), pp. 82–83.

70. Himes, *Medical History of Contraception*, pp. 5–10.

71. Rodrigue, "Black Community and the Birth Control Movement," p. 139; Brodie, *Contraception and Abortion*, pp. 52–54; Roberts, *Killing the Black Body*, p. 82.

72. *Afro-American Sentinel* (Omaha), June 6, 1896, p. 3.

73. *Atlanta Independent*, June 4, 1904, p. 6.

74. George Schuyler, "Quantity or Quality," *Birth Control Review* 16 (June 1932): 165–66; Jamie Hart, "Who Should Have the Children? Discussions of Birth Control among African-American Intellectuals, 1920–1939," *Journal of Negro History* 79 (Winter 1994): 71–84.

75. On differential fertility, see Susan Householder Van Horn, *Women, Work, and Fertility, 1900–1986* (New York: New York University Press, 1988), pp. 15–20; Tolnay, "Decline of Black Marital Fertility in the Rural South"; Engerman, "Changes in Black Fertility"; Grabill et al., *Fertility of American Women*; Hareven and Vinovskis, "Patterns of Childbearing"; Sallume and Notestein, "Trends in the Size of Families"; Earl Lomon Koos, "Class Differences in the Employment of Contraceptive Measures," *Human Fertility* 12 (December 1947): 97–101.

76. Roberts, *Killing the Black Body*, p. 84.

77. W. E. B. DuBois, "Black Folk and Birth Control," *Birth Control Review* (May 1938): 90. For a discussion of divisions within the black community, see Hart, "Who Should Have the Children?"

5. SALUTE TO PROPHYLAXIS

1. Josephus Daniels to W. L. Stoddard, February 12, 1915, box 2140, General Correspondence, Records of the Bureau of Medicine and Surgery, RG 52, National Archives; C. A. Setterstrom, "Development of Venereal Prophylaxis in the United States Navy," unpublished manuscript, circa 1925, box 421, General Correspondence, 1917–1927, Records of the Office of the Surgeon General, RG 112, National Archives; E. R. Stitt to Bureau of Navigation, May 2, 1921, box 421, General Correspondence, 1912–1925, Records of the Bureau of Medicine and Surgery.

2. Setterstrom, "Development of Venereal Prophylaxis."

3. Allan M. Brandt, *No Magic Bullet: A Social History of Venereal Disease in the United States since 1880* (New York: Oxford University Press, 1987), p. 166.

4. Setterstrom, "Development of Venereal Prophylaxis"; *The Merck Manual*, 17th ed. (Whitehouse Station, N.J.: Merck Research Laboratories, 1999), pp. 1323–33.

5. Arthur Parker Hitchens, "How the Army Protects Soldiers from Syphilis and Gonorrhea," and Joel T. Boone, "The Sexual Aspects of Military Personnel," both in *Journal of Social Hygiene* 27 (March 1941): 103–24; Brandt, *No Magic Bullet*, p. 97.

6. Brandt, *No Magic Bullet*, p. 98.

7. Vern L. Bullough, *Science in the Bedroom: A History of Sex Research* (New York: Basic Books, 1994), pp. 98–100; Brandt, *No Magic Bullet*, pp. 9–13, 40–41.

8. Brandt, *No Magic Bullet*, p. 12.

9. Ibid., pp. 11–13; Bullough, *Science in the Bedroom*, pp. 98–99.

10. Brandt, *No Magic Bullet*, pp. 40–41; Linda Gordon, *Woman's Body, Woman's Right: A Social History of Birth Control in America* (New York: Penguin, 1974), p. 205.

11. Setterstrom, "Development of Venereal Prophylaxis"; *Merck's 1899 Manual* (New York: Merck and Company, 1899), p. 59.

12. Setterstrom, "Development of Venereal Prophylaxis," pp. 2–3.

13. C. F. Stokes to Howard Hill, January 3, 1913, box 418, General Correspondence, Records of the Bureau of Medicine and Surgery; C. F. Stokes to Colin Ross, M.D., December 18, 1913, General Correspondence, Records of the Bureau of Medicine and Surgery; W. C. Braisted to Dr. Joseph Collins, April 21, 1915, box 418, General Correspondence, Records of the Bureau of Medicine and Surgery; Setterstrom, "Development of Venereal Disease"; Brandt, *No Magic Bullet*, p. 111.

14. W. C. Braisted to Dr. Joseph Collins, April 21, 1915; Setterstrom, "Development of Venereal Prophylaxis"; J. F. Siler, "Policies Relating to the Control of Venereal Diseases in the Army," p. 3, box 112, Correspondence 1928–1937, Records of the Office of the Surgeon General.

15. "Prophylactic Cream," *Drug and Cosmetic Industry* 4 (April 1934): 396; Brandt, *No Magic Bullet*, p. 111. The study reported a 99.6 percent efficacy rate against syphilis, gonorrhea, and chancroid when applied within three hours after sexual contact.

16. Brandt, *No Magic Bullet*, pp. 98, 111.

17. C. F. Stokes to Howard Hill, January 3, 1913, box 418, General Correspondence, Records of the Bureau of Medicine and Surgery; C. F. Stokes to Colin Ross, M.D.,

December 18, 1913, box 418, General Correspondence, Records of the Bureau of Medicine and Surgery; C. F. Stokes to Dr. W. R. Burns, February 28, 1913, box 418, General Correspondence, Records of the Bureau of Medicine and Surgery; C. F. Stokes to U.S. Public Health Service, December 15, 1913, box 418, General Correspondence, Records of the Bureau of Medicine and Surgery; Sanitube Company to the Bureau of Medicine and Surgery, March 21, 1918, and attached "Dear Doctor" letter, both in box 519, General Correspondence, Records of the Bureau of Medicine and Surgery; W. C. Braisted to Mr. A. F. Bond, July 11, 1918, box 421, General Correspondence, Records of the Bureau of Medicine and Surgery.

18. Daniels to Haines H. Lippincott, April 26, 1918, box 214, General Correspondence, Records of the Secretary of the Navy, RG 80, National Archives; Setterstrom, "Development of Venereal Prophylaxis."

19. Daniels to Stoddard, February 12, 1915.

20. Daniels to George Stout, December 17, 1917, box 418, General Correspondence, Records of the Bureau of Medicine and Surgery.

21. Quoted in Brandt, *No Magic Bullet*, p. 77.

22. Fred D. Baldwin, "The Invisible Armor," *American Quarterly* 16 (Autumn 1964): 434–45.

23. Edith Houghton Hooker, "The Case against Prophylaxis," *Social Hygiene* 5 (April 1919): 167.

24. Brandt, *No Magic Bullet*, pp. 102, 115; Hitchens, "How the Army Protects Soldiers from Syphilis and Gonorrhea," pp. 105, 111; Rodman circular; J. M. Enochs to Admiral Leigh, February 17, 1927, box 780, General Correspondence, 1925–1940, Records of the Bureau of Naval Personnel, RG 24, National Archives; United States Interdepartmental Social Hygiene Board, *Report of the United States Interdepartmental Social Hygiene Board for 1921* (Washington, D.C.: Government Printing Office, 1921), pp. 9–10.

25. Brandt, *No Magic Bullet*, p. 115.

26. "Live Straight If You Would Shoot Straight," United States Navy, circa 1917, box 421, Records of the Bureau of Medicine and Surgery; also see American Medical Association, *The Boy's Venereal Peril: Sex Hygiene* (Chicago: AMA, 1914), p. 37.

27. Quoted in Brandt, *No Magic Bullet*, p. 110.

28. Brandt, *No Magic Bullet*, p. 114.

29. Testimony of Merle Youngs, Transcript of Record, *Youngs Rubber Corporation* v. *C. I. Lee & Company, Inc.*, p. 29, Records of the U.S. Court of Appeals for the Second Circuit, National Archives, Regional Office, New York.

30. Brandt, *No Magic Bullet*, p. 99.

31. Jeannette Parisot, *Johnny Come Lately: A Short History of the Condom* (1985; reprint, Journeyman, 1987), p. 41; John Peel, "The Manufacture and Retailing of Contraceptives in England," *Population Studies* 17 (1963–1964): 122; www.durex.com.

32. Testimony of Merle Youngs, Transcript of Record, *Youngs Rubber Corporation* v. *C. I. Lee & Company, Inc.*, pp. 28–29, Records of the U.S. Court of Appeals for the Second Circuit.

33. Peel, "Manufacture and Retailing of Contraceptives in England," pp. 117, 120,

122; James S. Murphy, *The Condom Industry in the United States* (Jefferson, N.C.: McFarland and Company, 1990), p. 10; Parisot, *Johnny Come Lately*, pp. 37–41; www.durex.com; U.S. Patent Office, *Official Gazette*, January 13, 1931, p. 290, March 31, 1931, p. 75, May 26, 1931, p. 883; *Youngs Rubber Corporation* v. *C. I. Lee & Co., Inc.*, 45 *Federal Reporter*, 2nd ser., 103 (1930); Interview between George McClearly of Julius Schmid, Inc., and Clarence Gamble, September 30, 1940, box 64, folder 623, Planned Parenthood Federation of America Papers, Sophia Smith Collection, Smith College.

34. Alex. Sidney Rosenthal to William Braisted, November 22, 1916, box 418, General Correspondence, Records of the Bureau of Medicine and Surgery.

35. Brandt, *No Magic Bullet*, p. 115.

36. H. F. Hull to Bureau of Medicine and Surgery, June 2, 1916, box 519, General Correspondence, Records of the Bureau of Medicine and Surgery.

37. See, for instance, William H. McNeill, *The Pursuit of Power: Technology, Armed Force, and Society since* A.D. *1000* (Chicago: University of Chicago Press, 1982), n. 58, pp. 213–14; Jacques Dupaquier, "Problèmes demographiques de la France napoléonienne," *Annales historiques de la Révolution française* 42 (1970): 21; Gordon, *Woman's Body, Woman's Right*, p. 64.

38. Brandt, *No Magic Bullet*, p. 95.

39. W. C. Braisted to Dr. Joseph Collins, April 21, 1916, box 418, General Correspondence, Records of the Bureau of Medicine and Surgery; Setterstrom, "Development of Venereal Prophylaxis"; Hooker, "Case against Prophylaxis," pp. 163–64; Brandt, *No Magic Bullet*, p. 111.

40. Kahn quoted in H. H. Moore, "Four Million Dollars for the Fight against Venereal Disease," *Social Hygiene*, January 5, 1919, p. 16. Also see Hooker, "Case against Prophylaxis," and *Report of the United States Interdepartmental Social Hygiene Board*, pp. 7–12.

41. *The People of the State of New York* v. *Margaret H. Sanger*, Court of Appeals of New York, 118 N.E. 637.

42. Margaret Sanger, "Why I Went to Jail," *Together*, February 1960, p. 20; Elizabeth Stuyvesant, "The Brownsville Birth Control Clinic," *Birth Control Review* 1 (March 1917): 6–8; James Reed, *From Private Vice to Public Virtue: The Birth Control Movement and American Society since 1830* (New York: Basic Books, 1978), pp. 106–7.

43. *The People of the State of New York* v. *Margaret H. Sanger*, Court of Appeals of New York, 118 N.E. 637; Reed, *From Private Vice to Public Virtue*, pp. 106–8; Ellen Chesler, *Woman of Valor: Margaret Sanger and the Birth Control Movement in America* (New York: Simon and Schuster, 1992), pp. 159–60.

44. *The People of the State of New York* v. *Margaret H. Sanger*, Court of Appeals of New York, 118 N.E. 637; Transcript of Record, *Youngs Rubber Corporation* v. *C. I. Lee & Company*, Records of the U.S. Court of Appeals for the Second Circuit, pp. 34–35, 49, 54.

45. V. F. Calverton, *The Bankruptcy of Marriage* (New York: Macauley, 1928), pp. 132–33; "The Accident of Birth," *Fortune*, February 1938, p. 108.

46. Sanger, *Pivot of Civilization* (New York: Brentano's, 1922), p. 197.

47. Margaret Sanger, *The New Motherhood* (London: J. Cape, 1922), p. 120.

48. Chesler, *Woman of Valor*, chap. 4, pp. 154, 192–95; Parisot, *Johnny Come Lately*, pp. 33–36; Reed, *From Private Vice to Public Virtue*, pp. 83, 244–46; Andrea Tone, "Contraceptive Consumers: Gender and the Political Economy of Birth Control in the 1930s," *Journal of Social History* (Spring 1996): 492.

49. "Live Straight If You Would Shoot Straight," p. 14; also see United States Interdepartmental Social Hygiene Board, *Report of the United States Interdepartmental Social Hygiene Board*, p. 9.

50. Brandt, *No Magic Bullet*, p. 85; Carol McCann, *Birth Control Politics in the United States, 1916–1945* (Ithaca, N.Y.: Cornell University Press, 1994), p. 44.

51. W. E. Griffin to the U.S. Public Health Service, Secretaries Baker and Daniels, January 13, 1919, box 421, General Correspondence, Records of the Bureau of Medicine and Surgery.

52. Chesler, *Woman of Valor*, pp. 160–61.

53. H. A. Mary to Albert Gleaves, May 12, 1920, box 421, General Correspondence, Records of the Bureau of Medicine and Surgery.

54. W. N. Vernon to Commander, South China Patrol, March 1, 1927, box 780, General Correspondence, Records of the Bureau of Naval Personnel.

55. Annual report quoted in W. R. Dear, "Prevention and Control of Venereal Disease in the United States Army," December 29, 1936, unpublished manuscript, box 112, General Correspondence, Records of the Office of the Surgeon General.

56. Paul Preston, *Franco* (New York: Basic Books, 1994), p. 59.

57. Joel T. Boone, "The Sexual Aspects of Military Personnel," *Journal of Social Hygiene* 27 (March 1941): 114, 116; Dear, "Prevention and Control of Venereal Disease," p. 3.

58. J. A. Millspaugh, "The Prophylaxis of Venereal Disease," *U.S. Naval Medical Bulletin* 34 (January 1936): 34.

59. William Bisher, "Venereal Disease Control as Applied to the Army," *New York State Journal of Medicine*, October 1, 1943, p. 1833; Dear, "Prevention and Control of Venereal Disease," p. 10.

60. Dear, "Prevention and Control of Venereal Disease," pp. 9–10.

61. Millspaugh, "Prophylaxis of Venereal Disease," p. 33; Randolph Cautley, Gilbert W. Beebe, and Robert L. Dickinson, "Rubber Sheaths as Venereal Disease Prophylaxis: The Relation of Quality and Technique to Their Effectiveness," *American Journal of the Medical Sciences* 195 (1938): 155.

62. Bisher, "Venereal Disease Control as Applied to the Army," pp. 1833, 1835.

63. Leo A. Shifrin, "Venereal Diseases—A Navy Problem," *New York State Journal of Medicine*, October 1, 1943, p. 1832.

64. Harry Levin, "Commercial Distribution of Contraceptives in Developing Countries: Past, Present, and Future," *Demography* 5 (1968): 942.

65. Gilbert W. Beebe, "A Significant Invention," *Journal of Contraception* (1938): 92; "Prophylatic Sheaths," *Journal of Contraception* (May 1938): 111; "Standards for Rubber Prophylactics," *Journal of Contraception* (April 1938): 94; "Accident of Birth," *Fortune*, p. 108; Reed, *From Private Vice to Public Virtue*, pp. 244–46.

66. "Syphilis" script, "Film Scripts re: Venereal Disease," box 1, Records of the Center for Disease Control, RG 442, National Archives, Regional Office, Atlanta.

67. Dear, "Prevention and Control of Venereal Disease in the United States Army," p. 10.

6. A MEDICAL FIT

1. Sanger to Clarence Gamble, July 9, 1952, folder 3098, box 196, Clarence Gamble Papers, Countway Library of Medicine, Harvard Medical School, Boston, Mass.

2. Advertisement for Mizpah pessary in *National Police Gazette*, March 14, 1900, p. 14; Dorothy Bocker, *Birth Control Methods* (New York: Birth Control Clinical Research, 1924), pp. 6, 12–13, 18–20; Margaret Sanger, "Why I Went to Jail," *Together*, February 1960, p. 20; Robert L. Dickinson, "Contraception: A Medical Review of the Situation," *American Journal of Obstetrics and Gynecology* 8 (November 1924): 590–91; *Catalog of Drug Sundries* (Bridgeport, Conn.: Robert Dalton), box 785, Sex Collection, American Medical Association Health Fraud Archives, AMA Headquarters, Chicago; Ellen Chesler, *Woman of Valor: Margaret Sanger and the Birth Control Movement in America* (New York: Simon and Schuster, 1992), p. 151.

3. David M. Kennedy, *Birth Control in America: The Career of Margaret Sanger* (New Haven, Conn.: Yale University Press, 1970), pp. 20–21, 25–27; Chesler, *Woman of Valor*, p. 97; Andrea Tone, *Controlling Reproduction: An American History* (Wilmington, Del.: Scholarly Resources, 1997), pp. 155–56; James Reed, *From Private Vice to Public Virtue: The Birth Control Movement and American Society since 1830* (New York: Basic Books, 1978), pp. 97–99.

4. Margaret Sanger, *The Autobiography of Margaret Sanger* (1938; reprint, Elmsford, N.Y.: Maxwell Reprint Company, 1970), p. 142.

5. Ibid., p. 144.

6. Johannes Rutgers, "Clinics in Holland," *Birth Control Review* 4 (April 1920): 9; Bocker, *Birth Control Methods*, p. 26; Chesler, *Woman of Valor*, p. 145; Reed, *From Private Vice to Public Virtue*, p. 95. Advertisement for Mizpah pessary in *National Police Gazette*, March 14, 1900, p. 14; Sanger, *Autobiography*, pp. 142, 148; "Contraceptive Devices," *Human Fertility* 10 (September 1945): 69–70.

7. Margaret Sanger, "Suggestions for the Establishment of a Birth Control Clinic," p. 7, reel 29, Margaret Sanger Papers, Manuscripts Division, Library of Congress; Lovette Dewees and Gilbert W. Beebe, "Contraception in Private Practice: A Twelve Years Study," *Journal of the American Medical Association* 110 (April 9, 1938): 1169; Reed, *From Private Vice to Public Virtue*, p. 95; Chesler, *Woman of Valor*, p. 145; Dickinson, "Contraception," p. 591.

8. Reed, *From Private Vice to Public Virtue*, p. 97.

9. Bocker, *Birth Control Methods*, p. 19.

10. Quoted in Kennedy, *Birth Control in America*, p. 182; Reed, *From Private Vice to Public Virtue*, p. 113.

11. Reed, *From Private Vice to Public Virtue*, p. 113; Chesler, *Woman of Valor*, pp. 247–49; Kennedy, *Birth Control in America*, pp. 98–99.

12. Kennedy, *Birth Control in America*, p. 99; Chesler, *Woman of Valor*, p. 113.

13. R. Christian Johnson, "Feminism, Philanthropy, and Science in the Development of the Oral Contraceptive Pill," *Pharmacy in History* 19 (1977): 65; Bocker, *Birth Control Methods*, p. 6.

14. Bocker, *Birth Control Methods*, pp. 1, 5, 6, 19.

15. Sanger, "Suggestions for the Establishment of a Birth Control Clinic," pp. 6–7.

16. Slee quoted in Reed, *From Private Vice to Public Virtue*, p. 114.

17. Sanger, *Autobiography*, pp. 363–64; Bocker, *Birth Control Methods*, pp. 19–20, 26; James S. Murphy, *The Condom Industry in the United States* (Jefferson, N.C.: McFarland and Company, 1990), p. 10; "List of Reputable Manufacturers," Margaret Sanger Papers, reel 29; U.S. Patent Office, *Official Gazette*, January 13, 1931, p. 290, March 31, 1931, p. 75, May 26, 1931, p. 883; *Youngs Rubber Corporation v. C. I. Lee & Co., Inc.*, 45 *Federal Reporter*, 2nd ser., 103 (1930).

18. Anne Kennedy, "History of the Development of Contraceptive Materials in the United States," *American Medicine*, March 1935, p. 160; "Design Key Factor in New H-R Marketing Programs," *Drug and Cosmetic Industry* 94 (April 1964): 520–21; Herbert R. Simonds to Norman E. Himes, April 17, 1929, folder 320, box 29, Norman Himes Papers, Countway Library of Medicine; *New York City Directory 1933/34* (New York: R. L. Polk and Company, 1934), pt. 2., listing for Holland-Rantos Inc.

19. Kennedy, "History of Contraceptive Materials," p. 160.

20. Reed, *From Private Vice to Public Virtue*, p. 115; Lawrence Lader, *The Margaret Sanger Story and the Fight for Birth Control* (Garden City, N.Y.: Doubleday, 1955), p. 225.

21. Sanger marginalia on Percy Clark to Margaret Sanger, May 5, 1930, Sanger Papers, reel 30; *Youngs Rubber Corporation v. C. I. Lee & Co., Inc.*, 45 *Federal Reporter*, 2nd ser., 103 (1930).

22. As one obstetrician supportive of birth control remarked as late as 1940, "The medical profession['s] . . . lukewarm support, if not antipathy, in the past has been in part due to the overwhelming lay direction of the movement." Philip F. Williams, "Modern Contraceptives: Their Values and Limitations," *Human Fertility* 5 (February 1940): 14.

23. George Kosmak, "The Broader Aspects of the Birth Control Propaganda as It Should Interest the Physician," *American Journal of Obstetrics and Gynecology* 6 (1923): 276–85; Joyce M. Ray and F. G. Gosling, "American Physicians and Birth Control, 1936–1947," *Journal of Social History* (1985): 402–3. AMA opposition to birth control clinics is well detailed in Carol McCann, *Birth Control Politics in the United States, 1916–1945* (Ithaca, N.Y.: Cornell University Press, 1994), pp. 64–68.

24. Dickinson quoted in Chesler, *Woman of Valor*, p. 148.

25. Merriley Borell, "Biologists and the Promotion of Birth Control Research, 1918–38," *Journal of the History of Biology* 20 (Spring 1987): 65–72.

26. Sanger, *Autobiography*, p. 362.

27. Quoted in Lader, *Margaret Sanger Story*, p. 223.

28. Lader, *Margaret Sanger Story*, pp. 223–24; Chesler, *Woman of Valor*, p. 248.

29. Sanger, *Autobiography*, pp. 362–63; Reed, *From Private Vice to Public Virtue*, p. 161.

30. Margaret Sanger to James Cooper, October 10, 1925, box 6, folder 135, Florence Rose Collection, Sophia Smith Collection, Smith College.

31. Letter of D. Kenneth Rose, April 7, 1941, box 6, folder 134, Florence Rose Collection; Sanger, "Suggestions for the Establishment of a Birth Control Clinic," pp. 8–9.

32. Lader, *Margaret Sanger Story*, p. 225; Johnson, "Feminism, Philanthropy, and Science," p. 65.

33. "In re: Birth Control Movement," unpublished manuscript, circa 1932, box 1, folder 139, Rockefeller Family Archives, RG 2, Series Office, O.M.R., Rockefeller Archives, Tarrytown, New York; Herbert Simonds to Margaret Sanger, February 1926, box 6, folder 134, Florence Rose Collection; McCann, *Birth Control Politics*, p. 215.

34. Harry W. Hicks to Kenneth Rose, October 10, 1941, box 73, folder 696, Planned Parenthood Federation of America Papers, Sophia Smith Collection.

35. Planned Parenthood Federation of America 1943 study of the contraceptive industry by Foote, Cone & Belding, box 65, folder 647 (hereafter cited as PPFA 1943 study), Planned Parenthood Federation of America Papers, Sophia Smith Collection.

36. "The Accident of Birth," *Fortune*, February 1938, p. 108.

37. This ended in 1929 when one of the company's original officers, Dr. Le Mon Clark, a former professor of sociology and economics, defected to establish the Clinic Supply Company, manufacturers of diaphragms. In 1938, Clark's gross sales, including the sales of contraceptive jelly and cream, totaled thirty thousand dollars a year. But Clark's bid for market supremacy came too late. See "Accident of Birth," *Fortune*, p. 112.

38. Bocker, *Birth Control Methods*, p. 26.

39. Contraceptive Industry Report, p. 33, Planned Parenthood Federation of America Papers, Sophia Smith Collection; Holland-Rantos did not make profits a component of its advertisements to doctors, but it did to druggists, enlisting them in the campaign to solidify physician support. A retail drug advertising campaign in 1937 advised druggists "to let the physicians in your neighbourhood know that you can fill all of their Koromex prescriptions. Let us show you how you can become headquarters for the ethical business in your town." In an advertisement in *Drug Store Retailing*, a magazine for druggists, the company specified an ideal profit margin. It suggested that individual tubes of Koromex jelly purchased by the druggist for $.60 be sold to consumers for $1.50—a profit of 150 percent. "Merchandising News," *Drug and Cosmetic Industry* 41 (August 1937): 216; Rachel Lynn Palmer and Sarah Koslow Greenberg, *Facts and Frauds in Woman's Hygiene: A Medical Guide against Misleading Claims and Dangerous Products* (Garden City, N.Y.: Garden City Publishing Company, 1938), p. 256; Consumers Union of United States, "Analysis of

Contraceptive Materials," box 65, folder 646, Planned Parenthood Federation of America Papers, Sophia Smith Collection.

40. Dewees and Beebe, "Contraception in Private Practice," p. 1169.

41. Kennedy, "History of Contraceptive Materials," pp. 159–61; *New York City Directory 1933/34*, pt. 2, listing for Holland-Rantos Inc.

42. Holland-Rantos Co., Inc., *Report on Physicians' Replies to Questionnaire concerning Their Experience with the Vaginal Diaphragm and Jelly* (New York, 1929), pp. 16–17, 19; also see "Why the Diaphragm Is Strictly a Prescription Contraceptive," *Holland-Rantos Bulletin* 3 (January 1935), folder 319, box 29, Norman Himes Papers, Countway Library of Medicine.

43. Hannah M. Stone, "Maternal Health and Contraception: A Study of 2,000 Cases from Maternal Health Center, Newark, N.J.," *Medical Journal and Record*, April 19, 1933, pp. 7–15, and May 5, 1933, pp. 7–13. Bessie L. Moses, *Contraception as a Therapeutic Measure* (Baltimore, Md.: Williams and Wilkins Company, 1937). Also see Marie E. Kopp, *Birth Control in Practice* (New York: McBride, 1934); Dewees and Beebe, "Contraception in Private Practice, pp. 1169–72; Ruth A. Robishaw, "A Study of 4,000 Patients Admitted for Contraceptive Advice and Treatment," *American Journal of Obstetrics and Gynecology* 31 (March 1936): 426–35; Regine K. Stix, "Birth Control in a Midwestern City: A Study of the Clinics of the Cincinnati Committee on Maternal Health," *Milbank Memorial Fund Quarterly*, January 1939, pp. 69–91, April 1939, pp. 152–71, October 1939, pp. 392–423; Hannah M. Stone, "Therapeutic Contraception," *Medical Journal and Record*, March 21, 1928.

44. One study published in the *American Journal of Obstetrics and Gynecology* found that 3,514 of the 4,000 patients (88 percent) admitted to the Maternal Health Clinic of Cleveland between March 1928 and January 1934 were given the "diaphragm pessary used in conjunction with lactic acid jelly." Hannah Stone, Bocker's successor, estimated in 1936 that the combination was prescribed for more than 95 percent of patients at medically directed clinics nationwide. Hannah M. Stone, "Occlusive Methods of Contraception," *Journal of Contraception* (May 1937): 162. Her report was first presented at the Conference on Contraceptive Research and Clinical Practice, held in New York on December 29–30, 1936. Claude C. Pierce, "Contraceptive Services in the United States," *Human Fertility* 8 (September 1943): 92. Also see Sanger, "Suggestions for the Establishment of a Birth Control Clinic," p. 7.

45. "Merchandising News," *Drug and Cosmetic Industry* 41 (August 1937): 216; "Contraceptive," *Drug and Cosmetic Industry* 41 (July 1937): 75.

46. Sanger, *Autobiography*, p. 364.

47. Erick Kunnas to Mrs. Merlin Stoutenburgh, April 14, 1961, "Birth Control Products and Research, Holland-Rantos, 1956–1962," folder 8, box 4, Mary Steichen Calderone Papers, Schlesinger Library, Radcliffe Institute, Cambridge, Mass.

48. Kennedy, "History of Contraceptive Materials, p. 160.

49. Ibid., pp. 159–61; Le Mon Clark, "Two Types of Vaginal Diaphragms," *Journal of Contraception* (November 1938): 199–201; Abraham Stone, "Commercially Available Mechanical Devices for Use in Contraception," *Human Fertility* 10 (September

1945): 65–68; Bocker, *Birth Control Methods*, p. 20; Holland-Rantos, *Report on Physicians' Replies*, p. 29; H. J. Stern, "History," in C. M. Blow and C. Hepburn, eds., *Rubber Technology and Manufacture* (London: Butterworth Scientific, 1982), p. 7; Consumers Union of United States, *Analysis of Contraceptive Materials* (November 1937), pp. 14–17, box 65, folder 646, Planned Parenthood Federation of America Papers, Sophia Smith Collection; Holland-Rantos, *Suggestions for Contraceptive Practice* (New York, 1930), pp. 3–4.

50. Alan F. Guttmacher, "Conception Control and the Medical Profession: The Attitude of 3,381 Physicians toward Contraception and the Contraceptives They Prescribe," *Human Fertility* 12 (March 1947): 1–10; National Committee on Maternal Health, "Contraception, Sterilization, and Hygiene of Marriage in the Medical Curriculum," *American Journal of Obstetrics and Gynecology* 31 (January 1936): 165–68.

51. Dickinson, "Contraception," pp. 584–87.

52. Youngs Rubber Corporation Survey, pp. 1–2, National Committee on Maternal Health Papers, Countway Library of Medicine.

53. Guttmacher, "Conception Control and the Medical Profession," p. 8. Also see Marie Pichel Warner, "Contraception: A Study of Five Hundred Cases from Private Practice," *Journal of the American Medical Association* 115 (July 27, 1940): 279–85, and Robishaw, "Study of 4,000 Patients," pp. 426–35. Robishaw found that in four thousand birth control patients studied, the condom was recommended only once.

54. Bocker, *Birth Control Methods*, p. 5; Dickinson, "Contraception," p. 589.

55. Quoted in Judith Walzer Leavitt, *Brought to Bed: Childbearing in America, 1750 to 1950* (New York: Oxford University Press, 1986), pp. 179, 184. Also see McCann, *Birth Control Politics*, pp. 66–67.

56. Barton Cooke Hirst, "The Four Major Problems in Gynecology," *Journal of the American Medical Association* 101 (September 16, 1933): 900.

57. Thaddeus Montgomery, "Indications for Contraception from the Point of View of the Obstetrician and Gynecologist," *American Journal of Obstetrics and Gynecology* 32 (1936): 471.

58. The *Journal of Contraception* classified the following disorders as indications for contraception in 1936: systemic diseases (cardiac disease, nephritis, nephritic toxemias, severe anemia, hypertension, thyroid disease, diabetes, gall bladder disease, epilepsy, and so on); nervous and mental diseases (manic depression, anxiety neuroses, schizophrenia, mental defectiveness, constitutional inferiority, and so on); gynecological problems (recent pelvic repair, fistulas, extreme lacerations, repeated abortions [spontaneous or induced], adnexal disease, and so on); obstetrical problems (toxemias other than nephritic, repeated difficult deliveries, eclampsia, repeated cesarean sections, and so on); orthopedic and surgical problems (tuberculosis of spine or hip, osteomyelitis, fractured pelvis, recent operation, one kidney, kidney stones); venereal diseases (gonorrhea, syphilis, central nervous system syphilis); defects and deformities (spina bifida, various paralyses, congenital blindness, double vagina, and so on); multiparity (too many pregnancies or too frequent pregnancies

in a short period of time, often combined with general debility, malnutrition, anemia); indications of husbands (tuberculosis, epilepsy, postencephalitic condition, blindness, mental illness, lues, criminal alcoholism, and so on); eugenic problems (repeated defect in children, harelip in three children, three status lymphaticus deaths, family with Friedrich's ataxia, family with numerous institutionalized psychopaths); not strictly medical circumstances (marital disharmony, recent delivery, economic). See "Medical Indications for Contraception," *Journal of Contraception*, November 1936, p. 189.

59. The case was *United States v. One Package*, 13 F. Supp. 334 (1936); Birth Control Federation of America, *Questions and Answers about Birth Control* (New York, circa 1939), reel 10 of 26, Records of the National Association of Colored Women's Clubs, National Archives for Black Women's History, Washington, D.C.; Richard N. Pierson, Robert L. Dickinson, Ira S. Wile, and Woodbridge E. Morris, "Contraceptive Practice," *American Journal of Obstetrics and Gynecology* 41 (January 1941): 174–75; Ralph E. Brown, "The Legal Status of Contraception: A Practical Interpretation for the Doctor's Guidance," *American Medicine*, March 1935, pp. 167–70.

60. Owen Jones Toland, "Contraception—A Neglected Field for Preventive Medicine," *American Journal of Obstetrics and Gynecology* 27 (January 1934): 52. Toland's talk was first presented at a meeting of the Obstetrical Society of Philadelphia on May 4, 1933.

61. See Judith Walzer Leavitt, *Typhoid Mary: Captive to the Public's Health* (Boston: Beacon Press, 1996); James Jones, *Bad Blood: The Tuskegee Syphilis Experiment—A Tragedy of Race and Medicine* (New York: Free Press, 1981); Alan Kraut, *Silent Travelers: Germs, Genes, and the Immigrant Menace* (New York: Basic Books, 1994); Charles McClain, "Of Medicine, Race, and American Law: The Bubonic Outbreak of 1900," *Law and Social Inquiry* 13 (1988): 447–513; Vanessa Northington Gamble, "A Legacy of Distrust: African-Americans and Medical Research," *American Journal of Preventive Medicine* 9 (1993): 35–38. The Supreme Court's case on smallpox is *Jacobson v. Massachusetts*, 25 S.Ct. 358.

62. Galton quoted in F. H. Hankins, "The Interdependence of Eugenics and Birth Control," *Birth Control Review*, June 1931, p. 170; McCann, *Birth Control Politics*, p. 101. For a comprehensive history of the eugenics movement in the United States, see Daniel J. Kevles, *In the Name of Eugenics: Genetics and the Uses of Human Heredity* (New York: Alfred A. Knopf, 1985).

63. Hal Sears, *The Sex Radicals: Free Love in High Victorian America* (Lawrence: University Press of Kansas, 1977), p. 120; D'Emilio and Freedman, *Intimate Matters*, p. 165.

64. Violet Blair Janin, diary entry, December 31, 1878, Janin Family Collection, Huntington Library and Archives, San Marino, Calif.

65. Theodore Roosevelt, "Race Decadence," *Outlook*, April 8, 1911; E. S. Goodhue, "Race Suicide," *Medico-Legal Journal* 25 (June 1907): 251–56.

66. McCann, *Birth Control Politics*, pp. 103–5; Kevles, *In the Name of Eugenics*, pp. 44–54; Dorothy Roberts, *Killing the Black Body: Race, Reproduction, and the Meaning of Liberty* (New York: Vintage, 1997), pp. 59–63.

67. Hirst, "Four Major Problems in Gynecology," p. 900.

68. Paul Popenoe and Roswell Johnson, *Applied Eugenics* (New York: Macmillan Company, 1926), pp. 156–59, 284–85, 292, 297. Also see Roberts, *Killing the Black Body*, pp. 60–61.

69. Roberts, *Killing the Black Body*, p. 65.

70. M. A. Horn, ed., *Mother and Daughter* (Wilmington, Ohio: Hygienic Productions, 1947), p. 74.

71. Kevles, *In the Name of Eugenics*, pp. 90–94.

72. Roberts, *Killing the Black Body*, pp. 66–67; "Eugenic Sterilizations in the United States," *Journal of Contraception*, April 1938, pp. 81–83.

73. By 1906, doctors had performed an estimated 150,000 ovariectomies on American women under the guise of protecting their emotional stability and mental health. Tone, *Controlling Reproduction*, p. 65. Also see Barbara Ehrenreich and Deirdre English, *For Her Own Good: 150 Years of the Experts' Advice to Women* (Garden City, N.Y.: Anchor Press/Doubleday, 1978).

74. Norman Haire, "Sterilization of the Unfit," *Birth Control Review*, February 1922, pp. 10–11; "Eugenic Sterilizations in the United States," *Journal of Contraception*, pp. 81–82; E. H. F. Pirkner, "Prophylactic Salpingapotomy," *Medico-Legal Journal* 33 (March 1917): 14.

75. M. A. Horn, ed., *Father and Son* (Wilmington, Ohio: Hygienic Productions, 1947), p. 22.

76. "Contraception," *Medico-Legal Journal* 33 (April 1916): 10.

77. The Human Betterment Foundation, *Human Sterilization* (Pasadena, Calif.: The Human Betterment Foundation, circa 1930), pp. 5–6.

78. *Buck v. Bell*, 274 U.S. 200 (1927).

79. Of the 27,869 Americans sterilized between 1907 and 1937, 16,241 were women. "Eugenic Sterilizations in the United States," *Journal of Contraception*, p. 81.

80. For an especially good analysis of the complexities of the relationship between the eugenics and birth control movements, see McCann, *Birth Control Politics*, chap. 4.

81. Caroline Hadley Robinson, *Seventy Birth Control Clinics: A Survey and Analysis Including the General Effects of Control on Size and Quality of Population* (Baltimore, Md.: Williams and Wilkins Company, 1930), p. 246.

82. Human Betterment Foundation, *Human Sterilization*, p. 6.

83. Sanger quoted in McCann, *Birth Control Politics*, p. 107.

84. Sanger quoted in McCann, *Birth Control Politics*, p. 112.

85. "In re: Birth Control Movement," pp. 3–4, Rockefeller Archives; Roberts, *Killing the Black Body*, pp. 87–88; McCann, *Birth Control Politics*, chap. 5.

86. Sanger quoted in Roberts, *Killing the Black Body*, pp. 87–88.

87. Staupers quoted in Roberts, *Killing the Black Body*, p. 43.

88. Dickinson, "Contraception," p. 589.

89. Robert L. Dickinson and Louise Stevens Bryant, *Control of Conception: An Illustrated Medical Manual* (Baltimore, Md.: Williams and Wilkins Company, 1931), pp. 3, 67–68.

90. Ibid., p. 3.
91. "Discussion," *Journal of Contraception*, May 1937, p. 108.
92. "In re: Birth Control Movement," p. 4, Rockefeller Archives; Stone, "Maternal Health and Contraception."
93. Clinic experiences—the New York clinic was booked "three weeks in advance," she told one friend—demonstrated that "Birth Control assistance is proving a great blessing to the unemployed." Letter to Percy L. Clarke, October 31, 1931, Margaret Sanger Papers, reel 29.
94. "The Foam Powder Method," *Journal of Contraception*, May 1937, p. 108.

7. FEMININE HYGIENE

1. "The Accident of Birth," *Fortune*, February 1938, p. 84.
2. Ibid., p. 84; "Feminine Hygiene Products Face a New Marketing Era," *Drug and Cosmetic Industry* 37 (December 1935): 745; Harrison Reeves, "The Birth Control Industry," *American Mercury* 155 (November 1936): 287; "Birth Control Industry," *Drug and Cosmetic Industry* 46 (January 1940): 58; "Building Acceptances for Feminine Hygiene Products," *Drug and Cosmetic Industry* 38 (February 1936): 177.
3. As one advertising leaflet put it, "Feminine hygiene is the 'nice' term . . . invented for the care and cleanliness of the vaginal tract from its outer opening to the cervix." Quoted in Rachel Lynn Palmer and Sarah Koslow Greenberg, *Facts and Frauds in Woman's Hygiene: A Medical Guide against Misleading Claims and Dangerous Products* (Garden City, N.Y.: Garden City Publishing Company, 1938), p. 18.
4. Lee Rainwater, *And the Poor Get Children: Sex, Contraception, and Family Planning in the Working Class* (Chicago: Quadrangle Books, 1960), pp. 158–59.
5. "Accident of Birth," *Fortune*, pp. 84, 108.
6. The 1936 survey was sponsored by the American Institute of Public Opinion. Discussed in PPFA 1943 study, p. 13, Planned Parenthood Federation of America Papers, Sophia Smith Collection, Smith College. In 1938, *Ladies' Home Journal* reported similar findings in a subsequent investigation of the attitudes of American women. Henry F. Pringle, "What Do the Women of America Think about Birth Control?" *Ladies' Home Journal*, March 1938, pp. 14–15.
7. Dorothy Dunbar Bromley, "Birth Control and the Depression," *Harper's*, October 1934, p. 566; James Rorty, "What's Stopping Birth Control?" *New Republic*, February 3, 1932, p. 313.
8. Anonymous to Lindsey, May 12, 1925, Lindsey Papers, Manuscripts Division, Library of Congress.
9. Anonymous to Lindsey, May 24, 1925, Lindsey Papers.
10. Anonymous to Lindsey, n.d., Lindsey Papers.
11. "Accident of Birth," *Fortune*, p. 107. One guide reported in 1938 that "birth control clinics are still so few in number and situated so far apart that even when their location is generally known, a woman often cannot afford transportation to the nearest clinic." Palmer and Greenberg, *Facts and Frauds in Woman's Hygiene*, p. 225.

12. PPFA 1943 study, p. 27, Planned Parenthood Federation of America Papers, Sophia Smith Collection.

13. Earl Lomon Koos, "Class Differences in the Employment of Contraceptive Measures," *Human Fertility* 12 (December 1947): 99.

14. Rainwater, *And the Poor Get Children*, pp. 27–28.

15. Quoted in Palmer and Greenberg, *Facts and Frauds in Woman's Hygiene*, p. 225. On lack of training, see also Consumers Union of United States, *Analysis of Contraceptive Materials* (New York: Consumers Union of United States, 1937), p. 16.

16. Palmer and Greenberg, *Facts and Frauds in Woman's Hygiene*, pp. 11–12. Clinics, though anonymous, were not necessarily more inviting. A woman's "desire for reliable information must be very strong indeed to take her to a clinic where she has to meet several strangers, have her case history taken, answer many questions as to her health, marital history, pregnancies, [and] abortions." PPFA 1943 study, p. 29, Planned Parenthood Federation of America Papers, Sophia Smith Collection.

17. Quoted in Rainwater, *And the Poor Get Children*, p. 11.

18. Koos, "Class Differences," pp. 99–100. Also see Eric Matsner and Frederick Holden, *The Technique of Contraception*, 4th ed. (Baltimore, Md.: Williams and Wilkins Company, 1938), p. 13. In their discussion of diaphragm fitting and effectiveness, Matsner and Holden noted, "It should be pointed out that many failures are due to women purchasing diaphragms from drug stores and attempting self-fitting" (p. 13).

19. "Mailings: Questionnaire to Pharmacists," and "Results of a Questionnaire to Pharmacists on Birth Control," box 85, folder 812, Planned Parenthood Federation of America Papers, Sophia Smith Collection. The questionnaire was sent to a cross section of druggists in forty-one states and in communities of varying size. Of 1,000 sent questionnaires, 138 replied. When asked for contraceptive information, 36 percent recommended physician, 32 percent showed customer several products, 24 percent recommended a particular contraceptive, 5 percent avoided giving advice, 2 percent declined to give advice, 1 percent made it a practice to recommend a birth control clinic. When asked for the most reliable method, 63 percent recommended diaphragm and jelly, 23 percent condoms, 3 percent jelly and cream alone, 10 percent none. When asked how many customers seek help, 56 percent said that the proportion of regular customers asking for contraceptive advice at one time or another was approximately 30 percent of the total of regular customers. None of the replies indicates that less than 30 percent of the total of regular customers sought advice.

20. Robert A. Hatcher, Miriam Zieman, Alston Watt, Anita Nelson, Gary K. Stewart, Philip D. Darney, and Rachel B. Blankstein, *A Pocket Guide to Managing Contraception* (Tiger, Ga.: Bridging the Gap Foundation, 1998), p. 58.

21. Interview with Margaret Thorne, March 1998, transcript in author's possession. Also see Consumers Union of United States, *Analysis of Contraceptive Materials* (1937), pp. 14–16.

22. Dorrin F. Rudnick, "A New Type of Foreign Body in the Urinary Bladder," *Journal of the American Medical Association* 94 (May 17, 1930): 1565.

23. For a discussion of the consolidation of American consumer society in the 1920s and 1930s, see Richard Wrightman Fox, "Epitaph for Middletown: Robert S. Lynd and the Analysis of Consumer Culture," in Richard Wrightman Fox and T. J. Jackson Lears, eds., *The Culture of Consumption: Critical Essays in American History, 1880–1980* (New York: Pantheon Books, 1983); Daniel J. Boorstin, *The Americans, the Democratic Experience* (New York: Random House, 1973), especially part 2; Roland Marchand, *Advertising the American Dream: Making Way for Modernity, 1920–1940* (Berkeley: University of California Press, 1985); Stuart Ewen, *Captains of Consciousness: Advertising and the Social Roots of the Consumer Culture* (Toronto: McGraw-Hill, 1976); Gary Cross, *Time and Money: The Making of Consumer Culture* (London: Routledge, 1993), chap. 6; Liz Cohen, *Making a New Deal: Industrial Workers in Chicago, 1919–1939* (New York: Cambridge University Press, 1990).

24. See Susan Porter Benson, *Counter Cultures: Saleswomen, Managers, and Customers in American Department Stores* (Urbana: University of Illinois Press, 1986); Dana Frank, "Gender, Consumer Organizing, and the Seattle Labor Movement, 1919–1929," in Ava Baron, ed., *Work Engendered: Toward a New History of American Labor* (Ithaca, N.Y.: Cornell University Press, 1991); Kathy Peiss, "Making Faces: The Cosmetics Industry and the Cultural Construction of Gender, 1890–1930," *Genders* 7 (Spring 1990); William R. Leach, "Transformation in a Culture of Consumption: Women and Department Stores, 1890–1925," *Journal of American History* 71 (September 1984); Cynthia Wright, "Feminine Trifles of Vast Importance: Writing Gender into the History of Consumption," in Franca Iacovetta and Mariana Valverde, eds., *Gender Conflicts* (Toronto: University of Toronto Press, 1992).

25. Christine Frederick, *Selling Mrs. Consumer* (New York: Business Bourse, 1929), pp. 43–44. For general discussions of women and American advertising in the 1920s, see Nancy F. Cott, *The Grounding of Modern Feminism* (New Haven, Conn.: Yale University Press, 1987), pp. 170–74; Marchand, *Advertising the American Dream*, pp. 66–69, 179–85; and Ewen, *Captains of Consciousness*, pp. 159–76. Ruth Schwartz Cowan's insightful "The 'Industrial Revolution' in the Home: Household Technology and Social Change in the 20th Century," *Technology and Culture* 17 (1976), explores how household appliances were advertised to women in the 1920s. Advertisers in the 1920s consciously attempted to eradicate earlier, derisive perceptions of women's role as consumers by portraying female consumption as both psychologically fulfilling *and* economically functional. A sexual division of labor predating capitalist economic and social relations had designated the majority of household consumption women's work. The advance of industrial capitalism in the late eighteenth and early nineteenth centuries brought divisions between the household and the external market into sharper relief; in redefining "real" work as only that which possessed a tangible remunerative value, it amplified perceptions that women—largely excluded from wage labor—were dependent consumers rather than independent producers.

26. A poll published in *Ladies' Home Journal* in 1938 found that 79 percent of Ameri-

can women surveyed favored birth control. The most frequent argument given in its favor was economic considerations. See Pringle, "What Do the Women of America Think about Birth Control?" p. 15.

27. PPFA 1943 study, p. 28, Planned Parenthood Federation of America Papers, Sophia Smith Collection.

28. Koos, "Class Differences," p. 99.

29. Randolph Cautley, "Contraceptives in Advertising: An Economic Study of the Contraceptive Trade," January 15, 1934, unpublished manuscript, box 6, folder 233, National Committee on Maternal Health Papers, Countway Library of Medicine, Harvard Medical School, Boston, Mass.

30. Letter from John T. Mercer, M.D., to the Bureau of Information, American Medical Association, April 6, 1933, Birth Control Correspondence, box 86, American Medical Association Health Fraud Archives.

31. Quoted in PPFA 1943 study, p. 31, Planned Parenthood Federation of America Papers, Sophia Smith Collection.

32. For sample captions, see Bromley, "Birth Control and the Depression"; the advertisement captioned "The Fear That 'Blights' Romance and Ages Women Prematurely" is from McCall's, October 1932, p. 102.

33. "The Incompatible Marriage: Is It a Case for Doctor or Lawyer?" McCall's, May 1933, p. 107; "The Fear That 'Blights' Romance and Ages Women Prematurely," McCall's, p. 102.

34. Advertisement cited in Elizabeth Garrett, "Birth Control's Business Baby," New Republic, January 17, 1934, p. 271; "Incompatible Marriage," McCall's, p. 107.

35. "Incompatible Marriage," p. 107.

36. Ibid., p. 107; Garrett, "Birth Control's Business Baby," p. 271; Rorty, "What's Stopping Birth Control?" pp. 292–94.

37. Mary P. Ryan, "Reproduction in America," Journal of Interdisciplinary History 10 (Autumn 1979): 330; Joyce M. Ray and F. G. Gosling, "American Physicians and Birth Control, 1936–1947," Journal of Social History (1985): 405; Marchand, Advertising the American Dream, passim.

38. "Accident of Birth," Fortune, p. 112.

39. "The Serene Marriage . . . Should It Be Jeopardized by Needless Fears?" McCall's, December 1932, p. 87.

40. "The Fear That 'Blights' Romance and Ages Women Prematurely," McCall's, p. 64; "No Wonder Many Wives Fade Quickly with This Recurrent Fear," McCall's, August 1933, p. 64.

41. "Why Wasn't I Born a Man?" McCall's, May 1933, p. 93; "Marriage Is No Gambling Matter: Better Find Out, Better Be Sure about It," McCall's, March 1933, p. 107.

42. Garrett, "Birth Control's Business Baby," p. 270; Reeves, "Birth Control Industry," pp. 286–87; Bromley, "Birth Control and the Depression," p. 570; Anne Rapport, "The Legal Aspects of Marketing Feminine Hygiene Products," Drug and Cosmetic Industry 38 (April 1936): 474; Norman Himes, Medical History of Contraception

(Baltimore, Md.: Williams and Wilkins Company, 1936), p. 202; "Accident of Birth," *Fortune*, p. 85.

43. "Accident of Birth," *Fortune*, p. 112.

44. "Feminine Hygiene in the Department Stores," *Drug and Cosmetic Industry* 40 (April 1937): 482; "12 Ways to More Sales in Feminine Hygiene Products," *Chain Store Age*, June 1941, p. 54.

45. Zonite advertisements in *Chain Store Age*, January 1941, p. 5, and March 1941, p. 66; "12 Ways to More Sales in Feminine Hygiene Products," *Chain Store Age*, p. 19; "Feminine Hygiene Products Face a New Marketing Era," *Drug and Cosmetic Industry*, p. 747; H. C. Naylor, "Behind the Scenes Promotion Builds Feminine Hygiene Sales," *Chain Store Age*, March 1941, passim.

46. Garrett, "Birth Control's Business Baby," p. 269; Reeves, "Birth Control Industry," p. 287; David M. Kennedy, *Birth Control in America: The Career of Margaret Sanger* (New Haven, Conn.: Yale University Press, 1970), p. 212.

47. Ad quoted in Palmer and Greenberg, *Facts and Frauds in Woman's Hygiene*, p. 12.

48. "Accident of Birth," *Fortune*, p. 114.

49. Ibid., p. 114; Dorothy Dunbar Bromley, *Birth Control: Its Use and Misuse* (New York: Harper, 1934), p. 93; Dilex Institute to Mrs. M. Hoffman, August 31, 1931, Margaret Sanger Papers, reel 29, Library of Congress. The American Health Association (AHA) established a similar service. Like Dilex, the AHA borrowed a concept key to the burgeoning public health movement: household-by-household nursing visitations. The company hired women to be visiting nurses and equipped them with certificates of membership, badges of identification, and sacks full of AHA contraceptive merchandise. No training or experience was required to be a saleswoman, although each applicant had to pay thirty-five cents for "membership privileges" and sign a pledge of allegiance to the company and its mission. This the AHA articulated as bringing "healthful living through public education" to the masses. For the "millions and millions of wives who are just as needy but who are living on a farm, in a small town, or even in a larger city where no staff of visiting nurses has yet been organized" the company sent literature enabling women to buy its supplies through mail order. Federal Trade Commission to Norman Himes, March 15, 1938, folder 334, box 30, Norman Himes Papers, Countway Library of Medicine; Grace Naismith, "The Racket in Contraceptives," *American Mercury* 71 (July 1950): 7.

50. Lanteen Laboratories, *Birth Control: Plain Medical Information* (Chicago: Medical Bureaus of Information on Birth Control, 1929), in author's possession; Lanteen Laboratories, *Reliable Birth Control Preparations*, Margaret Sanger Papers, reel 29; Rudnick, "New Type of Foreign Body," pp. 1565–66; Consumers Union of United States, *Analysis of Contraceptive Materials* (1937), pp. 15, 18; Cautley, "Contraceptives in Advertising"; Naismith, "Racket in Contraceptives," pp. 7–8. On commercial birth control clinics in general, see Rose Holz, "Whose Business Is It Anyway? Commercial Contraceptive Clinics and the American Birth Control League in the 1930s," paper presented at the American Association of the History of Medicine, May 21, 2000, in author's possession.

51. Lanteen Laboratories, *Reliable Birth Control Preparations*, Margaret Sanger Papers,

reel 29; Lanteen Laboratories, *Birth Control: Plain Medical Information* (Chicago: Medical Bureaus of Information, 1936), in author's possession.

52. Rudnick, "New Type of Foreign Body," pp. 1565–66.

53. Lanteen Laboratories, *Birth Control: Plain Medical Information* (1936), p. 9.

54. "The Mythical 'Dr. Carr,' " *Journal of Contraception*, December 1937, p. 229; PPFA 1943 study, p. 32, Planned Parenthood Federation of America Papers, Sophia Smith Collection; Naismith, "Racket in Contraceptives," p. 8; "The Lanteen Laboratories, Inc.," *Journal of Contraception*, May 1939, pp. 116–18.

55. Form letters sent from the Bureau of Information, Birth Control Correspondence, box 86, American Medical Association Health Fraud Archives.

56. Letter from American Medical Association Bureau of Information to Mrs. R. F. Pease, September 26, 1932, Lysol and Zonite File, American Medical Association Health Fraud Archives.

57. J. J. Durrett, Chief, FDA Drug Division, to George Miller, June 20, 1938, Lehn & Fink—Lysol, vol. 1, carton 203, FDA History Office, Food and Drug Administration; "Accident of Birth," *Fortune*, p. 108; Palmer and Greenberg, *Facts and Frauds in Woman's Hygiene*, pp. 21–24.

58. National Committee on Maternal Health, "List of Contraceptive Jellies on the American Market," National Committee on Maternal Health Papers, Countway Library of Medicine; Consumers Union of United States, *A Report on Contraceptive Materials* (New York: Consumers Union of United States, 1945), pp. 18–20, 29–30; Palmer and Greenberg, *Facts and Frauds in Woman's Hygiene*, pp. 99, 123–36. Also see Royal I. Brown, "Changes of the Consistency of Contraceptive Preparations during Storage," *Human Fertility* 7 (December 1942): 161–63.

59. See Mary Calderone to William Kitay, December 9, 1963, folder 178, box 10, Mary Steichen Calderone Papers, Schlesinger Library, Radcliffe Institute, Cambridge, Mass.; Linda Gordon, *Woman's Body, Woman's Right: A Social History of Birth Control in America* (New York: Penguin, 1974), pp. 48–49, 62–64; Daniel Scott Smith, "Family Limitation, Sexual Control, and Domestic Feminism in Victorian America," *Feminist Studies* 1 (Winter–Spring 1973), passim. Pre-clinic contraceptive methods were well catalogued by physicians. See Marie E. Kopp, *Birth Control in Practice: Analysis of Ten Thousand Case Histories of the Birth Control Clinical Research Bureau* (New York: McBride, 1934); Raymond Pearl, "Contraception and Fertility in 4945 Married Women: A Second Report on a Study in Family Limitation," *Human Biology* 6 (1934); Hannah M. Stone, "Maternal Health and Contraception: A Study of 2,000 Cases from Maternal Health Center, Newark, N. J.," *Medical Journal and Record*, April 19, 1933, and May 5, 1933; "Feminine Hygiene Market," *Drug and Cosmetic Industry* 38 (May 1936): 647. The impact of the commercialization of contraception in the 1930s on contraceptive practice is documented by John Winchell Riley and Matilda White in "The Use of Various Methods of Contraception," *American Sociological Review* 5 (December 1940): 890–903, and discussed in Rainwater, *And the Poor Get Children*, p. 162; PPFA 1943 study, p. 28, Planned Parenthood Federation of America Papers, Sophia Smith Collection.

60. Robert L. Dickinson and Louise Stevens Bryant, *Control of Conception: An Illus-*

trated Medical Manual (Baltimore, Md.: Williams and Wilkins Company, 1931), pp. 78–80; Bromley, *Birth Control*, pp. 99–100; Palmer and Greenberg, *Facts and Frauds in Woman's Hygiene*, pp. 242–50.

61. Newark study quoted in Naismith, "Racket in Contraceptives," p. 5.

62. Lehn & Fink, *Lysol: Better Than Carbolic Acid* (New York: Lehn & Fink, 1913); "The Evolution of a Proprietary—Lysol," *Journal of the American Medical Association* 59 (December 14, 1912): 2173–74; advertisement in *New York Medical Journal*, July 12, 1919.

63. AMA Bureau of Information to Edward Wolkind, October 4, 1935, Lysol and Zonite folder, American Medical Association Health Fraud Archives; AMA Bureau of Information to Mrs. E. Davey, January 13, 1934, "Birth Control Correspondence," American Medical Association Health Fraud Archives; "The Evolution of a Proprietary—Lysol," *Journal of the American Medical Association*, pp. 2173–74; miscellaneous newspaper articles on Chicago suicides and homicides from Lysol poisonings are in the Lysol and Zonite folder, American Medical Association Health Fraud Archives; Palmer and Greenberg, *Facts and Frauds in Woman's Hygiene*, p. 95.

64. Dickinson and Bryant, *Control of Conception*, pp. 39–45, 69–74; Bromley, *Birth Control*, pp. 92–98; Palmer and Greenberg, *Facts and Frauds in Woman's Hygiene*, pp. 12–15, 142–51; Lysol ad from pamphlet by Dr. Emil Klarmann, *Formula L-F: A New Antiseptic and Germicide* (Lehn & Fink Inc.) appended to letter from Lehn & Fink to Margaret Sanger, November 24, 1931, Margaret Sanger Papers, reel 29; PX ad from Margaret Sanger Papers, box 232, folder "Commercial Advertisements, 1932–34."

65. "Effects of Corrosive Mercuric Chloride ('Bichloride') Douches," *Journal of the American Medical Association* 99 (August 6, 1932): 497.

66. "Accident of Birth," *Fortune*, pp. 110–12.

67. Letter from Edward H. Wolkind to Arthur J. Cramp, October 2, 1935, Lysol and Zonite folder, American Medical Association Health Fraud Archives.

68. Lehn & Fink to anonymous Iowa resident, September 22, 1941, Lehn & Fink—Lysol, vol. 1, carton 203, FDA History Office.

69. Memo from Division of Pharmacology to Bureau of Enforcement on new Lysol formulation, February 12, 1960, carton 221; A. J. Lehman to Edward Press, October 31, 1956, Edward Press to A. J. Lehman, October 23, 1956, and Harold O'Keefe to Sidney Kaye, May 19, 1954, all carton 203, Lehn & Fink—Lysol, FDA History Office; PPFA 1943 study, p. 28, Planned Parenthood Federation of America Papers, Sophia Smith Collection.

70. John Smith [name changed to protect the anonymity of the consumer] to FDA, August 13, 1961, Lehn & Fink to John Smith, August 22, 1961, FDA Establishment Inspection Report, September 18, 1961, all carton 221, Lehn & Fink—Lysol, vol. 6, FDA History Office.

71. "Pocket Book Los Angeles," *Southern California Business* 16 (November 1937): 21.

72. Morrow Mayo, *Los Angeles* (New York: Alfred A. Knopf, 1933), p. 270.

73. Ibid., p. 323.

74. *United States of America before Federal Trade Commission, Docket no. 3486, In the Matter of: Rosemarie Lewis, Trading as Certane Company, et al., Complaint* [hereafter *In the Matter of Rosemarie Lewis*], box 2590, Docketed case files 1915–1943, Records of the Federal Trade Commission, RG 122, National Archives.

75. Warren S. Thompson, *Growth and Changes in California's Population* (Los Angeles: Haynes Foundation, 1955), p. 25.

76. "Pocket Book Los Angeles," *Southern California Business* 15 (May 1936): 24; "The Picture Story of a Pay Envelope," *Southern California Business* 16 (December 1937): 12.

77. Ruth Milkman, "Women's Work and the Economic Crisis: Some Lessons from the Great Depression," in Nancy Cott and Elizabeth Pleck, eds., *A Heritage of Her Own: Toward a New Social History of American Women* (New York: Simon and Schuster, 1979), pp. 507–41.

78. "Working Wives in Los Angeles Set High Mark," *L.A. Examiner*, May 23, 1933, News Service, University of Southern California Library, Department of Special Collections, Regional History Center.

79. "Accident of Birth," *Fortune*, p. 208.

80. *In the Matter of Rosemarie Lewis*, p. 9.

81. Ibid., pp. 5–7, 55–56, 86.

82. Ibid., pp. 8–15, 27–28, 34, 36; Commission's Exhibit 2.

83. *In the Matter of Rosemarie Lewis*, pp. 9, 13, 58–61, 238.

84. Ibid., pp. 10, 51, 52, 56–57, 222, 323; Commission's Exhibit 8.

85. Transcript of Proceedings, *In the Matter of Charges against Rosemarie Lewis, Charles Luntz, and Max Lewis*, Fraud Order Hearing before the Solicitor of the Post Office Department, p. 32, box 159, Transcripts of Hearings on Fraud Cases, 1913–1945, Records of the Post Office Department, RG 28, National Archives.

86. Advertisements departed from script only when mentioning the firm's California roots: "Originally created to meet the requirements of critical Hollywood, CERTANE is now on sale at drug stores everywhere." *In the Matter of Rosemarie Lewis*, Brief of Counsel for the Commission, p. 6.

87. *In the Matter of Rosemarie Lewis*, pp. 10–11; Lewis to Federal Trade Commission, December 9, 1937 (also in FTC Transcript); PPFA 1943 study, p. 38, Planned Parenthood Federation of America Papers, Sophia Smith Collection.

88. Henry Miller, *Statutes and Decisions Pertaining to the Federal Trade Commission, 1914–29* (Washington, D.C.: Government Printing Office, 1930), pp. 1, 5–7.

89. Gabriel Kolko, *The Triumph of Conservatism* (New York: Free Press, 1963).

90. *United States v. One Package*, 13 F. Supp. 334; James Reed, *From Private Vice to Public Virtue: The Birth Control Movement and American Society since 1830* (New York: Basic Books, 1978), p. 121; Kennedy, *Birth Control in America*, pp. 242–52.

91. "New Legislation: The Federal Trade Commission Act," *Journal of Contraception*, May 1938, p. 116; Harriette H. Esch, *Statutes and Decisions Pertaining to the U.S. Federal Trade Commission*, vol. 3, 1939–1943 (Washington, D.C.: Government Printing Office, 1944), pp. 14–16.

92. Eric Matsner to the Certane Company, March 8, 1938, box 65, folder "Commercial Contraceptives Advertising," Planned Parenthood Federation of America Papers, Sophia Smith Collection.
93. *In the Matter of Rosemarie Lewis*, Brief of Counsel for the Commission, p. 7.
94. *In the Matter of Rosemarie Lewis*, pp. 81–104; Brief of Counsel for the Commission, pp. 6–9.
95. *In the Matter of Rosemarie Lewis*, Exhibit 26A.
96. *In the Matter of Rosemarie Lewis*, Brief of Counsel for the Commission; "Official Actions against the Misrepresentation of Contraceptive Products," *Human Fertility* (June 1941): 90–91.
97. *In the Matter of Charges against Rosemarie Lewis, Charles Luntz, and Max Lewis*, pp. 2–3, 7–31, box 159, Transcripts of Hearings on Fraud Cases, 1913–1945, Records of the Post Office Department.
98. Ibid., p. 50.
99. Garrett, "Birth Control's Business Baby," pp. 270–71; "Accident of Birth," *Fortune*, pp. 108, 110, 112; Bromley, "Birth Control and the Depression," p. 572; Reed, *From Private Vice to Public Virtue*, pp. 114, 244–46; Kennedy, *Birth Control in America*, p. 183; Palmer and Greenberg, *Facts and Frauds in Woman's Hygiene*, pp. 21–24; Naismith, "Racket in Contraceptives," pp. 4, 9.

8. CONDOM KINGS

1. V. F. Calverton, *The Bankruptcy of Marriage* (New York: Macauley, 1928), p. 131. It is possible the rate of growth was greater, for the author estimated prewar sales to be from "two or three million."
2. Ibid., pp. 129–33; Christina Simmons, "Modern Sexuality and the Myth of Victorian Repression," in Kathy Peiss and Christina Simmons, eds., *Passion and Power: Sexuality in History* (Philadelphia: Temple University Press, 1989), p. 161; Norman Himes, *Medical History of Contraception* (Baltimore, Md.: Williams and Wilkins Company, 1936), p. 205.
3. "The Accident of Birth," *Fortune*, February 1938, p. 108; Planned Parenthood Federation of America 1943 study of the contraceptive industry by Foote, Cone & Belding, box 65, folder 647 [hereafter cited as PPFA 1943 study], pp. 18–22, Planned Parenthood Federation of America Papers, Sophia Smith Collection, Smith College; Christopher Tietze and Clarence Gamble, "The Condom as a Contraceptive Method in Public Health Work," *Human Fertility* 9 (December 1944): 97–113; Grace Naismith, "The Racket in Contraceptives," *American Mercury* 71 (July 1950): 12.
4. Robert L. Dickinson and Louise Stevens Bryant, *Control of Conception: An Illustrated Medical Manual* (Baltimore, Md.: Williams and Wilkins Company, 1931), p. 65; Consumers Union of United States, *Analysis of Contraceptive Materials* (New York: Consumers Union of United States, 1937), p. 20.
5. "Accident of Birth," *Fortune*, p. 108; Naismith, "Racket in Contraceptives," p. 12.

6. Census Manuscripts of the Twelfth Census of the United States, Population Schedule, Queens County, New York, enumeration district 622, 1900, National Archives.

7. Julius Schmid Inc. to Margaret Sanger, November 11, 1933, Margaret Sanger Papers, reel 30, Manuscripts Division, Library of Congress.

8. U.S. Patent Office, *Official Gazette*, January 13, 1931, p. 290, March 31, 1931, p. 1075, May 26, 1931, p. 883, November 18, 1924, p. 562, July 21, 1925, p. 553.

9. James S. Murphy, *The Condom Industry in the United States* (Jefferson, N.C.: McFarland and Company, 1990), pp. 10–12.

10. Census Manuscripts of the Fourteenth Census of the United States, Population Schedule, Montgomery Township, Orange County, New York, enumeration district 131, 1920; Murphy, *Condom Industry in the United States*, pp. 10–11.

11. *New York State Manufacturers 1927* (New York: H. A. Manning Company, 1927), p. 1231; "Important Makers," *Drug and Cosmetic Industry*, December 1935, p. 746; Murphy, *Condom Industry in the United States*, pp. 10–11.

12. Trial Record, *Perry H. Stevens v. Carl Schmid, Inc.*, United States District Court for the Southern District of New York, April 22, 1932, Records of the U.S. District Court for the Southern District of New York, National Archives, Regional Office, New York; *R. L. Polk & Company's General Directory of New York City*, vol. 134 (New York: R. L. Polk & Company, Inc., 1925), p. 2016; *Polk's New York City Directory, 1933–1934* (New York: R. L. Polk & Company, 1932); "Important Makers," *Drug and Cosmetic Industry*, p. 746; Murphy, *Condom Industry in the United States*, pp. 10–11.

13. Julius Schmid Inc. to Margaret Sanger, November 11, 1933, reel 30, Margaret Sanger Papers; *Polk's New York City Directory, 1933–1934*; "Accident of Birth," *Fortune*, p. 108.

14. Testimony of Merle L. Youngs, Transcript of Record, *Youngs Rubber Corporation v. C. I. Lee & Company, Inc.*, pp. 28, 31, Records of the U.S. Court of Appeals for the Second Circuit, National Archives, Regional Office, New York.

15. Transcript of Record, *Youngs Rubber Corporation v. C. I. Lee & Company*, Records of U.S. Court of Appeals for the Second Circuit, pp. 3, 25–31.

16. Ibid., p. 31; Calverton, *Bankruptcy of Marriage*, p. 130; Himes, *Medical History of Contraception*, pp. 201–2; Harrison Reeves, "The Birth Control Industry," *American Mercury* 155 (November 1936): 286; "New Legislation," *Journal of Contraception*, August–September 1937, p. 165; "Accident of Birth," *Fortune*, p. 108; Randolph Cautley, Gilbert W. Beebe, and Robert L. Dickinson, "Rubber Sheaths as Venereal Disease Prophylactics," *American Journal of the Medical Sciences* (February 1938): 156; PPFA 1943 study, p. 25, Planned Parenthood Federation of America Papers, Sophia Smith Collection; "General Operation of the Prophylactic and Contraceptive Law in Oregon," *Journal of Contraception*, November 1937, p. 196; Anne Rapport, "The Legal Aspects of Marketing Feminine Hygiene Products," *Drug and Cosmetic Industry* 38 (April 1936): 474.

17. Testimony of Merle L. Youngs, Transcript of Record, *Youngs Rubber Corporation v.*

C. I. Lee & Company, pp. 28–31, Records of the U.S. Court of Appeals for the Second Circuit.

18. Dickinson and Bryant, *Control of Conception*, p. 65; Consumers Union of United States, *Analysis of Contraceptive Materials* (1937), pp. 20–21; PPFA 1943 study, p. 25, Planned Parenthood Federation of America Papers, Sophia Smith Collection; Consumers Union of United States, *Analysis of Contraceptive Materials* (New York: Consumers Union of United States, 1945), p. 28; Naismith, "Racket in Contraceptives," p. 12.

19. Dickinson and Bryant, *Control of Conception*, p. 65; Himes, *Medical History of Contraception*, pp. 201–5; Reeves, "Birth Control Industry," p. 286; Rachel Lynn Palmer and Sarah Koslow Greenberg, *Facts and Frauds in Woman's Hygiene: A Medical Guide against Misleading Claims and Dangerous Products* (Garden City, N.Y.: Garden City Publishing Company, 1938), pp. 271–72; "Accident of Birth," *Fortune*, p. 108; Cautley, Beebe, and Dickinson, "Rubber Sheaths as Venereal Disease Prophylactics," pp. 155–56; Consumers Union of United States, *Analysis of Contraceptive Materials* (1937), p. 13; House of Representatives, 72nd Congress, *Hearings before the Committee on Ways and Means*, May 19 and 20, 1932 (Washington, D.C.: Government Printing Office, 1932), p. 87.

    Himes's observation was corroborated by a major in the Medical Corps in 1937 who said he remembered "that one druggist in San Antonio, Texas, stated that he was able to pay his rent by his income from the sale of condoms." Memo, "Venereal Disease," from Charles G. Souder to Colonel Gentry, March 2, 1937, box 112, Correspondence, 1928–1937, Records of the Office of the Surgeon General, National Archives.

20. Transcript of Record, *Youngs Rubber* v. *C. I. Lee & Company*, pp. 31–35, Records of the U.S. Court of Appeals for the Second Circuit; Murphy, *Condom Industry in the United States*, pp. 11–12.

21. Transcript of Record, *Youngs Rubber* v. *C. I. Lee & Company*, p. 35–36, 49, 91–92, Records of the U.S. Court of Appeals for the Second Circuit; *Youngs Rubber Corporation* v. *C. I. Lee & Co.* 45 F. (2d), pp. 103–5.

22. U.S. Patent Office, *Official Gazette*, January 13, 1931, p. 290, March 31, 1931, p. 1075, May 26, 1931, p. 883.

23. See, for instance, Trojan advertisements in the January, February, March, April, and May 1931 volumes of the *Druggists' Circular* and the December 1931 volume of *American Druggist*.

24. Testimony of Merle L. Youngs, Transcript of Record, *Frank B. Killian and Company* v. *Allied Latex Corporation*, Civ. 43–404, April 4, 1949, p. 70, Records of the United States District Court for the Southern District of New York, National Archives, Regional Office, New York.

25. Transcript of Record, *Frank B. Killian and Company* v. *Allied Latex Corporation*, pp. 10, 61, 70, Records of the United States District Court for the Southern District of New York.

26. Testimony of Merle Youngs, Transcript of Record, *Frank B. Killian and Company* v.

Allied Latex Corporation, pp. 74–75, Records of the United States District Court for the Southern District of New York.

27. Transcript of Record, *Frank B. Killian and Company* v. *Allied Latex Corporation,* pp. 11–12, Records of the United States District Court for the Southern District of New York.

28. Transcript of Record, *Perry Stevens* v. *Carl Schmid,* pp. 282, 336–38, Records of the United States District Court for the Southern District of New York; "Accident of Birth," *Fortune,* p. 108; Transcript of Record, *Frank B. Killian and Company* v. *Allied Latex Corporation,* pp. 9–12, Records of the United States District Court for the Southern District of New York; U.S. Patent Office, patent no. 2,128,827, August 30, 1938.

29. Transcript of Record, *Frank B. Killian and Company* v. *Allied Latex Corporation,* pp. 9–12, 76, Records of the United States District Court for the Southern District of New York; Himes, *Medical History of Contraception,* pp. 202–4; Cautley, Beebe, and Dickinson, "Rubber Sheaths as Venereal Disease Prophylactics," pp. 155–56, 162; Christopher Tietze, *The Condom as a Contraceptive* (New York: National Committee on Maternal Health, 1960), pp. 6–10.

30. "Accident of Birth," *Fortune,* p. 108; Transcript of Record, *Frank B. Killian and Company* v. *Allied Latex Corporation,* p. 76, Records of the United States District Court for the Southern District of New York.

31. Transcript of Record, *Frank B. Killian and Company* v. *Allied Latex Corporation,* pp. 76–82, Records of the United States District Court for the Southern District of New York.

32. Cautley, Beebe, and Dickinson, "Rubber Sheaths as Venereal Disease Prophylactics," p. 155; "Accident of Birth," *Fortune,* p. 108.

33. Consumers Union of United States, *Analysis of Contraceptive Materials* (1937), pp. 12–13, 20–21; Consumers Union of United States, *Analysis of Contraceptive Materials* (1945), p. 22; Tietze, *Condom as a Contraceptive,* p. 6; PPFA 1943 study, p. 25, Planned Parenthood Federation of America Papers, Sophia Smith Collection; "Accident of Birth," *Fortune,* p. 110.

34. "Accident of Birth," *Fortune,* p. 110.

35. Dickinson and Bryant, *Control of Conception,* p. 65; Himes, *Medical History of Contraception,* pp. 201–2; "Accident of Birth," *Fortune,* p. 108; Cautley, Beebe, and Dickinson, "Rubber Sheaths as Venereal Disease Prophylactics," pp. 155–56.

36. Cautley, Beebe, and Dickinson, "Rubber Sheaths as Venereal Disease Prophylactics," pp. 156–58.

37. Ibid., p. 156.

38. Himes, *Medical History of Contraception,* p. 206; Cautley, Beebe, and Dickinson, "Rubber Sheaths as Venereal Disease Prophylactics," pp. 156–60; "Accident of Birth," *Fortune,* p. 100.

39. Transcript of Record, *Youngs Rubber* v. *C. I. Lee & Company,* p. 50, Records of the U.S. Court of Appeals for the Second Circuit.

40. Ibid., pp. 44–45.

41. "The Oregon Act on Contraception," *Journal of Contraception*, June–July 1937, pp. 142–43; "New Legislation," *Journal of Contraception*, p. 165; "The Idaho Law on Contraception," *Journal of Contraception*, November 1937, pp. 213–15; Murphy, *Condom Industry in the United States*, p. 9.

42. "Standards for Rubber Prophylactics," *Journal of Contraception*, April 1938, p. 94.

43. Transcript of Record, *Youngs Rubber* v. *Allied Latex*, April 13, 14, 15, 1950, Records of the U.S. Court of Appeals for the Second Circuit.

44. U.S. Patent Office, patent no. 2,213,113, August 27, 1940.

45. Transcript of Record, *Youngs Rubber* v. *Allied Latex*, p. 36, Records of the U.S. Court of Appeals for the Second Circuit.

46. "Information on Manufacturers of Prophylactics from the Administration Files," A.F. 19-186, box 178, FDA History Office; "The Adulteration and Misbranding of Prophylactics," *Journal of Contraception*, June–July 1937, p. 14; Consumers Union of United States, *A Report on Contraceptive Materials* (1945), p. 21.

47. "Adulteration and Misbranding of Prophylactics," *Journal of Contraception*, March 1939, p. 69.

48. "Information on Manufacturers of Prophylactics from the Administration Files," FDA History Office.

49. Tietze, *Condom as a Contraceptive*, p. 11.

50. Murphy, *Condom Industry in the United States*, p. 54.

51. Ibid., pp. 38–42. A report sponsored by Planned Parenthood Federation of America estimated in 1943 that roughly $75 million of the $100 million condom trade was carried out through "established drug channels." See PPFA 1943 study, Planned Parenthood Federation of America Papers, Sophia Smith Collection.

52. Interview between Mr. George McCleary of the sales department of Julius Schmid, Inc., and Clarence Gamble, September 30, 1940, box 64, folder 623, Planned Parenthood Federation of America Papers, Sophia Smith Collection; "Information on Manufacturers of Prophylactics from the Administration Files," p. 2; FDA Inspection Memo of 1-12-48, AF 19-186; "Prophylactics Memorandum," 6-18-1948; "Memorandum Report of Factory Inspection," 7-8-49, AF 19-186; "Factory Inspection Report," 5-11-55, AF 19-186; Establishment Inspection Report, 3-8-63, AF 19-186; "Memorandum of Interview," 10-30-1964, all FDA History Office; Murphy, *Condom Industry in the United States*, p. 12.

53. PPFA 1943 study, pp. 18–22, Planned Parenthood Federation of America Papers, Sophia Smith Collection; Tietze and Gamble, "Condom as a Contraceptive Method in Public Health Work," pp. 97–113; Naismith, "Racket in Contraceptives," p. 12.

54. According to *Fortune*, sales from condoms accounted for $38 million of the industry's annual $250 million sales. See "Accident of Birth," *Fortune*, p. 84; Naismith, "Racket in Contraceptives"; Ronald Freedman, Pascal K. Whelpton, and Arthur A. Campbell, *Family Planning, Sterility, and Population Growth* (New York: McGraw-Hill, 1959); Lee Rainwater, *And the Poor Get Children: Sex, Contraception, and Family Planning in the Working Class* (Chicago: Quadrangle Books, 1960), pp. 27–28.

9. DEVELOPING THE PILL

1. Elizabeth Siegel Watkins, *On the Pill: A Social History of Oral Contraceptives, 1950–1970* (Baltimore, Md.: Johns Hopkins University Press, 1998), p. 34.

2. Lawrence Lader, "Three Men Who Made a Revolution," *New York Times Magazine*, April 10, 1966.

3. James Reed, *From Private Vice to Public Virtue: The Birth Control Movement and American Society since 1830* (New York: Basic Books, 1978), pp. 334–36.

4. Ibid., pp. 334–39; Bernard Asbell, *The Pill: A Biography of the Drug That Changed the World* (New York: Random House, 1995), pp. 30–32; Watkins, *On the Pill*, pp. 26–27.

5. Reed, *From Private Vice to Public Virtue*, pp. 336–37.

6. Ellen Chesler, *Woman of Valor: Margaret Sanger and the Birth Control Movement in America* (New York: Simon and Schuster, 1992), p. 431; Reed, *From Private Vice to Public Virtue*, p. 337.

7. McCormick and Sanger quoted in R. Christian Johnson, "Feminism, Philanthrophy, and Science in the Development of the Oral Contraceptive Pill," *Pharmacy in History* 19 (1977): 72–73. The earliest surviving correspondence between the two women is from 1928.

8. Quoted in Paul Vaughan, *The Pill on Trial* (New York: Coward-McCann, Inc., 1972), p. 25.

9. Quoted in Asbell, *The Pill*, p. 9.

10. Watkins, *On the Pill*, p. 19.

11. Robert Sheehan, "The Birth-Control 'Pill,'" *Fortune*, April 1958, p. 155; Kim Yanoshik and Judy Norsigian, "Contraception, Control, and Choice: International Perspectives," in Kathryn Strother Ratcliff, ed., *Healing Technology: Feminist Perspectives* (Ann Arbor: University of Michigan Press, 1989), pp. 66–67; Huxley quoted in "Men or Maggots?" *Newsweek*, November 30, 1959.

12. Sheehan, "Birth-Control 'Pill,'" p. 155; Vogt quoted in Johnson, "Feminism, Philanthropy, and Science," p. 67. Also see Andrea Tone, "Violence by Design: Contraceptive Technology and the Invasion of the Female Body," in Michael Bellesiles, ed., *Lethal Imagination: Violence and Brutality in American History* (New York: New York University Press, 1999), pp. 378–79.

13. Quoted in Lara Marks, *Sexual Chemistry: An International History of the Pill* (New Haven, Conn.: Yale University Press, forthcoming), chap. 2, p. 11.

14. David Halberstam, *The Fifties* (New York: Villard Books, 1993), p. 289; "Gregory Pincus," *Triangle: The Sandoz Journal of Medical Science* 7 (1966): 194; Asbell, *The Pill*; Ruth Schwartz Cowan, *A Social History of American Technology* (New York: Oxford University Press, 1997), p. 320.

15. Quoted in Asbell, *The Pill*, p. 122.

16. Asbell, *The Pill*, p. 123.

17. Vaughan, *The Pill on Trial*, p. 51; F. B. Colton, "Steroids and 'The Pill': Early Steroid Research at Searle," *Steroids* 58 (December 1992): 624–30; Johnson, "Feminism, Philanthropy, and Science," pp. 69–70; www.searlehealthnet.com/searle.

18. Quoted in Carl Djerassi, *The Pill, Pygmy Chimps, and Degas' Horse: The Autobiography of Carl Djerassi* (New York: Basic Books, 1992), pp. 33–34.
19. Djerassi, *The Pill, Pygmy Chimps, and Degas' Horse*, p. 38.
20. Asbell, *The Pill*, p. 117; Djerassi, *The Pill, Pygmy Chimps, and Degas' Horse*, p. 48.
21. Quoted in Asbell, *The Pill*, p. 118.
22. Quoted in Steven M. Spencer, "The Birth Control Revolution," *Saturday Evening Post*, January 15, 1966, p. 23; Vaughan, *The Pill on Trial*, p. 23.
23. Planned Parenthood Federation of America, *Research in Human Reproduction*, p. 9, 1948 pamphlet, folder 1948, box 18, Planned Parenthood Federation of America Papers, Sophia Smith Collection, Smith College.
24. Watkins, *On the Pill*, p. 26; Memo from NIH Consultants to Dr. David Price, 1961, container 49, Pincus Papers, Manuscripts Division, Library of Congress.
25. In 1956, the Dickinson Research Memorial was sponsoring ten separate birth control studies, including ones on spermatotoxins, chimpanzee radiation, cervical mucus, and steroidal sterilization. Planned Parenthood Federation of America, *The Control of Human Reproduction* (New York, 1957), pp. 5, 11, container 28, Pincus Papers.
26. Marks, *Sexual Chemistry*, chap. 2, p. 2.
27. H. H. Simmer, "On the History of Hormonal Contraception," *Contraception* 1 (January 1970): 3–44; Watkins, *On the Pill*, p. 22; Robert A. Hatcher, James Trussell, Felicia Stewart, Gary K. Stewart, Deborah Kowal, Felicia Guest, Willard Cates, Jr., and Michael S. Policar, *Contraceptive Technology*, 16th rev. ed. (New York: Irvington, 1994), p. 286; Djerassi, *The Pill, Pygmy Chimps, and Degas' Horse*, p. 51.
28. Marks, *Sexual Chemistry*, chap. 3, pp. 1–2.
29. Quoted in Lader, "Three Men Who Made a Revolution"; Watkins, *On the Pill*, p. 22; Cowan, *Social History of American Technology*, pp. 320–21.
30. Quoted in Asbell, *The Pill*, pp. 92, 104.
31. Quoted in Halberstam, *The Fifties*, p. 290.
32. Asbell, *The Pill*, p. 124.
33. Halberstam, *The Fifties*, p. 602.
34. Pincus to Dr. Abraham Stone, January 25, 1952, container 12, Pincus Papers.
35. Marks, *Sexual Chemistry*, chap. 3, p. 13; Johnson, "Feminism, Philanthropy, and Science," p. 71.
36. Richard Lincoln and Lisa Kaeser, "Whatever Happened to the Contraceptive Revolution?" *Family Planning Perspectives* 20 (January/February 1988): 20–24; Marjorie A. Koblinsky, Frederick S. Jaffe, and Roy O. Creep, "Funding for Reproductive Research: The Status and the Needs," *Family Planning Perspectives* 8 (September/October 1976): 212–13.
37. Quoted in "The Administration: About-Face on Birth Control," *Time*, December 9, 1966, p. 31.
38. Quoted in William H. Robertson, "Contraception: Past, Present, and Future," *Alabama Journal of Medical Sciences* 12 (October 1975): 318; Watkins, *On the Pill*, p. 68.

39. Spencer, "Birth Control Revolution"; Robertson, "Contraception," p. 319; Watkins, *On the Pill*, p. 68.

40. "Contraceptive Technology: Advances Needed in Fundamental Research," *Science* 168 (May 15, 1970): 805. In contrast, the Ford and Rockefeller Foundations and the Population Council contributed $4.8 million and the drug industry $17.2 million.

41. Watkins, *On the Pill*, pp. 17, 25–26; Koblinsky, Jaffe, and Creep, "Funding for Reproductive Research," pp. 212–13.

42. Quoted in Marks, *Sexual Chemistry*, chap. 3, p. 14.

43. Asbell, *The Pill*, pp. 126–27.

44. Halberstam, *The Fifties*, p. 601; Lader, "Three Men Who Made a Revolution."

45. John Rock, "The Scientific Case against Rigid Legal Restrictions on Medical Birth-Control Advice," *Clinics* 1 (April 1943): 1598–602.

46. Quoted in Lader, "Three Men Who Made a Revolution."

47. Oscar Hechter quoted in Halberstam, *The Fifties*, p. 601.

48. Quoted in Asbell, *The Pill*, p. 128.

49. Quoted in Djerassi, *The Pill, Pygmy Chimps, and Degas' Horse*, pp. 51–63; Vaughan, *The Pill on Trial*, pp. 16–17; Cowan, *Social History of American Technology*, p. 321; Asbell, *The Pill*, p. 110.

50. "Procedure for Progesterone Tests," 1954 [n.d.], container 17, Pincus Papers; Vaughan, *The Pill on Trial*, pp. 30–31; Halberstam, *The Fifties*, p. 602.

51. Quoted in Vaughan, *The Pill on Trial*, p. 6.

52. McCormick to Sanger, July 21, 1954, Margaret Sanger Papers, Sophia Smith Collection. Also see Lara Marks, " 'A "Cage" of Ovulating Females': The History of the Early Oral Contraceptive Pill Clinical Trials, 1950–1959," in Soraya De Chadarevain and Harmke Kamminga, eds., *Molecularizing Biology and Medicine: New Practices and Alliances, 1930s–1970s* (Reading, U.K.: Harwood Academic Press, 1997).

53. McCormick to Sanger, May 31, 1955, Margaret Sanger Papers, Sophia Smith Collection.

54. Lader, "Three Men Who Made a Revolution."

55. "Procedure for Progesterone Tests," 1954 [n.d.], container 17, "Long-Term Administration of Vilane to Human Subjects," April 1957, container 109, Pincus to I. C. Winter, October 21, 1957, container 109, all Pincus Papers; "Regulating Pregnancy," *Time*, October 21, 1957, p. 70; Lara Marks, "Human Guinea Pigs? The History of the Early Oral Contraceptive Trials," *History and Technology* 15 (1999): 270–71.

56. Carmen R. De Alvarado and Christopher Tietze, "Birth Control in Puerto Rico," *Human Fertility* 12 (March 1947): 15; "A Study of Contraceptive Services in Puerto Rico," *Human Fertility* (December 1942): 184; Doone Williams and Greer Williams, *Every Child a Wanted Child: Clarence James Gamble, M.D., and His Work in the Birth Control Movement* (Boston: Harvard University Press, 1978), pp. 159–61.

57. De Alvarado and Tietze, "Birth Control in Puerto Rico"; "A Study of Contraceptive Services in Puerto Rico," *Human Fertility*, pp. 15–16.

58. Pincus to McCormick, March 5, 1954, container 17, Pincus Papers; Family Planning Association of Puerto Rico, "Application for a Family Planning Project to the Office of Economic Opportunity," September 1965, container 90, Pincus Papers; "A Study of Contraceptive Services in Puerto Rico," *Human Fertility*; De Alvarado and Tietze, "Birth Control in Puerto Rico."

59. Pincus to McCormick, March 5, 1954, container 17, Pincus Papers.

60. Ibid.

61. Ibid.

62. Marks, "Human Guinea Pigs?" p. 272.

63. Albert Q. Maisel, "New Hope for Childless Women," *Ladies' Home Journal*, August 1957.

64. Gregory Pincus, "Field Trials with Norethynodrel as an Oral Contraceptive," pp. 1–3, paper presented at the Sixth International Conference on Planned Parenthood, New Delhi, February 1959, John Rock Papers, Countway Library of Medicine, Harvard Medical School, Boston, Mass.; Manuel E. Paniagua, "Report on Oral Contraceptive," container 28, Pincus Papers; Asbell, *The Pill*, p. 145. A double-blind study using placebos and Enovid in Puerto Rico to determine the "true" incidence of side effects is discussed in Pincus to Lee D. van Antwerp, July 4, 1958, container 110, Pincus Papers.

65. Pincus, "Field Trials with Norethynodrel as an Oral Contraceptive," pp. 1–3; Pincus to McCormick, December 28, 1955, container 17, Pincus Papers; Reed, *From Private Vice to Public Virtue*, p. 359.

66. Translation from *El Imparcial*, April 21, 1956, container 22, Pincus Papers.

67. Adaline Pendleton Satterthwaite to Gamble, December 2, 1959, folder 819, box 50, Clarence Gamble Papers, Countway Library of Medicine.

68. Rice-Wray cited in Asbell, *The Pill*, p. 147; Manuel E. Paniagua, "Report on Oral Contraceptive," p. 28, Pincus Papers.

69. Lader, "Three Men Who Made a Revolution"; Pincus to Edris Rice-Wray, June 14, 1956, container 22, Pincus Papers. Emphasis added. Also see Pincus to Margaret Sanger, July 22, 1957, container 29, and Pincus to Lee D. van Antwerp, July 4, 1958, container 110, Pincus Papers.

70. Adaline Pendleton Satterthwaite to Gamble, June 21, 1957, and July 17, 1957, both in folder 797, box 49, Clarence Gamble Papers.

71. Edris Rice-Wray to Gregory Pincus, June 11, 1956, container 22, Pincus Papers.

72. Gregory Pincus, Celso R. Garcia, John Rock, Manuel Paniagua, Adaline Pendleton, Felix Laraque, Rene Nicholas, Raymond Borno, and Verginiaud Pean, "Effectiveness of an Oral Contraceptive," *Science* 130 (July 10, 1959): 81.

73. Albert Raymond to Pincus, October 4 and 17, 1957, container 109, Pincus Papers.

74. Quoted in Vaughan, *The Pill on Trial*, pp. 49–50.

75. Letter to Pincus, October 27, 1960, container 43, Pincus Papers.

76. Letter to Pincus, March 17, 1960, container 43, Pincus Papers.

77. Letter to Pincus, October 31, 1957, container 25, Pincus Papers.

78. Pincus to Sanger, July 22, 1957, container 29, Pincus Papers.

79. McCormick quoted in Asbell, *The Pill*, p. 159.

80. Letter from Ruth Crozier for Gregory Pincus, June 14, 1958, container 31, Pincus Papers.

81. Irwin Winter, "Industrial Pressure and the Population Problem—The FDA and the Pill," *Journal of the American Medical Association*, May 11, 1970, p. 1067.

82. Ibid.

83. Watkins, *On the Pill*, p. 12.

84. Asbell, *The Pill*, p. 157; Watkins, *On the Pill*, p. 24.

85. Quoted in Asbell, *The Pill*, pp. 159–60.

86. Djerassi, *The Pill, Pygmy Chimps, and Degas' Horse*, p. 63; Mary Steichen Calderone to Pincus, June 19, 1959, and Pincus to Calderone, June 22, 1959, container 40, Pincus Papers.

87. Irwin Winter to Pincus, December 29, 1958, container 110, Pincus Papers.

88. Sheehan, "The Birth-Control 'Pill,' " p. 222.

89. The FDA approved the sedative Librium, for instance, tested on 1,163 patients, within months of approving Enovid. The Librium tests involved a greater patient total, but the total itself fails to reveal the separate clinical trials, each conducted to evaluate a separate use of Librium, which constituted the whole. Hence though all of the 897 enrolled in the Pill trial were involved in determining Enovid's safety as a contraceptive, patients in the Librium tests spanned the pharmaceutical landscape: 570 patients tested its benefits as an antipsychotic, but only 3 tested its usefulness for epilepsy. But when the FDA approved Librium, it did so for both of these indications, and more. As the historian Lara Marks has argued, judging the wisdom of FDA action by a crude attention to numbers "distorts the kinds of evidence that investigators and pharmaceutical regulators were looking for." See Marks, "Human Guinea Pigs?" p. 281.

90. Quoted in Asbell, *The Pill*, p. 167.

10. THE PILL IN PRACTICE

1. Sharon Snider, "The Pill: 30 Years of Safety Concerns," *FDA Consumer*, December 1990, p. 9; Elizabeth Siegel Watkins, *On the Pill: A Social History of Oral Contraceptives, 1950–1970* (Baltimore, Md.: Johns Hopkins University Press, 1998), p. 34.

2. Author interview with Elizabeth Linden, March 6, 1998, Pasadena, California. Name changed to protect anonymity. Transcript in author's possession.

3. Ibid.

4. Letter to Pincus, n.d., container 52, letter to Pincus, June 29, 1963, container 60, Mrs. Jack Feit to Pincus, April 24, 1962, container 52, all in Pincus Papers, Manuscripts Division, Library of Congress.

5. Barbara Seaman, *The Doctors' Case against the Pill: 25th Anniversary Edition* (Alameda, Calif.: Hunter House, 1995), p. 56.

6. "The Pill," words and music by Lorene Allen, Don McHan, and T. D. Bayless,

recorded by Loretta Lynn, Science News Service, Smithsonian Institution, Washington, D.C.

7. These women's stories are discussed in Seaman, *Doctors' Case against the Pill*, pp. 48–51.

8. Steven M. Spencer, "The Birth Control Revolution," *Saturday Evening Post*, January 15, 1966, p. 21.

9. Louis Lasagna, "Caution on the Pill," *Saturday Review*, November 2, 1968; Seaman, *Doctors' Case against the Pill*, p. 45.

10. Lasagna, "Caution on the Pill"; Seaman, *Doctors' Case against the Pill*, p. 45.

11. Ruth Schwartz Cowan, *A Social History of American Technology* (New York: Oxford University Press, 1997), p. 322.

12. Snider, "The Pill: 30 Years of Safety Concerns," p. 10; Robert Sheehan, "The Birth-Control 'Pill,' " *Fortune*, April 1958, p. 222.

13. Sheehan, "Birth-Control 'Pill,' " p. 155. Also see Carl Djerassi, *The Pill, Pygmy Chimps, and Degas' Horse: The Autobiography of Carl Djerassi* (New York: Basic Books, 1992), pp. 118–19.

14. Leroy Pope, "Will Birth Control Hit Economy?" *New York World Telegram*, June 16, 1964.

15. Pincus to Arthur Ogren, February 16, 1960, container 43, Pincus Papers.

16. Letter from John Rock, October 10, 1961, John Rock Papers, Countway Library of Medicine, Harvard Medical School, Boston, Mass.

17. Quoted in Lawrence Lader, "Three Men Who Made a Revolution," *New York Times Magazine*, April 10, 1966.

18. Patricia McBroom, "The Pill Has Brought No Revolution in Morals," January 10, 1968, Science News Service, Smithsonian Institution.

19. "Birth Control: The Pill and the Church," *Newsweek*, July 6, 1964, pp. 51–52; John Rock, "Let's Be Honest about the Pill," *Journal of the American Medical Association* 192 (May 3, 1965): 401–2; John Rock, "We Can End the Battle over Birth Control!" *Good Housekeeping*, July 1961.

20. "Birth Control: The Pill and the Church," *Newsweek*, p. 52.

21. Watkins, *On the Pill*, p. 47.

22. "Oral Contraceptives—U.S.," Remarks of Alejandro Zaffaroni, Ph.D., President of Syntex Research, News Release, July 15, 1965, Science News Service, Smithsonian Institution.

23. "Searle Will Cut Dose, Price of Contraceptive Pills If FDA Approves," *Wall Street Journal*, July 10, 1962, p. 6; Mary C. Stokes, news release, August 6, 1963, Science News Service, Smithsonian Institution; *New York World Telegram*, July 20, 1963; Lader, "Three Men Who Made a Revolution"; Linda Grant, *Sexing the Millennium: Women and the Sexual Revolution* (New York: Grove Press, 1994), p. 54.

24. "Mexican Maker Says It Has Cut Cost of Drug for Birth-Control Pills," *Wall Street Journal*, October 8, 1962; Bernard Asbell, *The Pill: A Biography of the Drug That Changed the World* (New York: Random House, 1995), p. 169.

25. "Sequential Oral Contraceptives," *Medical Letter on Drugs and Therapies*, Septem-

ber 24, 1965. Unlike the older oral contraceptives, which contained a fixed amount of estrogen and progestin, the sequential pills contained two differently formulated tablets: estrogen-only pills, taken during the first phase of the menstrual cycle, and combined estrogen-progestin pills for the remainder.

26. Jane Brody, "The Pill: A Revolution in Birth Control since Its Introduction," *New York Times*, May 31, 1966; G. D. Searle, *Looking Back at 30 Years of Birth Control*, Science News Service, Smithsonian Institution; G. D. Searle, *Contraception: From Antiquity to Science through Research in the Service of Medicine*, Science News Service, Smithsonian Institution; "Pill Makers See No Loss of Sales," Science News Service, Smithsonian Institution; Harry Levin, "Commercial Distribution of Contraceptives," *Demography* 5 (1968): 934.

27. Andrea Tone, *Controlling Reproduction: An American History* (Wilmington, Del.: Scholarly Resources, 1997), pp. 183–86; also see *Griswold* v. *Connecticut* 381 U.S. 479 (1965) and *Eisenstadt* v. *Baird* 405 U.S. 438 (1972).

28. Author telephone interview with Birgit Haus, August 2000. The name of the interviewee has been changed to protect her privacy.

29. Mary Calderone to Case Canfield, December 6, 1961, box 4, folder 50, Mary Steichen Calderone Papers, Schlesinger Library, Radcliffe Institute, Cambridge, Mass.

30. "Industry: In the Shadows," *Time*, February 15, 1963; Alfred D. Sollins and Raymond L. Belsky, "Commercial Production and Distribution of Contraceptives," *Reports on Population/Family Planning* 4 (June 1970): 3.

31. "Pill Makers See No Loss of Sales," Science News Service, Smithsonian Institution.

32. Sollins and Belsky, "Commercial Production and Distribution of Contraceptives," pp. 3, 5, 10; "Industry: In the Shadows," *Time*.

33. Testimony of John Madry in U.S. House of Representatives, Committee on Government Operations, *Regulation of Medical Devices (Intrauterine Contraceptive Devices)*, 93rd Cong., 1st sess. (Washington, D.C.: Government Printing Office, 1973), pp. 5–6.

34. Andrea Tone, "Violence by Design: Contraceptive Technology and the Invasion of the Female Body," in Michael Bellesiles, ed., *Lethal Imagination: Violence and Brutality in American History* (New York: New York University Press, 1999), p. 381; Mary Ryan, "Reproduction in American History," *Journal of Interdisciplinary History* 10 (1979): 330.

35. S. S. Spivack, "The Doctor's Role in Family Planning," *Journal of the American Medical Association* 188 (1964): 152; Morton A. Silver, "Birth Control and the Private Physician," *Family Planning Perspectives* 4 (April 1972): 43.

36. Lois R. Chevalier and Leonard Cohen, "The Terrible Trouble with the Birth-Control Pills," *Ladies' Home Journal*, July 1967, pp. 44–45.

37. Interview with Jack Linden, February 16, 1998, Pasadena, California. Transcript of interview in author's possession. The interviewee's name has been changed to protect his privacy.

38. Ibid.

39. Pincus to Warren Nelson, December 21, 1961, container 49, Pincus Papers.

40. John G. Searle, press release, August 9, 1962, Science News Service, Smithsonian Institution.

41. Quoted in Watkins, *On the Pill*, p. 82.

42. "Drug Amendments of 1962—Federal Food, Drug, and Cosmetic Act: A Summary," *Journal of New Drugs* 2 (September–October 1962): 315–18; U.S. Food and Drug Administration, *From Test Tube to Patient: Improving Health through Human Drugs* (Washington, D.C.: FDA, 1999), p. 37.

43. John G. Searle, news release, August 9, 1962, Science News Service, Smithsonian Institution.

44. Watkins, *On the Pill*, p. 82.

45. Elizabeth Mirel, "Risks of Birth Control Pill Seen for Women over 35," August 2, 1963, Science News Service, Smithsonian Institution; "Enovid Defended by Medical Group," *New York Times*, August 9, 1962; U.S. Department of Health, Education, and Welfare, Food and Drug Administration, press release, August 4, 1963, container 64, Pincus Papers; "Searle Agrees to Warn Doctors, Pharmacists on Use of Enovid Pill," *Wall Street Journal*, August 19, 1962; Watkins, *On the Pill*, p. 82.

46. Quoted in Watkins, *On the Pill*, p. 86.

47. Paul Vaughan, *The Pill on Trial* (New York: Coward-McCann, Inc., 1972), p. 91; Watkins, *On the Pill*.

48. Claudia Dreifus, foreword to *Doctors' Case against the Pill*, by Seaman, p. viii.

49. Seaman, *Doctors' Case against the Pill*, p. 45.

50. Ibid., p. 19.

51. Spencer, "Birth Control Revolution," p. 24. A 1970 study found that most women who quit oral contraceptives did so because of adverse effects they experienced, such as nausea, weight gain, headaches, and fatigue. See Watkins, *On the Pill*, p. 100.

52. "Oral Contraceptives—U.S.," Remarks of Alejandro Zaffaroni, July 15, 1965; "The Pill: Do Its Benefits Outweigh Its Hazards?" *Consumer Reports*, May 1970, p. 319; "The Pill at 40: Renewed, Improved, and in Its Prime," *New York Times*, October 20, 1988; author interview with Elizabeth Linden.

53. B. Burt Gerstman, Thomas P. Gross, Dianne L. Kennedy, Ridgely C. Bennett, Dianne K. Tomita, and Bruce Stadel, "Trends in the Content and Use of Oral Contraceptives in the United States, 1964–1988," *American Journal of Public Health* 81 (January 1991): 90–96. The reasons behind manufacturers' dosing changes were threefold. First, they made oral contraceptives cheaper to make and sell. Second, medical studies found that contraceptive efficacy was not diminished by a lower estrogen content. Third, lower-dosed pills were in keeping with medical reports that linked estrogen to many of the Pill's troubling side effects, including blood clots.

54. Letter to John Rock, March 22, 1965, Rock Papers.

55. Letter to Gregory Pincus, April 12, 1966, container 95, Pincus Papers.

56. Letter to Rock, January 16, 1963, Rock Papers.

57. Letter from Rock, January 22, 1964, Rock Papers.

58. Letter of Gregory Pincus, April 14, 1965, container 95, Pincus Papers.

59. Susan Douglas, *Where the Girls Are: Growing Up Female with the Mass Media* (New York: Times Books, 1994).

60. Lara Marks, *Sexual Chemistry: An International History of the Pill* (New Haven, Conn.: Yale University Press, forthcoming), chap. 6, p. 17; Nelson quoted in Watkins, *On the Pill*, p. 107.

61. Watkins, *On the Pill*, pp. 105–8.

62. Douglas, *Where the Girls Are*, p. 172; Watkins, *On the Pill*, pp. 109–16.

63. Ortho Pharmaceutical Corporation, press release, "Gallup Poll Indicates the Pill Is Coming Back," April 1970, Science News Service, Smithsonian Institution; Gerstman et al., "Trends in the Content and Use of Oral Contraceptives," p. 90; "Poll Finds . . . ," *New York Times*, February 2, 1970; Watkins, *On the Pill*, p. 115.

64. "Washington Women's Liberation Statement on Birth Control Pills," U.S. Senate, Subcommittee on Monopoly of the Select Committee on Small Business, *Competitive Problems in the Drug Industry: Present Status of Competition in the Pharmaceutical Industry; Oral Contraceptives*, 91st Cong., 2nd sess. (Washington, D.C.: Government Printing Office, 1970), vol. 3: pt. 17, pp. 7283–84.

65. Letter quoted in Watkins, *On the Pill*, p. 123.

66. *Competitive Problems in the Drug Industry*, pt. 15, p. 5924.

67. Ibid., pt. 15, p. 6151.

68. Dr. Frederick Robbins, quoted in Seaman, *Doctors' Case against the Pill*, p. 11.

69. *Competitive Problems in the Drug Industry*, pt. 16, p. 6269.

70. Marks, *Sexual Chemistry*, chap. 6, p. 19; Watkins, *On the Pill*, p. 126.

71. Jennifer Macleod, "How to Hold a Wife: A Bridegroom's Guide," *Village Voice*, February 11, 1971, p. 5.

72. "The Pill," *Redbook*, January 1966, p. 76.

73. Robert W. Kistner, "What the Pill Does to Husbands," *Ladies' Home Journal*, January 1969, p. 68.

74. Ibid.

75. D. J. Patanelli, "Male Fertility Control," paper presented at the Eleventh National Medicinal Chemistry Symposium of the American Chemical Society, June 25, 1968, Quebec City, Canada, Science News Service, Smithsonian Institution.

76. Letter of John Rock, May 17, 1966, Rock Papers.

77. Sheldon J. Segal, "Contraceptive Research: A Male Chauvinist Plot?" *Family Planning Perspectives* 4 (July 1972): 22–26.

78. Ibid., p. 22.

79. McCormick quoted in Marks, *Sexual Chemistry*, chap. 2, p. 11.

80. "Contraceptive for Men Cheaper Than Aspirin," *Washington Post*, April 3, 1963; Leslie Aldridge, "7,000,000 American Women Take the Pill," *Esquire*, January 1969, p. 93; "Male Pill," *Newsweek*, April 15, 1963, p. 94, Science News Service, Smithsonian Institution; "Industry: In the Shadows," *Time*, p. 85.

81. Segal, "Contraceptive Research," pp. 22–23; Aldridge, "7,000,000 American Women Take the Pill," p. 93.

82. Carl T. Rowan, " 'Genocide' Fear Deserves Study," *Evening Star* (Washington, D.C.), June 24, 1970.

83. Dorothy Roberts, *Killing the Black Body: Race, Reproduction, and the Meaning of Liberty* (New York: Vintage, 1997), p. 99.

84. "NAACP 57th Annual Convention Resolutions," "NAACP Correspondence from 1962" folder, Planned Parenthood Federation of America Papers, Sophia Smith Collection.

85. Dick Gregory, "My Answer to Genocide," *Ebony*, October 1971, p. 66.

86. Wylda Cowles to Alan Guttmacher, March 28, 1966, "Black Attitudes from 1962" folder, Planned Parenthood Federation of America Papers, Sophia Smith Collection.

87. Roberts, *Killing the Black Body*, p. 99.

88. Beal quoted in ibid., p. 100. Also see Simone M. Carn, "Birth Control and the Black Community in the 1960s: Genocide or Power Politics?" *Journal of Social History* (Spring 1998): 549.

89. Toni Cade, "The Pill: Genocide or Liberation?" in Toni Cade, ed., *The Black Woman: An Anthology* (New York: New American Library, 1970), pp. 163–64.

90. "The Pill," *Redbook*, p. 78.

91. "Birth Control: Losing Support of Negroes?" *U.S. News & World Report*, August 7, 1967, p. 13.

92. Watkins, *On the Pill*, p. 56.

93. Roberts, *Killing the Black Body*, p. 101.

94. Charles F. Westoff, "The Modernization of U.S. Contraceptive Practice," *Family Planning Perspectives* 4 (1972): 9–12; "An Analysis of Some Select Findings," in "Birth Control Methods: General Correspondence" folder, Planned Parenthood Federation of America Papers, Sophia Smith Collection.

95. Spencer, "Birth Control Revolution," p. 22; William I. Searle to Mary Calderone, August 16, 1960, Planned Parenthood Federation of America Papers, Sophia Smith Collection; Sheehan, "Birth-Control 'Pill,' " p. 222.

96. Letter to Planned Parenthood, January 25, 1965, Planned Parenthood Federation of America Papers, Sophia Smith Collection.

97. Maurice Sagoff to J. William Crosson, February 16, 1961, Planned Parenthood Federation of America Papers, Sophia Smith Collection.

98. Watkins, *On the Pill*, pp. 34–35, 41.

99. Spencer, "Birth Control Revolution," p. 22.

100. For an excellent analysis of the history of Pill packaging, see Patricia Peck Gossel, "Packaging the Pill," in Robert Budd, Bernard Finn, and Helmut Trischler, eds., *Manifesting Medicine: Bodies and Machines* (New York: Harwood Academic Publishers, 1999), pp. 105–21.

101. Rice-Wray quoted in *Time*, March 20, 1964; similar findings are discussed in Naomi Thomas Gary, "Programming to Meet Family Planning Needs of Low-Income Negroes," paper presented at the 1965 Annual Forum of the National Conference on Social Welfare, Atlantic City, N.J., May 25, 1965, Ophelia Egypt Papers, Manuscripts Division, Moorland-Spingarn Research Center, Howard University.

102. Quoted in Rickie Solinger, *Wake Up Little Susie: Single Pregnancy and Race before Roe v. Wade* (New York: Routledge, 1992), p. 41; also see Sidney Furie, "Birth Control and the Lower-Class Unmarried Mother," *Social Work* 11 (January 1966): 42–49; Rose Bernstein, "Are We Still Stereotyping the Unmarried Mother?" *Social Work* 5 (July 1960): 22–28.

103. Alan Guttmacher, "Where Is Science Taking Us?" *Saturday Review*, February 6, 1960, pp. 50–51.

104. Davis quoted in Nicole Grant, *The Selling of Contraception: The Dalkon Shield Case, Sexuality, and Women's Autonomy* (Columbus: Ohio State University Press, 1992), p. 31.

11. SEARCHING FOR SOMETHING BETTER

1. Richard Lincoln and Lisa Kaeser, "Whatever Happened to the Contraceptive Revolution?" *Family Planning Perspectives* 20 (January/February 1988): 20–24.

2. Ibid., p. 20.

3. Hugh Davis, "Intrauterine Contraceptive Devices: Present Status and Future Prospects," *American Journal of Obstetrics and Gynecology* 114 (1972): 135.

4. "Now It's Official: U.S. Backs Birth-Control Aid," *U.S. News & World Report*, March 22, 1965.

5. "Oral Contraceptives: Government Supported Programs Are Questioned," *Science*, February 7, 1969.

6. "A National Plan on Curbing Births," *U.S. News & World Report*, July 28, 1969, p. 4; "About Face on Birth Control," *Time*, December 9, 1966, p. 30; "Oral Contraceptives: Government Supported Programs Are Questioned," *Science*.

7. "Now It's Official: U.S. Backs Birth-Control Aid," *U.S. News & World Report*, p. 66.

8. "Family-Planning Campaign—The Louisiana Story," *U.S. News & World Report*, July 28, 1969.

9. "Now It's Official: U.S. Backs Birth-Control Aid," *U.S. News & World Report*, p. 64.

10. Davis, "Intrauterine Contraceptive Devices," pp. 134–35; Howard Tatum, "Intrauterine Contraception," *American Journal of Obstetrics and Gynecology* 112 (1972): 1000–1; Andrea Tone, "Violence by Design: Contraceptive Technology and the Invasion of the Female Body," in Michael Bellesiles, ed., *Lethal Imagination: Violence and Brutality in American History* (New York: New York University Press, 1999), p. 377.

11. Davis, "Intrauterine Contraceptive Devices," pp. 134–35; Tatum, "Intrauterine Contraception," pp. 1000–1.

12. Caryl Potter, "Complications Following the Use of the Gold Spring Pessary," *American Journal of Surgery*, October 1930, p. 143; Howard C. Clark, "Foreign Bodies in the Uterus," *American Journal of Surgery*, March 1938, p. 631; Davis, "Intrauterine Contraceptive Devices," p. 135.

13. "IUD—The New Contraceptive," transcript of radio broadcast, March 1965, Station WBAI, New York City, box 123, Population Council Records, Rockefeller Archives; FDA Advisory Committee on Obstetrics and Gynecology, *Report on Intrauterine Contraceptive Devices* (Washington, D.C.: Government Printing Office, 1968), pp. 1, 6; Population Council, *Preliminary Report: 1962 Conference on Intrauterine Devices*, pp. 13–14; U.S. Patent Office, patent 3,200,815, August 17, 1965; Tatum, "Intrauterine Contraception," p. 1001; Tone, "Violence by Design," p. 382; W. Oppenheimer, "Prevention of Pregnancy by the Gräfenberg Ring Method," *American Journal of Obstetrics and Gynecology* 78 (August 1959): 446–54.

14. Tone, "Violence by Design," p. 381.

15. *Population Council: 1952–64* (New York, 1965), p. 41, and *The Population Council Annual Report for the Year Ended December 31, 1966* (New York), p. 17, boxes 87 and 88, Population Council Records, Rockefeller Archives.

16. Nicole Grant, *The Selling of Contraception: The Dalkon Shield Case, Sexuality, and Women's Autonomy* (Columbus: Ohio State University Press, 1992), p. 47.

17. *The Population Council, Report for 1962 & 1963*, box 88, Population Council Records, Rockefeller Archives.

18. Christopher Tietze, "History of Contraceptive Methods," *Indiana Journal of Public Health* 12 (1968): 43; "Projects on Intrauterine Devices, July, 1963," box 123, Population Council Records, Rockefeller Archives.

19. Jack Lippes to Alan Guttmacher, March 4, 1965, box 124, Population Council Records, Rockefeller Archives.

20. *Population Council: 1952–64*, box 87, Population Council Records, Rockefeller Archives; Lippes to Guttmacher, March 4, 1965, box 124, Population Council Records, Rockefeller Archives; Steven M. Spencer, "The Birth Control Revolution," *Saturday Evening Post*, January 15, 1966, p. 25; Population Council, *IUD Handbook*, pp. 1, 7, box 123, and *Population Council Annual Report for the Year Ended December 31, 1966*, p. 17, box 88, both in Population Council Records, Rockefeller Archives.

21. "Oral Contraceptives: Government Supported Programs Are Questioned," *Science*; "Now It's Official: U.S. Backs Birth-Control Aid," *U.S. News & World Report*, pp. 64, 66; Morton Mintz, *At Any Cost: Corporate Greed, Women, and the Dalkon Shield* (New York: Pantheon Books, 1985), p. 4; FDA Medical Device and Drug Advisory Committees on Obstetrics and Gynecology, *Second Report on Intrauterine Contraceptive Devices* (Washington, D.C.: Government Printing Office, 1978), p. 12; "A. H. Robins to Collect Unused IUDs in U.S., Slates a Modification," *Wall Street Journal*, January 21, 1975, p. 12.

22. "IUD—The New Contraceptive"; Charles F. Westoff, "The Modernization of U.S. Contraceptive Practice," *Family Planning Perspectives* 4 (1972): 10–12. Westoff's study, which explored trends in birth control use among married couples of childbearing age, found a 1965 IUD adoption rate of .7 percent among whites and 1.7 percent among blacks, and a 1970 adoption rate of 4.8 percent among whites and 4.5 percent among blacks. These percentages included all couples of childbearing

age, even those not practicing birth control. A separate calculation of methods of contraception in 1970 by wife's education and by color, excluding couples not using birth control, revealed an IUD adoption rate of 8.4 percent among white women with a college education and 9.3 percent among black women without a high school education. These represented the highest rate in each racial group.

23. Spencer, "Birth Control Revolution," p. 25.

24. Winfield Best, "Something New in Birth Control," *McCall's*, February 1965.

25. Emphasis added. U.S. Patent Office, patent 3,675,647, July 11, 1972; patent 3,633,574, January 11, 1972; patent 3,364,927, January 23, 1968. For an excellent analysis of the gendered biases of seemingly objective scientific accounts of women's reproductive organs, see Emily Martin, *The Woman in the Body: A Cultural Analysis of Reproduction* (Boston: Beacon Press, 1987).

26. U.S. Patent Office, patent 3,598,115, August 10, 1971.

27. Grant, *Selling of Contraception*, p. 73.

28. "IUD—The New Contraceptive."

29. Alan Guttmacher to John Searle, December 29, 1964, "Searle & Co. Correspondence from 1964," Planned Parenthood Federation of America Papers, Sophia Smith Collection.

30. Robert McG. Thomas, Jr., "Hugh J. Davis, Gynecologist Who Invented Dalkon Shield," *New York Times*, October 26, 1996; Mintz, *At Any Cost*, pp. 23–24.

31. Testimony of Hugh J. Davis, U.S. Senate, Subcommittee on Monopoly of the Select Committee on Small Business, *Competitive Problems in the Drug Industry: Present Status of Competition in the Pharmaceutical Industry; Oral Contraceptives*, 91st Cong., 2nd sess. (Washington, D.C.: Government Printing Office, 1970), pp. 5926–41; Mintz, *At Any Cost*, pp. 23–24.

32. *Competitive Problems in the Drug Industry*, p. 5941.

33. Mintz, *At Any Cost*, pp. 27–28.

34. Richard Sobol, *Bending the Law: The Story of the Dalkon Shield Bankruptcy* (Chicago: University of Chicago Press, 1991), p. 3.

35. Ibid., p. 3.

36. FDA Inspection Report of 6/14–21/1973, A. H. Robins Company Files, AF 16-375, box 195, FDA History Office; Mintz, *At Any Cost*, pp. 45–47; Sobol, *Bending the Law*, p. 5.

37. Grant, *Selling of Contraception*, pp. 43–44; Sobol, *Bending the Law*, pp. 5–6.

38. Sobol, *Bending the Law*, p. 2.

39. Ibid., pp. 2, 7.

40. U.S. House of Representatives, Committee on Government Operations, *Regulation of Medical Devices (Intrauterine Contraceptive Devices)*, 93rd Cong., 1st sess. (Washington, D.C.: Government Printing Office, 1973), pp. 2, 180–81.

41. Sobol, *Bending the Law*, p. 6.

42. Testimony of Major Russel J. Thomsen, *Regulation of Medical Devices (Intrauterine Contraception Devices)*, p. 52; FDA Records, AF 16-375, box 195, FDA History Office.

43. *Wall Street Journal*, May 29, 1974; Morton Mintz, "Questions Arose Early on Contraceptive's Safety," *Washington Post*, April 7, 1985; Thomas, "Hugh J. Davis"; Sobol, *Bending the Law*, p. 7; *Biomedical News*, June 1970, p. 15.

44. Testimony of Major Russel J. Thomsen, *Regulation of Medical Devices (Intrauterine Contraceptive Devices)*, p. 49.

45. Ibid., pp. 51–52.

46. FDA Inspection Report of 6/14–21/73, A. H. Robins Company Files, AF 16-375, box 195, FDA History Office.

47. Consumer complaint, May 31, 1973, A. H. Robins Company Files, AF 16-375, box 195, FDA History Office.

48. Letter to Representative Benjamin S. Rosenthal, June 1, 1973, A. H. Robins Company Files, AF 16-375, box 195, FDA History Office.

49. *Wall Street Journal*, May 29, 1974, and September 26, 1980, p. 12; Thomas, "Hugh J. Davis."

50. *Wall Street Journal*, August 26, 1974, p. 14; Grant, *Selling of Contraception*, p. 66.

51. *Wall Street Journal*, May 29, 1974; testimony of Dr. Jack Freund, vice president of A. H. Robins, *Regulation of Medical Devices (Intrauterine Contraceptive Devices)*, p. 305; Sobol, *Bending the Law*, pp. 9–11.

52. *Wall Street Journal*, September 26, 1980, p. 12.

53. *Wall Street Journal*, March 17, 1980, p. 19.

54. Mintz, *At Any Cost*, p. 14.

55. Mintz, "Questions Arose Early on Contraceptive's Safety"; Sobol, *Bending the Law*, p. 23; Mintz, *At Any Cost*, p. 7.

56. Mintz, *At Any Cost*, pp. 200–2.

57. Sobol, *Bending the Law*, p. 15.

58. Judge Miles W. Lord, courtroom statement, February 29, 1984, in Mintz, *At Any Cost*, pp. 264–67.

59. Mintz, "Questions Arose Early on Contraceptive's Safety"; Sobol, *Bending the Law*, pp. 22–23.

60. Thomas, "Hugh J. Davis"; Sobol, *Bending the Law*, passim.

EPILOGUE: THE CONTRACEPTIVE CONUNDRUM

1. Danise Kafka and Rachel Benson Gold, "Food and Drug Administration Approves Vaginal Sponge," *Family Planning Perspectives* 15 (May/June 1983): 146–48; "Farewell to the Sponge," *New Woman*, June 1995, p. 81; "The Return of the Sponge," *New Woman*, July 1999, p. 30.

2. Denise Grady, "Female Condom: A Market Wallflower," *New York Times*, November 17, 1998; Robert A. Hatcher, Miriam Zieman, Alston Watt, Anita Nelson, Gary K. Stewart, Philip D. Darney, and Rachel B. Blankstein, *A Pocket Guide to Managing Contraception* (Tiger, Ga.: Bridging the Gap Foundation, 1998), p. 52.

3. Hatcher et al., *Pocket Guide to Managing Contraception*, p. 129; Joy Fishel, "Contraceptive Technologies: How Much Choice Do We Really Have?" *ZPG Reporter*, March/April 1997, pp. 3–6.

4. Ellen Sweet, "A Failed Revolution," Ms., March 1985, p. 75.

5. Linda J. Piccinino and William D. Mosher, "Trends in Contraceptive Use in the United States, 1982–1995," Family Planning Perspectives 30 (January/February 1998): 1–15.

6. Fishel, "Contraceptive Technologies," p. 2; Michael Klitsch, "Still Waiting for the Contraceptive Revolution," Family Planning Perspectives 27 (November/December 1995): 246.

7. Jacqueline Darroch Forrest, "The End of IUD Marketing in the United States: What Does It Mean for American Women?" Family Planning Perspectives 18 (March/April 1986): 52; "U.S. Birth Control R & D Lags," Wall Street Journal, February 13, 1990; Shari Roan, "The Chill in Birth Control Research," Los Angeles Times, March 23, 1998; Carl Djerassi, The Pill, Pygmy Chimps, and Degas' Horse: The Autobiography of Carl Djerassi (New York: Basic Books, 1992), p. 119.

8. Richard Lincoln and Lisa Kaeser, "Whatever Happened to the Contraceptive Revolution?" Family Planning Perspectives 20 (January/February 1988): 22.

9. Linda E. Atkinson, Richard Lincoln, and Jacqueline Darroch Forrest, "The Next Contraceptive Revolution," Family Planning Perspectives 18 (January–February 1986): 25.

10. Lincoln and Kaeser, "Whatever Happened to the Contraceptive Revolution?" pp. 21–22; Atkinson, Lincoln, and Forrest, "Next Contraceptive Revolution," pp. 19–26.

11. Roan, "Chill in Birth Control Research."

12. Sweet, "Failed Revolution," p. 79.

13. Carl Djerassi, "Birth Control after 1984," Science, September 4, 1970, p. 949.

14. Warren Leary, "Variety of Obstacles Is Blocking New Contraceptives a Medical Panel Says," New York Times, May 29, 1996.

15. Roan, "Chill in Birth Control Research."

16. Robert A. Hatcher, James Trussell, Felicia Stewart, Gary K. Stewart, Deborah Kowal, Felicia Guest, Willard Cates, Jr., and Michael S. Policar, Contraceptive Technology, 16th rev. ed. (New York: Irvington, 1994), pp. 575–77; Fishel, "Contraceptive Technologies," p. 1.

17. Boston Women's Health Book Collective, The New Our Bodies, Ourselves (New York: Simon and Schuster, 1992), p. 292.

18. Interview with Lorraine Fletcher, March 1999, transcript in author's possession. Interviewee's name has been changed to protect her privacy.

19. Diane Lore, "Insurers Slow to See Benefits of the Pill," Atlanta Journal-Constitution, May 9, 2000; Charlotte F. Muller, "Insurance Coverage of Abortion, Contraception, and Sterilization," Family Planning Perspectives 10 (March/April 1978): 71, 73; Allisa J. Rubin, "Lawmakers Put Focus on Family Planning Coverage," Los Angeles Times, June 24, 1998; Tamar Lewin, "Effort to Cover Contraception Likely to Fail," Los Angeles Times, March 23, 1998; Piccinino and Mosher, "Trends in Contraceptive Use," pp. 1–15; Tamar Lewin, "Suit Seeks Insurance Coverage for Contraceptives," Atlanta Journal-Constitution, July 20, 2000.

Index

363.9609 Tone, Andrea,
T   1964-

          Devices and desires :
          a history of
          contraceptives in
          America.

Hi Lile d thru oul 6/12 om

DATE			